Psychiatry and Mental Health

Psychiatry and Mental Health

Editor: Laurel Harper

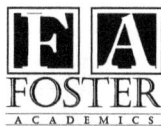

FOSTER
ACADEMICS

www.fosteracademics.com

www.fosteracademics.com

FA FOSTER
ACADEMICS

Cataloging-in-Publication Data

Psychiatry and mental health / edited by Laurel Harper.
    p. cm.
Includes bibliographical references and index.
ISBN 978-1-63242-787-8
    1. Psychiatry. 2. Mental health. 3. Medicine and psychology. 4. Psychology, Pathological.
I. Harper, Laurel.
RC454 .P79 2019
616.89--dc23

Foster Academics,
118-35 Queens Blvd., Suite 400,
Forest Hills, NY 11375, USA

ISBN 978-1-63242-787-8 (Hardback)

Contents

Preface

This book was inspired by the evolution of our times; to answer the curiosity of inquisitive minds. Many developments have occurred across the globe in the recent past which has transformed the progress in the field.

Psychiatry is a field of science and medicine. It is concerned with the diagnosis, prevention and treatment of mental disorders. It deals with various disorders related to mood, perception, behavior and cognition. The process of assessing a patient's mental condition begins with a case history and mental status examination. Mental health is one's state of psychological well-being, where one is functioning at a satisfactory level of emotional and behavioral adjustment. All diagnosable mental health conditions related to mood, behavior and thoughts are categorized as mental illness. Cognitive behavioral therapy, psychoanalysis, systemic therapy, electroconvulsive therapy, psychosurgery, art therapy, antipsychotics, anxiolytics and antidepressants are some of the common treatment methods useful in the treatment of mental illnesses. This book unfolds the innovative aspects of psychiatry and mental health which will be crucial for the progress of these fields in future. It studies, analyzes and upholds the pillars of psychiatry and mental health and their utmost significance in modern times. Those in search of information to further their knowledge will be greatly assisted by this book.

This book was developed from a mere concept to drafts to chapters and finally compiled together as a complete text to benefit the readers across all nations. To ensure the quality of the content we instilled two significant steps in our procedure. The first was to appoint an editorial team that would verify the data and statistics provided in the book and also select the most appropriate and valuable contributions from the plentiful contributions we received from authors worldwide. The next step was to appoint an expert of the topic as the Editor-in-Chief, who would head the project and finally make the necessary amendments and modifications to make the text reader-friendly. I was then commissioned to examine all the material to present the topics in the most comprehensible and productive format.

I would like to take this opportunity to thank all the contributing authors who were supportive enough to contribute their time and knowledge to this project. I also wish to convey my regards to my family who have been extremely supportive during the entire project.

Editor

Children's mental health problems and their relation to parental stress in foster mothers and fathers

Arnold Lohaus[1]*, Sabrina Chodura[1], Christine Möller[1], Tabea Symanzik[1], Daniela Ehrenberg[2], Ann-Katrin Job[2], Vanessa Reindl[3], Kerstin Konrad[3] and Nina Heinrichs[2]

Abstract

Background: This study focuses on children living in foster families with a history of maltreatment or neglect. These children often show adverse mental health outcomes reflected in increased externalizing and internalizing problems. It is expected that these adverse outcomes are associated with increased parental stress levels experienced by foster mothers as well as foster fathers.

Methods: The study sample included 79 children living in foster families and 140 children living in biological families as comparison group. The age of the children ranged from 2 to 7 years. Mental health problems were assessed with the Child Behavior Checklist, while parenting stress was measured with a parenting stress questionnaire including subscales on the amount of experienced stress and the amount of perceived support. The Child Behavior Checklist assessments were based mainly on maternal reports, while the parental stress assessments were based on maternal as well as paternal reports.

Results: As expected the results showed increased externalizing and internalizing scores for the foster children accompanied by increased parental stress experiences in the foster family sample (however only in the maternal, but not in the paternal stress reports). The stress differences between the foster and biological family groups disappeared, when the children's mental health problem scores were included as covariates. Moreover, especially the externalizing scores were strong predictors of parental stress in both, the groups of foster and biological parents. The amount of perceived social support was associated with reduced parental stress, but only in the group of biological fathers.

Conclusion: The emergence of parental stress in biological as well as foster parents is closely related to child characteristics (mainly externalizing child problems). Possible implications for the reduction of parental stress are discussed as a consequence of the present results.

Keywords: Parental stress, Foster families, Mental health problems, Internalizing behavior, Externalizing behavior

Background

When children are allocated to a foster family, they often look back at a history of maltreatment experiences during the time when they lived in their biological families. Childhood maltreatment is associated with a range of emotional and behavioral problems. Maltreated children show significantly more externalizing and internalizing symptoms, more discipline problems in school and more symptoms of depression than children without such experiences [1, 2]. As a consequence, foster parents are confronted with increased demands, which may induce parental stress as an aversive psychological reaction to the demands of being a parent [3].

Several previous studies showed associations between parental stress and child mental health problems in non-foster parents. For example, a study by Mesman and Koot [4] found significant relations between parental stress and

---

*Correspondence: arnold.lohaus@uni-bielefeld.de
[1] Faculty of Psychology and Sports Sciences, University of Bielefeld, P.O. Box 10 01 31, 33501 Bielefeld, Germany
Full list of author information is available at the end of the article

the extent of externalizing and internalizing symptoms in children aged 10–11. The association to parental stress was closer for externalizing in comparison to internalizing symptoms. This is also underlined by studies addressing attention deficit hyperactivity disorder (ADHD) problems. As a meta-analysis by Theule et al. [5] showed, parents of children with ADHD reported more parenting stress than parents of nonclinical controls. Moreover, the severity of the ADHD symptoms was associated with parenting stress, especially in combination with conduct problems (e.g., oppositional behavior). Associations to parental stress were also found for children with developmental delays [6], for children with autism spectrum disorders [7], for children with sleep disturbances [8] and for children with chronic diseases [9]. In general, mental as well as somatic problems are typically associated with increased demands for parents, which are often reflected in increased parental stress perceptions.

Parenting might in some respects be even more demanding for foster parents. On the one hand, foster children may exhibit increased emotional and behavioral problems as a result of previous maltreatment experiences [10]. On the other hand, children and foster parents are unfamiliar with each other when the children enter their new families. This means that emotional ties and familiar behavior patterns may emerge over time, but are not available from the beginning. This is an important difference to many other challenging child conditions, because, in general, children with mental or somatic problems live in their familiar environment. Thus, the perceived parental stress may even be increased in foster parents, because they are confronted with an unfamiliar child with potential mental health problems.

Increased perceived parental stress may be associated with reduced parenting capacities. As a study by Farmer, Lipscombe and Moyers [11] for foster caregivers of adolescents showed, conduct problems, hyperactivity, and violent behavior shown by the adolescents increased caregivers' strain. Increased caregivers' strain, on the other hand, was associated with significantly higher disruption rates (which indicates increased mutual interaction problems). Thus, increased parental stress may reduce the quality of the parent–child-interaction and thus may contribute to an increase of child problems. The authors also found that the perceived strain was reduced when caregivers received help from friends and local professionals, which underlines the role of social support in reducing stress experiences.

Although relations between challenging child characteristics and parental stress have been addressed in previous studies, most of these studies were related to non-foster contexts, while empirical studies focusing on stress perceptions of foster parents—especially in

children—are scarce. Previous studies used parenting stress as outcome measure in parent training for foster parents [12], included parenting stress as control variable in studying parenting practices of foster parents [13] or were related to specific subgroups, e.g. parenting stress in adolescent mothers in foster care [14]. A study by Jiménez et al. [15] is related to parental stress in kinship foster families, which, however, are only in part comparable to the situation of non-kinship foster families addressed in the current study. One of the few studies which are directly related to parental stress in foster parents is a study of Nadeem et al. [16] with repeated assessments of foster children's mental health problems and their foster parent's parental stress. This study showed associations between children's problems and parental stress and, moreover, changes of parenting stress across repeated assessments (at 2 months, 12 months and 5 years postplacement), but included no comparison group. The current study is directly related to comparing the parenting stress of non-kinship foster parents with biological parents. The focus is on stress perceptions of both foster mothers and foster fathers. Although fathers are also involved in parenting, the majority of previous studies focused on mothers only, because they are typically the primary reference persons for children. To our knowledge, this is the first study that does not only include foster mothers, but also foster fathers.

It is hypothesized that the perceived level of stress in foster parents and also the extent of children's mental health problems are increased in comparison to control parents living exclusively with their biological children (Hypothesis 1) and that the differences between the stress levels of foster and biological parents are expected to disappear by controlling for the extent of the children's mental health problems (Hypothesis 2). In addition, it is assumed that the level of perceived parental stress is closely related to the extent of the children's mental health problems (in foster as well as biological families) and that social support perceived by the parents decreases the level of perceived parental stress (Hypothesis 3). Because little is known about the relation between children's mental health problems and parenting stress in preschool and elementary school age children (especially in foster families), the focus of the current investigation is on young children aged 2–7 years.

Methods
Sample
The data of the current investigation are obtained from the GROW&TREAT foster family study, funded by the Federal Ministry of Education and Research. The total sample of the GROW&TREAT project consisted of 94 foster children and 157 children living in their biological

families. Only non-kinship foster care families were included in the foster sample. Most foster families were recruited from youth welfare offices at three regions in Germany (up to 200 km around Aachen, Bielefeld, and Braunschweig). The biological parents were recruited from the same regions with postings or at parents' evenings in nursery and elementary schools. If the foster or the biological families had more than one child in the target age, they were asked to select one child as the target child (based on a random choice). However, in some cases, more than one child of a foster or biological family was selected as target child. This was the case for 15 foster and 17 biological families. To avoid dependencies within the data set, these families were excluded from the analyses reported in this study. Thus, the final sample of this study included 79 children living in foster families and 140 children living in biological families. In the final sample, the age of the children varied between 2 and 7 years [$M = 3.49$ ($SD = 1.32$) for the foster children and $M = 4.40$ ($SD = 1.41$) for the biological children]. A t test indicated a significant age difference between the two groups $t = 4.65$, $df = 217$, $p < .001$, but there were no significant differences with regard to the children's sex. Because of the significant age difference, all statistical analyses in the "Results" section included age as covariate. The foster children lived in their foster families since $M = 17.72$ months ($SD = 8.61$). The most important sample characteristics are provided in Table 1. Participation of the foster families required the permission of the foster parents, the youth welfare office, and the biological mother or the legal guardian. The procedure and assessments were approved by an independent ethics committee. The foster as well as the biological families received 30 Euros as incentive for participation at the assessments included in this study. For more information on the GROW&TREAT project and on the complete assessments see http://www.grow-and-treat.de.

Measures

Parental stress was assessed by the Parental Stress Questionnaire [17], which includes a 17-item subscale (Parental Distress Subscale) related to the degree of experienced parental stress (item example: "I struggle a lot with my child"). Moreover, there are subscales related to perceived social support in general (item example: "I have people in my surrounding who might watch my child") and to perceived social support by the partner (item example: "My partner supports me in the education of our child"). The latter subscale had to be completed only if a partner was available. A forth subscale of the Parental Stress Questionnaire (Role Restriction) was not provided in the context of this study. All items had to be assessed on a 4-point Likert scale (0 = "strongly disagree", 1 = "disagree", 2 = "agree" and 3 = "strongly agree"). For further analyses sum scores were calculated for the three subscales (separately for mothers and fathers). It should be noted that there are two versions of the parental distress subscale for parents of preschool and school children. Thus, the parents were asked to complete the school version if their child already attended a school. Five items of the parental distress subscale are reformulated in the school version to meet the specific demands of parents of older children. As a consequence, the scale values of the two versions were z-standardized (across the foster and non foster groups, but separately for the preschool and school versions and separately for mothers and fathers) to adjust the values to comparable ranges. The calculations in the "Results" section are based on these z values. The mothers as well as the fathers in foster and biological families were asked to complete the subscales. Data for the parental stress subscale were available from 72 foster mothers. For the general social support and the partner support subscale, data were provided from 76 respectively 70 foster mothers. The respective sample sizes for foster fathers were 66, 69, and 68. In the case of biological families, the sample sizes were 130, 131, and 121 (mothers) and 111, 116, and 114 (fathers). The internal consistencies of the subscales are provided in Table 2. Across samples, the correspondence between the assessments of fathers and mothers was $r = .38$, $p < .001$ for the parental distress subscale. The respective values for the general social support and the partner support subscale were $r = .51$, $p < .001$, and $r = .35$, $p < .001$.

Table 1 Sample characteristics of the recruited samples (children living in foster and biological families)

	Foster families	Biological families	Statistical test
Children's age	$M = 3.49$ ($SD = 1.32$)	$M = 4.40$ ($SD = 1.41$)	$t = 4.65$, $df = 217$, $p < .001$
Children's sex	39 female, 40 male	76 female, 64 male	$\chi^2 = .49$, $p = .484$
Age of the mother	$M = 40.54$ ($SD = 6.81$)	$M = 35.38$ ($SD = 5.40$)	$t = 6.17$, $df = 217$, $p < .001$
Age of the father	$M = 44.01$ ($SD = 6.73$)	$M = 38.62$ ($SD = 6.01$)	$t = 5.96$, $df = 209$, $p < .001$
Time in foster family (in months)	$M = 17.72$ ($SD = 8.61$)		

Table 2 Internal consistencies for the questionnaire scales included in this study

	Foster families	Biological families	Total
Maternal distress—pre-school	.88	.89	.89
Maternal distress—school	.93	.90	.92
Mothers' perceived social support—general	.78	.80	.79
Mothers' perceived social support—partner	.80	.83	.82
Paternal distress—pre-school	.88	.89	.88
Paternal distress—school	.95	.85	.87
Fathers' perceived social support—general	.79	.68	.73
Fathers' perceived social support—partner	.45	.76	.71
CBCL—total score—age range 2–4	.95	.97	.96
CBCL—externalizing problems—age range 2–4	.89	.89	.90
CBCL—internalizing problems—age range 2–4	.91	.81	.90
CBCL—total score—age range 5–7	.94	.89	.91
CBCL—externalizing problems—age range 5–7	.89	.86	.89
CBCL—internalizing problems—age range 5–7	.74	.76	.75

Psychological symptoms of the children were assessed using German versions of the Child Behavior Checklist (CBCL). For children in an age range from 2 to 4 years, the CBCL 1½–5 was used [18], while the CBCL 4–18 was used in the age range from 5 to 7 [19]. The CBCL reports were typically only provided by the mothers (in 81.2% of the cases), while 7.7% of the assessments were provided by fathers and 11.1% completed the CBCL jointly. In line with the manual's instructions, a total problem score was calculated as well as scores for the broad-band scales for internalizing and externalizing syndromes. As previously described for parenting stress, the scale values for the CBCL 1½–5 and the CBCL 4–18 were z-standardized separately to adjust the values of the different versions to comparable ranges. The internal consistencies are provided in Table 2. The externalizing and internalizing scale values correlated $r = .65$, $p < .001$ across samples.

Statistical analyses

The comparisons of the perceived level of stress and the extent of children's mental health problems between the groups of foster and biological parents were based on analyses of variance (Hypothesis 1). In the case of externalizing and internalizing problems, multivariate analysis of variance was used to account for the substantial correlations between these dependent variables. Hypothesis 2 was tested by including the extent of the children's mental health problems as a covariate in the analysis of variance addressing parenting stress differences between foster and biological parents. Hierarchical regression analyses were used to analyze the contribution of children's mental health problems and perceived social support (in general and by the partner) to parental stress (Hypothesis 3). Because of missing data in some assessments, the sample sizes may vary across the analyses, as can be seen by the degrees of freedom or by the sample sizes reported in the Tables.

Results

Children's mental health problems and parental stress in foster vs. biological families

To address Hypothesis 1, a univariate analysis of variance was calculated with family type (foster vs. biological) as independent variable and the total CBCL score as dependent variable. The age of the children was included as covariate. The results indicated a significant difference for the total CBCL score ($F_{1,209} = 29.30$, $p < .001$, $\eta^2 = .123$) with increased values in the foster children (see Table 3). There was no additional age effect ($F_{1,209} = .93$, $p = .337$, $\eta^2 = .004$).

A multivariate analysis of variance with the internalizing and externalizing CBCL scales as dependent variables and age as covariate underlines the result for the total score. There is a significant multivariate difference ($F_{2,208} = 13.57$, $p < .001$, $\eta^2 = .115$). Moreover, the univariate analyses indicated significant differences for both the internalizing ($F_{1,209} = 14.27$, $p < .001$, $\eta^2 = .070$) and the externalizing scale ($F_{1,209} = 26.30$, $p < .001$, $\eta^2 = .112$). Again, there was no significant age effect. In both cases, the Child Behavior Checklist scores are increased for the group of foster children (see Table 3).

Analyses of variance were calculated for the parental distress subscale as dependent variable for mothers and fathers separately. The age of the children was again included as covariate. The results for the mothers indicated significant effects for the parental distress subscale ($F_{1,199} = 10.04$, $p = .002$, $\eta^2 = .048$) indicating increased parental stress in the group of foster mothers (see Table 3). The results for the fathers revealed no significant differences for the parenting distress subscale. Moreover, there was no effect of age as covariate.

To summarize, the parents noticed increased mental health problems in foster care children and especially the foster mothers perceived in addition increased parental stress. To address the question, whether the parental stress differences between foster and biological mothers

Table 3 CBCL and parental stress scores in foster and biological families (based on z values)

	Foster families			Biological families		
	Mean z value	SD	n	Mean z value	SD	n
CBCL total score	.47	1.20	78	−.24	.75	134
CBCL externalizing score	.47	1.19	78	−.24	.78	134
CBCL internalizing score	.33	1.24	78	−.19	.74	134
Maternal parental distress (scale)	.28	.98	72	−.16	.98	130
Paternal parental distress (scale)	.06	1.00	66	−.04	1.00	111

are due to increased mental health problems in foster children, the analyses of variance, which were calculated to address Hypothesis 1, were recalculated including the total CBCL scores as covariate (in addition to age). Confirming Hypothesis 2, the analysis of variance did not indicate any parental stress difference between foster and biological mothers. These calculations were repeated using the externalizing and the internalizing problem scores as covariates (in separate analyses). Again, the differences between the two groups disappeared after including the child behavior problem scores in the analyses.

Relation between children's mental health problems and parental stress

Table 4 shows the Pearson correlations between the CBCL scores and the parental stress indicators. As can be seen, there are substantial correlations between both variable sets. As can be expected, the stress experienced by the parents was increased if they noticed mental health problems in their children (in foster as well as in biological parents). In general, the correlations seem to be increased for externalizing in comparison to internalizing problems.

To analyse the relative contribution of externalizing and internalizing problems to parental stress, hierarchical regression analyses were calculated. In the first step

of the analyses, externalizing and internalizing scores were included as predictors, in the second step the general social support and social support by the partner were added as predictors to be able to analyse the role of perceived social support for parental stress (Hypothesis 3). The results are shown in Table 5 for maternal and in Table 6 for paternal stress.

As the results for step 1 show, externalizing problems were the most important predictor for maternal as well as paternal stress (in both foster and biological families). Internalizing problems did not additionally contribute to the explanation of variance in parental stress. If the social support variables were included, there was no significant increase in the explanation of maternal stress. This result was comparable for foster fathers, but there was a significant stress decrease in biological fathers if they experienced increased support by their partners.

To summarize, there are substantial relations between parental stress and children's externalizing CBCL scores, and a contribution of perceived social support could only be identified for biological fathers.

Discussion
According to Abidin [20] there are many possible sources of parental stress. Relevant stressors are related to work, environment, marital relationship, daily hassles, life events, parent characteristics, and child characteristics.

Table 4 Correlations between CBCL and parental stress scores in foster and biological families and in the total sample

	CBCL total score	CBCL externalizing score	CBCL internalizing score
Total sample			
Maternal parental distress (scale)	.52*** (n = 198)	.57*** (n = 198)	.34*** (n = 198)
Paternal parental distress (scale)	.33*** (n = 172)	.38*** (n = 172)	.16* (n = 172)
Foster families			
Maternal parental distress (scale)	.43*** (n = 69)	.48*** (n = 69)	.30* (n = 69)
Paternal parental distress (scale)	.34** (n = 63)	.36*** (n = 63)	.17 (n = 63)
Biological families			
Maternal parental distress (scale)	.55*** (n = 124)	.61*** (n = 124)	.33*** (n = 124)
Paternal parental distress (scale)	.33*** (n = 106)	.40*** (n = 106)	.13 (n = 106)

* p < .05, ** p < .01, *** p < .001

Table 5 Prediction of maternal stress in foster and biological families by CBCL scores (externalizing and internalizing) and perceived social support

	B	SE B	β	p	Δr^2	Significance of Δr^2
Foster families—maternal stress						
Step 1—predictors					.387	<.001
CBCL externalizing score	.808	.114	.640	<.001		
CBCL internalizing score	−.045	.127	−.043	.726		
Step 2—predictors					.014	.274
CBCL externalizing score	.776	.118	.615	<.001		
CBCL internalizing score	−.052	.127	−.037	.681		
Social support—general	.100	.070	.107	.153		
Social support—partner	−.077	.077	−.078	.319		
Biological families—maternal stress						
Step 1—predictors					.198	.001
CBCL externalizing score	.354	.115	.440	.006		
CBCL internalizing score	.005	.106	.007	.961		
Step 2—predictors					.012	.628
CBCL externalizing score	.337	.119	.419	.006		
CBCL internalizing score	.002	.119	.002	.988		
Social support—general	−.047	.116	−.048	.682		
Social support—partner	−.096	.109	−.103	.380		

n = 67 in foster families and n = 117 in biological families

Table 6 Prediction of paternal stress in foster and biological families by CBCL scores (externalizing and internalizing) and perceived social support

	B	SE B	β	p	Δr^2	Significance of Δr^2
Foster families—paternal stress						
Step 1—predictors					.139	.009
CBCL externalizing score	.364	.129	.428	.007		
CBCL internalizing score	−.079	.120	−.100	.514		
Step 2—predictors					.046	.188
CBCL externalizing score	.331	.129	.390	.013		
CBCL internalizing score	−.082	.118	−.104	.492		
Social support—general	−.037	.115	−.038	.748		
Social support—partner	−.295	.163	−.212	.075		
Biological families—paternal stress						
Step 1—predictors					.167	<.001
CBCL externalizing score	.600	.141	.469	<.001		
CBCL internalizing score	−.186	.159	−.129	.244		
Step 2—predictors					.122	<.001
CBCL externalizing score	.491	.135	.384	<.001		
CBCL internalizing score	−.228	.151	−.158	.132		
Social support—general	.086	.090	.083	.342		
Social support—partner	−.333	.080	−.369	<.001		

n = 65 in foster families and n = 105 in biological families

This study focused mainly on emotional and behavioral problems as specific child characteristics, which may be associated with increased parental stress. As the results for Hypothesis 1 show, there is evidence that parents of foster children are confronted with increased levels of child behavioral and emotional problems. It is well known from previous studies that children in foster care usually show higher levels of behavioral and emotional problems compared to children living with their biological parents [21, 22]. While many previous studies focused on elementary school aged children and on adolescents, the present study shows that these results may also be extended to preschool age children.

At the same time, especially foster mothers reported increased parental stress. However, the differences between the stress levels of foster and biological mothers disappeared when the children's mental health problems were included as covariates in the analyses. Thus, our findings support the assumption that large contributions to the emergence of stress in foster families may be related to child characteristics (especially behavioral and emotional problems), at least in foster mothers. It is, however, unclear how this relation emerges, because it is also possible that parents perceiving increased strain are less effective in parenting and caregiving which may also result in a close relation between children's problems and parental stress. Thus, it is possible that there are bidirectional relations between parental stress and child characteristics. Independent of the direction, it might—as a consequence—be helpful to support foster parents in caring for children with such problems in order to reduce parental stress.

It is interesting to note that the association of parental stress to child characteristics is lower for internalizing than externalizing problems [23]. The reason may be that internalizing problems are hardly identified by external observations—an effect well known from studies on cross-informant discrepancies [24–26]. Similar results were shown in a previous study by Mesman and Koot [4] who found closer associations between externalizing problems and parental stress than between internalizing problems and parental stress. According to Mesman and Koot [4] externalizing behavior problems are not only more observable for parents, but they also require more attention. As a consequence, this relation is shown not only in foster parents, but also in biological parents, although foster parents may be confronted with even more child behavior problems. The decreased observability may also explain the insignificant correlations between internalizing problems and paternal stress in Table 4 (in foster families as well as in biological families). In many families, the mothers spend more time with their children than the fathers, which may lead to an increased chance for mothers to perceive internalizing problems. Although the regression analyses underline that externalizing problems are generally more closely associated with parental stress than internalizing problems, it should be noted that this study is restricted to young children and that externalizing behavior may be more salient for

parents at this age. Thus, it is unclear whether the contribution of externalizing problems to parental stress in comparison to internalizing problems will change, when the children grow older.

Although a significant contribution of perceived social support to the reduction of parental stress was assumed, this could only be found for biological fathers. In this case, perceived social support by the partner contributed to decreased parental stress. It should, however, be noted that social support may not only lead to decreased parental stress, but that increased parental stress may also lead to increased social support to cope with a demanding situation. Thus, there may be a mutual influence in both directions, which may explain the absence of substantial relations between both variable sets in most analyses. The situation may also be different in foster parents who receive, at least in some communities in Germany, additional professional social support by foster family support groups or supervisory meetings, etc.

It is additionally interesting to note that there were no sex differences regarding the results of this study. It is well known from the literature that externalizing problems are typically more often shown by boys and internalizing problems by girls. These differences emerge, however, more clearly during early adolescence, but seem to be less prominent during childhood [27, 28]. This could explain the absence of sex influences in the included age range.

Conclusions

In sum, our results indicate that there is a close association between children's mental health problems and parental stress and that this is true for biological as well as for foster families. Assuming a bidirectional relationship between parental stress and child behavior problems, there might be at least three possible implications of the current study results for the reduction of parental stress: (1) interventions with a focus on the parent (training of coping strategies, strengthening parental resources etc.), (2) interventions with a focus on the child (interventions treating children's mental health problems to indirectly influence parental stress), and (3) interventions related to parent–child interactions (to improve the mutual adjustment of parents and their children). Although all three approaches may be promising in reducing parental stress and improving a child's well-being, it may depend on the specific situation of the family and of the target child, which strategy is most appropriate. An intervention example is the keeping foster parents trained and supported (KEEP) approach [29], which equips foster parents with strategies to manage externalizing behavior problems. The program has been shown to be effective in reducing children's problem behavior and in reducing parental stress levels.

According to Chamberlain et al. [30] the number of child problem behaviors is linearly related to the risk of placement disruption during subsequent years. The perceived parental stress may be an important mediator variable in this relationship. On the other hand, placement disruptions increase the risk for child problem behaviors. To avoid vicious circles it is important to provide appropriate interventions at early stages of the development of problem behavior. Foster parents need support because of their duties and challenges on many different levels. Therefore they have to be well prepared and trained and the social services should provide easy accessible structures of help to support foster parents. Generally, a close collaboration between social services and clinical child and adolescent psychological services should be strengthened. Further research is needed to identify specific stressors in the context of parental stress and to develop appropriate prevention and intervention support programs.

A possible weakness of this study may be seen in the recruitment of the samples, because there might be self-selection effects, which may reduce the representativeness of the samples. It should, however, be noted that the mean CBCL-T values of the control children were 49.71 for externalizing and 50.31 for internalizing problems which is very close to the $T = 50$ value expected for the total population. However, the T value calculations had to be based on American norm data, because there are no specific German norm data for the CBCL-version used for younger children. Based on the available norm data, there is no indication that the children from the biological families represent a specific population with improved mental health. It should also be noted that the foster families may be representative for a relatively highly educated sample. This, however, represents the typical living conditions of foster children after a placement in a new family in Germany, because most foster families are well educated with a specific interest in improving the well-being of children.

A specific strength of the current study is that it compares parental stress and children's mental health problems in comparably large samples of foster and biological parents. Previous studies were typically related to the role of child characteristics for parental stress in non-foster samples, while few studies were directly related to parental stress in foster family samples comparing the parental stress of foster and biological parents at early stages of their children's life. Moreover, there are very few studies focusing not only on maternal stress, but also on paternal stress. To our knowledge, there was no previous study including paternal stress in a foster family sample. Thus, the study at hand has broadened the knowledge about

the relations between children's behavior problems and parental stress especially in foster families.

Abbreviations
ADHD: attention deficit hyperactivity disorder; CBCL: Child Behavior Checklist; KEEP: keeping foster parents trained and supported.

Authors' contributions
AL, KK and NH are principle investigators responsible for the organization of the study in the regions of Bielefeld, Aachen and Braunschweig. SC, CM, TS, DE, AKJ and VR are responsible for the data collections and data documentation in the study sites. All authors participated in reading and preparing the manuscript. All authors read and approved the final manuscript.

Author details
[1] Faculty of Psychology and Sports Sciences, University of Bielefeld, P.O. Box 10 01 31, 33501 Bielefeld, Germany. [2] University of Braunschweig, Institute of Psychology, Humboldtstr. 33, 38106 Brunswick, Germany. [3] Department for Child and Adolescent Psychiatry, University Hospital Aachen, Neuenhoferweg 21, 52074 Aachen, Germany.

Competing interests
The authors declare that they have no competing interests.

Funding
This research was funded by the German Federal Ministry of Education and Research (Bundesministerium für Bildung und Forschung, BMBF, FKZ: 01KR1302C).

References
1. Éthier LS, Lemelin JP, Lacharité C. A longitudinal study of the effects of chronic maltreatment on children's behavioral and emotional problems. Child Abuse Negl. 2004;28:1265–78.
2. Oswald SH, Heil K, Goldbeck L. History of maltreatment and mental health problems in foster children: a review of the literature. J Pediatr Psychol. 2010;35:462–72.
3. Deater-Deckard K. Parenting stress and child adjustment: some old hypotheses and new questions. Clin Psychol Sci Pract. 1998;5:314–32.
4. Mesman J, Koot HM. Common and specific correlates of preadolescent internalizing and externalizing psychopathology. J Abnorm Psychol. 2000;109:428–37.
5. Theule J, Wiener J, Tannock R, Jenkins JM. Parenting stress in families of children with ADHD: a meta-analysis. J Emot Behav Disord. 2010;21:3–17.
6. Neece CL, Green SA, Baker BL. Parenting stress and child behavior problems: a transactional relationship across time. Am J Intellect Dev Disabil. 2012;117:48–66.
7. Hayes SA, Watson SL. The impact of parenting stress: a meta-analysis of studies comparing the experience of parenting stress in parents of children with and without Autism Spectrum Disorder. J Autism Dev Disord. 2013;43:629–42.
8. Meltzer LJ, Mindell JA. Relationship between child sleep disturbances and maternal sleep, mood, and parenting stress: a pilot study. J Fam Psychol. 2007;21:67–73.
9. Cousino MK, Hazen RA. Parenting stress among caregivers of children with chronic illness: a systematic review. J Pediatr Psychol. 2013;38:809–28.
10. Clausen JM, Landsverk J, Ganger W, Chadwick D, Litrownik A. Mental health problems of children in foster care. J Child Fam Stud. 1998;7:283–96.
11. Farmer E, Lipscombe J, Moyers S. Foster carer strain and its impact on

parenting and placement outcomes for adolescents. Br J Soc Work. 2005;35:237–53.

12. Chamberlain P, Price J, Leve LD, Laurent H, Landsverk JA, Reid JB. Prevention of behavior problems for children in foster care: outcomes and mediation effects. Prev Sci. 2008;9:17–27.

13. Linares LO, Montalto D, Rosbruch N, Li M. Discipline practices among biological and foster parents. Child Maltreat. 2006;11:157–67.

14. Budd KS, Holdsworth MJA, HoganBruen KD. Antecedents and concomitants of parenting stress in adolescent mothers in foster care. Child Abuse Negl. 2006;30:557–74.

15. Jiménez JM, Mata E, León E, Muñoz A. Parental stress and children adjustment in kinship foster families. Span J Psychol. 2013;16:1–10.

16. Nadeem E, Waterman J, Foster J, Paczkowski E, Belin TR, Miranda J. Long-term effects of pre-placement risk factors on children's psychological symptoms and parenting stress among families adopting children from foster care. J Emot Behav Disord. 2016. doi:10.1177/1063426615621050.

17. Domsch H, Lohaus A. Elternstressfragebogen (ESF) [Parental Stress Questionnaire]. Göttingen: Hogrefe; 2010.

18. Achenbach TM, Rescorla LA. CBCL/1,5-5 & TRF/1,5-5 profiles. Burlington: University of Vermont, Department of Psychiatry; 2000.

19. Achenbach TM. Manual of the child behavior checklist/4-18 and 1991 profile. Burlington: University of Vermont, Department of Psychiatry; 1991.

20. Abidin RR. The determinants of parenting behavior. J Clin Child Psychol. 1992;21:407–12.

21. Woods SB, Farineau HM, McWey LM. Physical health, mental health, and behaviour problems among early adolescents in foster care. Child Care Health Dev. 2013;39:220–7.

22. Clausen JM, Landsverk J, Ganger W, Chadwick D, Litrownik A. Mental health problems of children in foster care. J Child Fam Stud. 1998;7:283–96.

23. Morgan J, Robinson D, Aldridge J. Parenting stress and externalizing child behaviour. Child Fam Soc Work. 2002;7:219–25.

24. John OP, Robins RW. Determinants of interjudge agreement on personality traits: the Big Five domains, observability, evaluativeness, and the unique perspective on the self. J Personal. 1993;61:521–51.

25. Comer JS, Kendall PC. A symptom-level examination of parent–child agreement in the diagnosis of anxious youths. J Am Acad Child Adolesc Psychiatry. 2004;43:878–86.

26. Vierhaus M, Lohaus A, Shah I. Internalizing behaviour during the transition from childhood to adolescence: separating age from retest effects. Eur J Psychol Assess. 2010;26:187–93.

27. Scaramella LV, Conger RD, Simons RL. Parental protective influences and gender-specific increases in adolescent internalizing and externalizing problems. J Res Adolesc. 1999;9:111–41.

28. Zahn-Waxler C, Klimes-Dougan B, Slattery M. Internalizing problems of childhood and adolescence: prospects, pitfalls, and progress in understanding the development of anxiety and depression. Dev Psychopathol. 2000;12:443–66.

29. Price JM, Roesch S, Walsh NE, Landsverk J. Effects of the KEEP foster parent intervention on child and sibling behavior problems and parental stress during a randomized implementation trial. Prev Sci. 2015;16:685–95.

30. Chamberlain P, Price JM, Reid JB, Landsverk J, Fisher PA, Stoolmiller M. Who disrupts from placement in foster and kinship care? Child Abuse Negl. 2006;30:409–24.

2

Mobilizing agencies for incidence surveys on child maltreatment: successful participation in Switzerland and lessons learned

Andreas Jud[1,2]* , Céline Kosirnik[3], Tanja Mitrovic[2], Hakim Ben Salah[3], Etienne Fux[4], Jana Koehler[4], Rahel Portmann[2] and René Knüsel[3]

Abstract

Background: Many countries around the world lack data on the epidemiology of agency response to child maltreatment. They therefore lack information on how many children in need get help and protection or if children stand equal chances across regions to get services. However, it has proven difficult to commit child protection agencies to participation in incidence studies.

Methods: The Optimus Study invested in a continuous collaborative effort between research and practice to develop a data collection for the first national study on the incidence of agency responses to all forms of child maltreatment in Switzerland. An innovative approach of utilizing individual agencies' standardized data reduced work burden for participation respectably: any arbitrary excerpt of data on new cases between September 1 and November 30, 2016, could be uploaded to a secured web-based data integration platform. It was then mapped automatically to fit the study's definitions and operationalizations.

Results: This strategy has led to a largely successful participation rate of 76% of agencies in the nationwide sample. 253 agencies from the social and health sector, public child protection, and the penal sector have provided data.

Conclusions: Valuing agencies context-specific knowledge and expertise instead of viewing them as mere providers of data is a precondition for representativeness of incidence data on agency responses to child maltreatment. Potential investigators of future similar studies might benefit from the lessons learned of the presented project.

Keywords: Child maltreatment, Incidence, Administrative data, Knowledge mobilization

Background

There is widespread agreement that in order to make progress in the prevention and reduction of child maltreatment it is important for policy-makers and administrators to have information on its scope and characteristics [1]. The worldwide number of efforts to nationally collect administrative data on agencies' knowledge of child maltreatment is, however, rare [1–3]. Countries' instable financial situations are not the only contributor to blame as also many high-income countries

lack a system of child maltreatment surveillance [3]. In many continental European countries, for example, there is no mandate for organizations in the child protection system to investigate and substantiate allegations of child maltreatment. Administrative data collection in these countries has so far primarily focused on the services provided. Another reason for lacking data are complex, federally organized child protection systems. Jud et al. [3] discuss reasons for lacking child maltreatment surveillance in high-income countries in detail. Anyhow, with lacking information on who enters the child protection systems, policy-makers and administrators do lack information about how to best allocate scarce resources to the ones most in need, change practices in assessment and intervention, train professionals, and reorganize

*Correspondence: andreas.jud@hslu.ch
[2] School of Social Work, Lucerne University of Applied Sciences and Arts, Lucerne, Switzerland
Full list of author information is available at the end of the article

systems for better responses [1]. So far, many research-ers around the world have responded to this need using surveys to count the prevalence of child sexual victimiza-tion or physical maltreatment in the general population. The prevalence of psychological maltreatment and child neglect has been less intensely studied. Furthermore, general population surveys do not inform policy-makers about the services or agencies in their jurisdictions that have knowledge of (alleged) child maltreatment, and what they are doing or not doing when they encounter it. Such data is gathered trough "agency surveys" or by ana-lyzing administrative data. For agency surveys, frontline workers provide information on their cases by complet-ing questionnaires. All of these studies cover the respec-tive country's public child protection organizations, some additionally sentinels like schools or agencies in the (mental) health sector [e.g. 4, 5].

To counter the lack of data on agency responses to child maltreatment, the World Health Organization provided a toolkit for researchers [6]. It assembles the lessons learned from previous studies on agencies' knowledge of child maltreatment. In all of theses studies, a knowledge mobilization approach has been essential for agency par-ticipation [7]. This approach does not consider agencies and frontline workers as mere informants and provid-ers of data. Instead, they are viewed as trusted partners in a mutual relationship with researchers; their local and context-specific knowledge is valued [e.g. 8, 9]. Research staff acknowledges that child protection practice will only commit to participation if the research initiative is per-ceived as being both relevant and credible. Major barriers to overcome are agencies' concerns on the confidentiality of data, concerns of being evaluated and compared, and, probably most importantly, work burden: Extra work for data collection will conflict with work time for clients or with the worker's free time [7].

This article adds to the literature by presenting an inno-vative study design to counter the lack of national data on agency response to child maltreatment. It describes how a large participation rate of agencies has been reached using this approach in Switzerland, and provides lessons learned. Despite of being one of the world's wealthiest countries, Switzerland lacks uniform and comparable data on child maltreatment incidents known to agencies. It therefore lacks data on how (frequently) and which vic-timized children receive support and protection [10].

Child protection in Switzerland
The child protection and child welfare systems in Swit-zerland are structured according to the political prin-ciples of federalism and subsidiarity which include the goals of organizing service systems on the cantonal (provincial) level and providing services—whenever

possible—at the lowest political level, the municipali-ties [11]. Consequently, there are 26 cantonal variations of organizing mandated and voluntary support for chil-dren in need. Further variations occur within cantons. This complexity on a relatively small scale of 8.5 million inhabitants is amplified by Switzerland's cultural and lin-guistic variety of three major languages, German, French, and Italian. Three sectors are essential for child protec-tion in Switzerland [11]:

- *Public child protection* The Swiss Civil Code empow-ers the child protection authorities to enact child protection orders if parents are unable or unwilling to remedy a situation of child endangerment. In most cases, they issue a general and unspecified mandate to a social worker in a specialized or general social service appointing him/her a deputy to the child. In more severe cases, the authorities can place the child in out-of-home care or finally withdraw parental cus-tody. At a subsidiary level, child welfare services have to offer help and counseling to children and fami-lies free-of-charge. Child protection orders are only enacted if this support is not deemed sufficient to counter an endangerment.
- *Penal sector* In severe cases of child maltreatment, prosecution and conviction of the perpetrator(s) can be a part of protecting the child from further harm. This goal is accompanied by the societal or individual need for dispensing justice and convicting felonies. Penal authorities handling cases of criminally liable child maltreatment include the police forces, the agencies of prosecution, and the criminal courts plus specialized juvenile courts and juvenile prosecution organizations to enforce juvenile criminal law.
- While a huge variety of organizations offer help and support to children and families with difficulties, some public and private bodies have established *spe-cialized agencies supporting children affected by child maltreatment*. They particularly include interdiscipli-nary child protection teams (in hospitals or region-ally administered), private counseling centers focused on support for victims of child sexual victimization, and publicly funded victim aid agencies.

For more details and a discussion of the role of sen-tinel agencies, see Jud and Knüsel [11], a framework for mapping child protection agencies is suggested in Trocmé et al. [12]. Much of the debate on professional-izing and improving child protection in Switzerland still falls within these sectorial or disciplinary silos. Data col-lection is even more fragmented and far from being uni-form or harmonized across or even within sectors. While most agencies still gather standardized information in an idiosyncratic approach for their agency, a few national efforts to collect child protection-relevant data at a national level nevertheless exist. These efforts include the federal annual reports of Police Criminal Statistics [e.g. 13, 14] and of services by victim aid agencies [15], the annual report on newly enacted and ongoing child protection orders [e.g. 16], and a national data set for cases of hospital child protection teams [e.g. 17, 18]. Agencies' participation in the latter two is, however, not mandatory; incomplete or missing data regularly occur. An initiative aiming at sharing uniform data across sectors has been lacking so far.

Obtaining agency participation in Switzerland: the Optimus Study[1]

The Optimus Study Switzerland addresses the paucity of incidence data on child maltreatment. A first cycle both included a population and agency survey on sexually victimized children and adolescents [19–21]. The population survey among adolescents highlighted the large amount of peer-to-peer sexual violence [20]. For the agency survey, weighted estimates indicate that 2.68 children per 1000 children in the population are reported to agencies based on an alleged incident of child sexual abuse. Unfortunately, the agency survey was bothered by low participation rates, especially in the French- and Italian-speaking parts of Switzerland [21]. Furthermore, it has been criticized that, for a child protection system, a focus on child sexual victimization is an isolated view. The different agencies and organizations not only intervene when sexual violence has been allegedly perpetrated, but as well to protect and support victims of neglect, physical and psychological violence. Multiple victimization is not the exception, but rather the rule [e.g. 22, 23].

To address these criticisms and to boost participation in a future wave of data collection, cycle 2 of the Optimus Study Switzerland reached out to stakeholders in the field of child protection—both administrators and policy-makers at the national, regional and municipal level, as well as frontline workers. The goal of this knowledge mobilization effort was to share and operationalize definitions of child maltreatment and its subtypes across sectors, to find solutions for addressing work burden for participating agencies, and creating a practice-validated and therefore relevant and credible questionnaire. It resulted in the first Swiss study on agency response to all forms of child maltreatment.

Establishing a multisite and multidisciplinary research team

Establishing familiarity with the different linguistic, regional, and disciplinary contexts has been a first step to present child protection practitioners with a trustworthy research team. Much like in other linguistically diverse countries such as Belgium or Canada, agencies in the linguistic minority parts of Switzerland feel easily dominated by organizations representing the major language region. It has therefore been essential to locate the research team both in Lausanne (French-speaking part) and in Lucerne (German-speaking part). Furthermore, the team assembles researchers of different disciplinary backgrounds relevant to the field. Their affiliations, Observatory on Child Maltreatment at University of Lausanne and Lucerne School of Social Work, are well known for their projects and continuing education on child protection.

The team was complemented with several collaborators, e.g. in the Italian-speaking part and from the penal sector as not all linguistic regions and disciplinary backgrounds were covered. These experts in their region and field helped as facilitators of access to individual agencies and regional or federal stakeholders in the field of child protection (see "Facilitating participation" section).

A practice-validated set of variables

Based on the assumption that practitioners are more ready to commit to participating in an epidemiological study on child protection if the variables of the data set are perceived as relevant and feasible, administrators, frontline workers and other stakeholders in child protection were invited to develop the set of study variables in a Delphi-type approach. First, a sample of agencies from different sectors were asked to provide their set of variables for standardized data entry, their definitions-in-use for child maltreatment and its subtypes. These lists of variables were then systematically compared with each other to identify uniform data elements. They were further compared to a minimum data set for child maltreatment surveillance developed in a pan-European project [24]. Next, the resulting set of variables was presented to around 50 stakeholders in child protection. In the German-speaking part of Switzerland, half-day workshops were offered in four different cities; in the more top-down organized Latin parts of Switzerland, various administrators were visited in their offices. Stakeholders discussed advantages and disadvantages of child maltreatment definitions and operationalization, commented on their priorities of including presented or additional variables in the data set, and on the feasibility of data collection. Based on this feedback, the research team created a pre-final

---

[1] The label "Optimus Study" encompasses projects on child sexual abuse and child maltreatment epidemiology in different countries around the world, namely in China, South Africa and Switzerland. All projects have been sponsored by the private UBS Optimus Foundation, Switzerland.

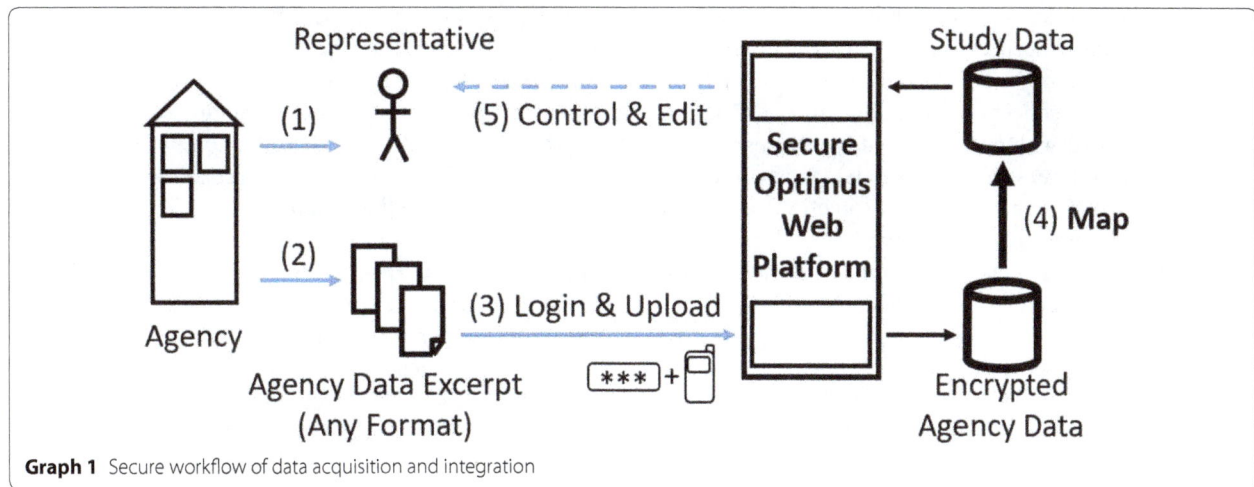

Graph 1 Secure workflow of data acquisition and integration

draft of the set of variables, their definitions and operationalization that was, once again, commented by our collaborators (see "Establishing a multisite and multidisciplinary research team" section). This process resulted in 25 variables on the caseworkers (age, gender, profession, job experience), report specifications (date, source, prior report), the maltreatment incidents (type(s), onset and frequency), child characteristics (gender, age, canton of residence, disabilities, household situation, number of siblings, socioeconomic status), the perpetrators (number of perpetrators, relation to victim, age, gender), services provided, and referrals. While both researchers and practitioners agreed that it would have been important to collect information on child maltreatment severity, caregiver demographics and family risk factors, these variables were rarely available in a standardized way across sectors or operationalized too differently to map on common definitions. They could therefore not be included in this minimum data set.

Mapping agencies' administrative data on the study data set

Practitioners readily embraced the idea of shared uniform data across sectors of child protection in the workshops. They however expressed concerns that the work burden of manually completing forms would decrease participation respectably and advocated for valuing agencies' efforts of data collection. This led to an innovative approach of mapping the agencies' pre-existing administrative data onto the study data set. We have added computer science specialists to our team who developed a procedure both guaranteeing user-friendliness and data security. Data acquisition and integration proceeded within a secure workflow (see Graph 1):

1. Each participating agency determined a representative who was registered with the web-based data integration platform.
2. In the ideal case, the representative was able to create an anonymized excerpt from the agency's standardized data collection that corresponded with the reference period of September 1, 2016 to November 30, 2016.[2] However, the excerpt could also contain original data covering longer periods if cantonal data protection law allowed for the transfer of such data.
3. He/she then uploaded these excerpts to the secure web-based platform using two-factor authentication (username/password and code via SMS). The study's platform was able to anonymize and process any arbitrary format of excerpts.
4. Once uploaded, data was encrypted and removed from the web platform immediately. Algorithms mapped the agency's individual data set onto the study data set with uniform definitions and operationalization. Variables not corresponding with the study data set were filtered out, as were any potential personal identifiers that had not already been removed before uploading. Any leftover personal identifiers were deleted immediately.
5. After mapping, agency representatives were able to complete missing data manually through a secure web interface. Most of the participating agencies lacked one or more of the study variables in their individual set of standardized administrative data. However, many agencies had information on the missing standardized data available from individual notes in the case files.

---

[2] A 3-month reference period for data collection has both been chosen to reduce work burden and for correspondence with previous agency surveys 2 [4].

During data collection, a multilingual helpline was offered to support agencies and address all their questions. The workflow was defined within a detailed 15-page security concept and architecture document. It was established with and reviewed by the responsible ethics committee and all 26 cantonal data protection officers (plus five municipal data protection officers of large cities) to ensure conformity with ethical guidelines, federal and cantonal legislation on data protection, and to disperse any potential concern of confidentiality.

Facilitating participation

In addition to the practice-validated data set and the innovative and timesaving approach to data collection, further steps were implemented to facilitate agencies' participation. Several of these steps pertain to the invitation to participate: first, many agencies and stakeholders were contacted informally by our collaborators to introduce the study to their peers. Credibility and relevance of the formal invitation letter was considerably increased through support letters from the federal office responsible for coordinating child protection and several supracantonal organizations. To guarantee a clear, concise and non-academic style in the invitation letter, the invitation letter was reviewed both by communication experts and several stakeholders from child protection practice. The invitation letter addressed major concerns such as confidentiality of data and the concern of being evaluated or compared. To counter the latter, we have guaranteed that individual agencies will not be identified once results will be presented. Furthermore, the invitation had been sent out well in advance of data collection to allow for addressing potential concerns and all letters were addressed individually rather than just anonymously "to whom it may concern".

If the agency did not respond to the invitation letter, we have followed-up by several telephone calls. Once an agency accepted to participate, an individual contact person was identified that would upload the excerpts from their agency's software (see "Mapping agencies' administrative data on the study data set" section). To further guarantee a constant exchange with agencies and other stakeholders, we have provided a biannual newsletter on the project's progress.

For some agencies, the work burden to participate was reduced dramatically if a national data set had already been established for their type of organization (see "Child protection in Switzerland" section). They either had to give us (written) consent of accessing their data in the national data set. For the two national data sets in responsibility of the Federal Statistical Office (FSO), rights had already been transferred to the FSO, so we had access to all police and victim aid agency data via contract with

the FSO. In addition, some data was directly exported and uploaded from the IT systems of a software vendor whose products are in use by a number of agency. An agency only needed to charge the vendor with the upload who then worked directly with the computer specialists of the study team. Obviously, this procedure called for a budget to reimburse the vendor.

Participation rate of agencies in Optimus Study 3

All these different measures culminated in a largely successful agency participation rate of 76% in total, or 253 participating agencies out of 334 sampled. The population of agencies in the three essential sectors for child protection in Switzerland summed up to 545 agencies at the time of data collection. With 46% of all organizations in these three sectors, our sample of 253 participating agencies accounts for a large proportion of agencies in the Swiss child protection system.

Participation was largely comparable in the German-speaking part (78%) and in the Latin parts of Switzerland (70%). Both access to data via direct uploads of agencies individual administrative data or indirectly via access to national data sets contributed essentially to participation (see Table 1).

The reason for non-participation was rarely rejection. Instead, the 57 actively declining agencies did not collect standardized administrative data at all or only in a very basic way and were therefore not able to create excerpts. Another main reason for declining participation was excessive agency workload—including agencies that first accepted to participate, but later did not upload their data. Finally, 24 out of 81 non-participating agencies have been considered declining after five unsuccessful telephone calls (in different weeks at different times) to contact the agency's director.

Discussion

Epidemiological studies on agency responses to child maltreatment are still much needed [1]. To achieve a high agency participation rate in such a research initiative, an approach that views the child protection practice as partners instead of informants is essential, but not sufficient. Researchers have also to address work burden as a major barrier to participation. The second wave of data collection of the Optimus Study Switzerland adequately included these pillars of agency participation in their project to reach a highly satisfying overall participation rate of 76% of the sample. Advantages and caveats of the study design are discussed, so readers might be able to potentially use our procedure as an example of "good practice".

Primarily, work burden has to be addressed as a major barrier to participation as agencies are already struggling

Table 1 Participating organizations by region and type of participation

	Number of agencies						Grand total
	German-speaking part			Latin parts			
	Public child protection	Penal sector[a]	Social and health sector	Public child protection	Penal sector[a]	Social and health sector	
	n (%)	n (%)	n (%)	n (%)	n (%)	n (%)	
Sample	152	22	60	51	8	41	334
Participation (total)	117 (77)	22 (100)	44 (73)	31 (61)	8 (100)	31 (76)	253 (76)
Uploading agency's individual administrative data	69	8	18	22	6	20	143
Giving access to own data in national data set	48	14	26	9	2	11	110
Non-participation (total)	35 (23)	0 (0)	16 (27)	20 (39)	0 (0)	10 (24)	81 (24)
Do not participate to the study	29	0	12	10	0	6	57
Communication failed	6	0	4	10	0	4	24

[a] Agencies included in the penal sector are police forces

to allocate scarce resources to the most urgent problems and many child protection workers will complain that they are overworked [7]. While producing a data export for a 3-month reference period and uploading it onto a secured web-infrastructure was indeed a timesaving way of participating in an epidemiological study for a majority of agencies, some software environments did not allow for an easy processing: The export function was restricted to a few variables or the software lacked an export function completely.

The innovative design of mapping a multitude of different administrative data formats onto the study data set (see "Mapping agencies' administrative data on the study data set" section) not only reduced work burden for agencies, but was also a means to appreciate agencies' previous efforts. Somewhat surprisingly, some agency representatives deemed the process of exporting data from their software as too tedious and preferred to collect data manually instead. So we additionally created an excel form with the study data set to for manual completion and easy upload onto the web-based platform. The excel form came also in handy for those small agencies that did not collect standardized administrative data at all.

Confidentiality is without any doubt an important ethical precondition for research on agency response to child maltreatment. Dealing with almost three dozen data protection officers and their feedback, however, was a time-consuming endeavor. Based on our insights into data storage of agencies, it is obvious that the security of our study data sometimes largely exceeds data security of agencies. Literacy in information technologies was at a low level for many agencies, only large agencies employ their own IT specialists. Some small agencies even had tools in use that store their data on servers in the US—outside of Swiss legislation and potentially accessible to unwanted third parties.

While it is obvious that participation will benefit from the efforts presented in this article, this procedure of knowledge mobilization is associated with an extensive temporal investment of the research team and therefore considerable budgetary resources. Our first contacts with stakeholders took place in 2012; data collection was completed in 2017. For many researchers it will be challenging to convince a scientific foundation to support a lot of exchange with participants that will not directly and/or timely lead to data and findings—we also had to invest a lot in advocating our study to our funder. Furthermore, a knowledge mobilization approach may challenge a researcher's career goals as much of the work cannot easily be transferred into written output.

The innovative and timesaving approach is also challenged by missing data. While gender and age of the victim and the type of violence he or she suffered are available for the majority of cases, data on the perpetrator(s), child and caregiver risk factors are collected quite differently by the various agencies in different sectors—if collected at all. An implicit goal of this study was also to identify shortcomings in agencies' individual data collection in order to define strategies towards a more uniform and shared approach to data collection on children and families in need.

Conclusion: on the road to child maltreatment surveillance

Representatives from the relevant federal offices and supra-cantonal bodies welcomed the Optimus Study as a bottom-up initiative; administrators readily committed to the goal of shared uniform data, but perceived a lack of political will to establish a national surveillance of child maltreatment incidents. The present research initiative will identify gaps in providing support and protection to maltreated children, an especially vulnerable group of citizens. Administrators expressed their hope that the identified gaps will help convincing policy-makers to take steps towards establishing a national surveillance procedure.

Our study was also accompanied by advocacy efforts to improve the sustainability of our approach and to further pave the ground for a nationwide child maltreatment surveillance. We have reached out to policy-makers in advance of publishing our findings. An advocacy company supports and overviews all our communication activities. Dissemination efforts will comprise short presentations for individual agencies and (supra-)cantonal stakeholders, a practice-oriented research brief, press releases, etc. This strategy guarantees that dissemination of the findings not only reaches academics, but also has its impact on policy-makers so that epidemiological research can have an impact on children's lives.

Authors' contributions
AJ is the principal investigator and project coordinator in the German-speaking-Part. He developed the study design, drafted, edited and finalized the manuscript. CK, TM and RP have been responsible for operationalizing the data set; CK and TM have joined AJ in drafting the manuscript. EF and JK developed the web-infrastructure and secure workflow of data acquisition and integration. They have drafted and edited the respective sections of the manuscript. RK and HBS are principle investigator and project manager for the Latin part. They have joined in editing the manuscript. All authors read and approved the final manuscript.

Author details
[1] Child and Adolescent Psychiatry/Psychotherapy, University of Ulm, Ulm, Germany. [2] School of Social Work, Lucerne University of Applied Sciences and Arts, Lucerne, Switzerland. [3] Observatory on Child Maltreatment, University of Lausanne, Lausanne, Switzerland. [4] School of Information Technology, Lucerne University of Applied Sciences and Arts, Rotkreuz, Switzerland.

Acknowledgements
The study team thanks Camille Sigg for her work on the Optimus-Study until April, 2017.

Competing interests
The authors declare that they have no competing interests.

Funding
The study is funded by the UBS Optimus Foundation, Switzerland.

References
1. Jud A, Fegert JM, Finkelhor D. On the incidence and prevalence of child maltreatment: a research agenda. Child Adolesc Psychiatry Ment Health. 2016;10:17.
2. Krüger P, Jud A. Overview of previous agency surveys and national administrative data sets. In: Jud A, Jones L, Mikton C, editors. Toolkit on mapping legal, health and social services responses to child maltreatment. Geneva: World Health Organization; 2015. p. 4–9.
3. Jud A, Fluke J, Alink LR, Allan K, Fallon B, Kindler H, Lee BJ, Mansell J, van Puyenbroek H. On the nature and scope of reported child maltreatment in high-income countries: opportunities for improving the evidence base. Paediatr Int Child Health. 2013;33:207–15.
4. Fallon B, Trocmé N, Fluke J, MacLaurin B, Tonmyr L, Yuan Y-Y. Methodological challenges in measuring child maltreatment. Child Abuse Negl. 2010;34:70–9.
5. Euser S, Alink LR, Pannebakker F, Vogels T, Bakermans-Kranenburg MJ, Van IMH. The prevalence of child maltreatment in the Netherlands across a 5-year period. Child Abuse Negl. 2013;37:841–51.
6. Jud A, Jones LM, Mikton C. Toolkit on mapping legal, health and social services responses to child maltreatment. Geneva: World Health Organization; 2015.
7. Jud A, AlBuhairan F, Ntinapogias A, Nikolaidis G. Obtaining agency participation. In: Jud A, Jones L, Mikton O, editors. Toolkit on mapping legal, health and social services responses to child maltreatment. Geneva: World Health Organization; 2015. p. 55–62.
8. Trocmé N, Esposito T, Laurendeau C, Thomson W, Milne L. La mobilisation des connaissances en protection de l'enfance. Criminologie. 2009;42:33–59.
9. Lomas J. Using 'linkage and exchange' to move research into policy at a Canadian foundation. Health Aff (Millwood). 2000;19:236–40.
10. UN Committee on the Rights of the Child. Concluding observations on the combined second to fourth periodic reports of Switzerland. New York: UN Committee on the Rights of the Child; 2015.
11. Jud A, Knüsel R. Structure and challenges of child protection in Switzerland. In: Merkel-Holguin L, Fluke J, Krugman, R, editors. National systems of child protection: understanding the international context for developing policy and practice. Springer, Dordrecht (in press).
12. Trocmé N, Akesson B, Jud A. Responding to child maltreatment: a framework for mapping child protection agencies. Child Indic Res. 2015;9(4):1029–41.
13. Bundesamt für Statistik (BFS). Polizeiliche Kriminalstatistik (PKS): Jahresbericht 2015. Neuchâtel: BFS; 2016.
14. Bundesamt für Statistik (BFS). Polizeiliche Kriminalstatistik (PKS): Jahresbericht 2016. Neuchâtel: BFS; 2017.
15. Bundesamt für Statistik (BFS). Beratungsfälle, nach Straftat, Geschlecht, Alter und Nationalität 2000–2016. Neuchâtel: BFS; 2017.
16. Konferenz für Kindes- und Erwachsenenschutz (KOKES). KOKES-Statistik 2015: Anzahl Personen mit Schutzmassnahmen. Zeitschrift für Kindes- und Erwachsenenschutz. 2015;2016(71):313–5.
17. Wopmann M. Gleichbleibend hohe Anzahl von Fällen von Kindsmisshandlung an schweizerischen Kinderkliniken. Baden: Schweizerische Gesellschaft für Pädiatrie, Fachgruppe Kinderschutz der schweizerischen Kinderkliniken; 2016.
18. Wopmann M. Erneute Zunahme der Fälle von Kindsmisshandlungen an Schweizerischen Kinderkliniken. Baden: Schweizerische Gesellschaft für Pädiatrie, Fachgruppe Kinderschutz der schweizerischen Kinderkliniken; 2017.
19. Averdijk M, Müller-Johnson K, Eisner M. Sexual victimization of children and adolescents in Switzerland: final report for the UBS Optimus Foundation. Zürich: UBS Optimus Foundation; 2012.

20. Mohler-Kuo M, Landolt MA, Maier T, Meidert U, Schönbucher V, Schnyder U. Child sexual abuse revisited: a population-based cross-sectional study among Swiss adolescents. J Adolesc Health. 2014;54:304–11.

21. Maier T, Mohler-Kuo M, Landolt MA, Schnyder U, Jud A. The tip of the iceberg. Incidence of disclosed cases of child sexual abuse in Switzerland: results from a nationwide agency survey. Int J Public Health. 2013;58:875–83.

22. Dong M, Anda RF, Felitti VJ, Dube SR, Williamson DF, Thompson TJ, Loo CM, Giles WH. The interrelatedness of multiple forms of childhood abuse, neglect, and household dysfunction. Child Abuse Negl. 2004;28:771–84.

23. Romano E, Bell T, Billette JM. Prevalence and correlates of multiple victimization in a nation-wide adolescent sample. Child Abuse Negl. 2011;35:468–79.

24. Ntinapogias A, Gray J, Durning P, Nikolaidis G. CAN-MDS policy and procedures manual. Athens: Institute of Child Health; 2015.

3

A multi-national comparison of antipsychotic drug use in children and adolescents, 2005–2012

Luuk J. Kalverdijk[1*], Christian J. Bachmann[2], Lise Aagaard[3], Mehmet Burcu[4], Gerd Glaeske[5], Falk Hoffmann[6], Irene Petersen[7], Catharina C. M. Schuiling-Veninga[8], Linda P. Wijlaars[7,9] and Julie M. Zito[4]

Abstract

Over the last decades, an increase in antipsychotic (AP) prescribing and a shift from first-generation antipsychotics (FGA) to second-generation antipsychotics (SGA) among youth have been reported. However, most AP prescriptions for youth are off-label, and there are worrying long-term safety data in youth. The objective of this study was to assess multinational trends in AP use among children and adolescents. A repeated cross-sectional design was applied to cohorts from varied sources from Denmark, Germany, the Netherlands, the United Kingdom (UK) and the United States (US) for calendar years 2005/2006–2012. The annual prevalence of AP use was assessed, stratified by age group, sex and subclass (FGA/SGA). The prevalence of AP use increased from 0.78 to 1.03% in the Netherlands' data, from 0.26 to 0.48% in the Danish cohort, from 0.23 to 0.32% in the German cohort, and from 0.1 to 0.14% in the UK cohort. In the US cohort, AP use decreased from 0.94 to 0.79%. In the US cohort, nearly all ATP dispensings were for SGA, while among the European cohorts the proportion of SGA dispensings grew to nearly 75% of all AP dispensings. With the exception of the Netherlands, AP use prevalence was highest in 15–19 year-olds. So, from 2005/6 to 2012, AP use prevalence increased in all youth cohorts from European countries and decreased in the US cohort. SGA were favoured in all countries' cohorts.

Keywords: Adolescents, Children, Antipsychotic drugs, Atypical, Denmark, Germany, Netherlands, UK, USA, Pharmacoepidemiology

Introduction

During the past decades, antipsychotic drugs (AP) have gained popularity as a treatment for psychiatric disorders in young people in most developed countries [1]. AP can be divided in two groups: first generation (typical) antipsychotics (FGA) and second-generation (atypical) antipsychotics (SGA) [2, 3]. Efficacy of AP in youth has been demonstrated for psychotic symptoms [4], bipolar disorder [5], irritability in autistic children [6], tics [7], and some forms of (severe) aggressive behaviour [8, 9]. Ample use of AP drugs has been described in children with a mental handicap and behavioral symptoms [10]. But only few antipsychotic drugs are licensed for those indications and for children and there is a lack of long-term efficacy and safety data [11]. Therefore, the treatment of youth with antipsychotics is subject to debate among clinicians, scientists and health policy makers [12].

Numerous reports from Western countries have described an increase in AP use, especially SGA, over recent years [1, 13–17]. These studies differ in terms of studied time period, age groups and other methodological features, thus hampering comparability. While there are some multinational studies comparing antidepressant or ADHD medication use in children and adolescents [18–20], updating patterns of AP use across countries and regions is warranted.

The objective of this study is therefore to determine recent trends in AP use from 2005/2006 through 2012 in 0- to 19 year-olds from five Western countries.

*Correspondence: l.j.kalverdijk@umcg.nl
[1] Department of Psychiatry, University of Groningen, University Medical Center Groningen, Groningen, The Netherlands
Full list of author information is available at the end of the article

Methods

Data sources

Denmark

We employed data from the Danish Registry of Medicinal Products Statistics (RMPS). The RMPS is a national prescription database, which encompasses all outpatient pharmacy-dispensed prescription medications in Denmark (5.53 million inhabitants). Each prescription record contains detailed information on the drug dispensed (incl. ATC code). Any drug utilisation prevalence can be calculated using an estimation of the underlying population as denominator.

Germany

To perform this study, claims data of the single largest German health insurance company, the BARMER GEK (about 9.1 million insurees, representing more than 10% of the German population) was used. Each prescription record contains detailed information on the prescribed drug, including ATC code. In relation to the complete German population, the BARMER GEK has a slightly higher proportion of female insurees, but there are no differences in terms of socioeconomic status (as measured by education level) [21]. The German data of this study have been published before in a German publication [16].

The Netherlands

The data used for this study are pharmacy dispensing data extracted from the IADB.nl database [22]. The IADB.nl database contains all prescription drug dispensing data since 1994 from about 60 community pharmacies. The corresponding population consists of about 600,000 persons from the North East Netherlands. In the Netherlands, patients are generally registered at one pharmacy, and there is an exchange of dispensing data between pharmacies. As a result, a single pharmacy can provide a complete listing of each registered subject's prescribed drugs history, with the exception of over-the-counter drugs and in-hospital prescriptions. The IADB.nl database population is representative for the whole Dutch population [22].

United Kingdom

We used primary care prescribing data from The Health Improvement Network (THIN) primary care database. In the UK National Health Service, primary care doctors (GP's) are the gatekeepers of referral to both secondary and tertiary care. Children, including those with severe forms of mental disorders, are either not referred for assessment to specialist services or followed up in primary care. THIN holds information on prescriptions issued in general practices (GPs) in all four UK nations.

The database covers approximately 6% of the UK population and is broadly representative of the UK population in terms of demographics and consultation behaviour [23]. In this study, we only included practices that had achieved good quality data recording in terms of patient mortality, and average number of records per patient per year [24, 25]. In total, we included 552 practices that contributed data between 2005 and 2012. Overall, prescriptions recorded in THIN reflect redeemed prescriptions, with an average redemption rate of 98.5% in 2008. However, the redemption rate is slightly lower for AP prescriptions at 85.1% in 2008 [26].

United States

We used computerized Medicaid administrative claims for the calendar years 2006 through 2012 from a narrowly-defined population of youth (0–19 years) in a mid-Atlantic state enrolled in Children's Health Insurance Program (CHIP). These children and adolescents are eligible for Medicaid coverage due to family income (upper limit: three times the federal poverty level [27]. The cohort consisted of over 131,000 youth in 2006 and of over 105,000 youth in 2012. Youth who were on Medicaid due to (1) disability; (2) foster care status or (3) family income below poverty level were excluded. Thus the population was similar to privately-insured youth in the US in terms of general health status, age distribution, race and family composition, with moderately lower parental education, employment, and income [28]. Each individual was assigned an encrypted identification number, which was then used to link the enrollment data files to prescription drug claim files.

Study variables and statistical analysis

Antipsychotics were defined as: all substances designated as class N05A (except Lithium) by the Anatomical Therapeutic Chemical (ATC) Code [29]. Of all AP the following drugs were considered second generation antipsychotics: Amisulpride, aripiprazole, asenapine, clozapine, iloperidone, lurasidone, olanzapine, paliperidone, quetiapine, risperidone, sertindole, sulpiride, ziprasidone and zotepine. The remaining antipsychotic drugs were considered first generation (e.g. chlorprotixene, chlorpromazine, haloperidol and pipamperone).

Annual AP use prevalence was defined as the percentage of youth (0–19 years at the time of prescription) with one or more AP dispensings or prescriptions among continuously enrolled youths in a given calendar year in the 2005/6–2012 period. Rates were not adjusted for age - or sex composition across the cohorts. Relative differences between years were calculated as the difference in prevalence, divided by the prevalence in the first year. The data were stratified by age groups (0–4, 5–9, 10–14,

15–19 years) and gender. The 95% confidence interval for the prevalence rates was calculated with the score method, with continuity correction for small proportions [30]. Differences were considered significant at $p < .05$.

Results

Trends in total use by country and according to age group

From 2005/6 to 2012 the annual prevalence for AP use for youth increased in four of the five countries under study (Fig. 1). This increase was as follows: in Denmark 0.26 to 0.48% (83.9% relative increase), in the German cohort 0.23 to 0.32% (40.8% increase), in the Netherlands' cohort (0.78 to 1.03% (31.7% increase), and in the UK cohort 0.11 to 0.14% (29.3% increase). A decrease from 0.94 to 0.79% was observed in the US cohort (− 15.6%).

When comparing the prevalence of AP use between countries' cohorts, large differences were observed (Table 1). In 2012, the highest AP use was observed in the Netherlands' cohort (1360/131,954; 1.03%), which was eight-fold higher than in the country with the lowest prevalence (UK; 0.14%).

With the exception of the Netherlands' cohort, AP use was higher in older age cohorts, with 15–19 year-olds showing the highest prevalence (2012: Denmark cohort 1.33%, German cohort 0.54%, Netherlands' cohort 1.47%,

UK cohort 0.31%, US 2.53%). Only in the Netherlands' cohort AP use prevalence was highest in 10–14 year olds (2012: 1.59%). For 0–4 year olds, after 2008 AP use remained lower than 1 per 1000 in all cohorts.

Trends in AP use by gender

In all studied cohorts, the prevalence of AP use was higher in boys than in girls (Table 2). In 2012, the male/female ratio ranged from an almost threefold higher use by boys in the Netherlands' data (2.87) to 1.38 in Denmark.

Across countries, AP use in girls was at or below 0.5% in contrast to AP use in boys that peaked at 1.54% in the Netherlands' data and 1.05% in the US data. From 2005/6 to 2012 use in boys increased relatively more than in girls in the German cohort, while the opposite was observed in the Netherlands' and in the UK cohort. In the US data, use in boys decreased more than in girls (− 19.9% vs. − 5.3%). In Denmark, the increase in boys and girls was comparable.

Patterns in FGA use vs. SGA use by country

In all cohorts except the US cohort the proportion of SGA relative to FGA prescriptions increased (Fig. 2). In the US regional cohort, SGA were almost the only class

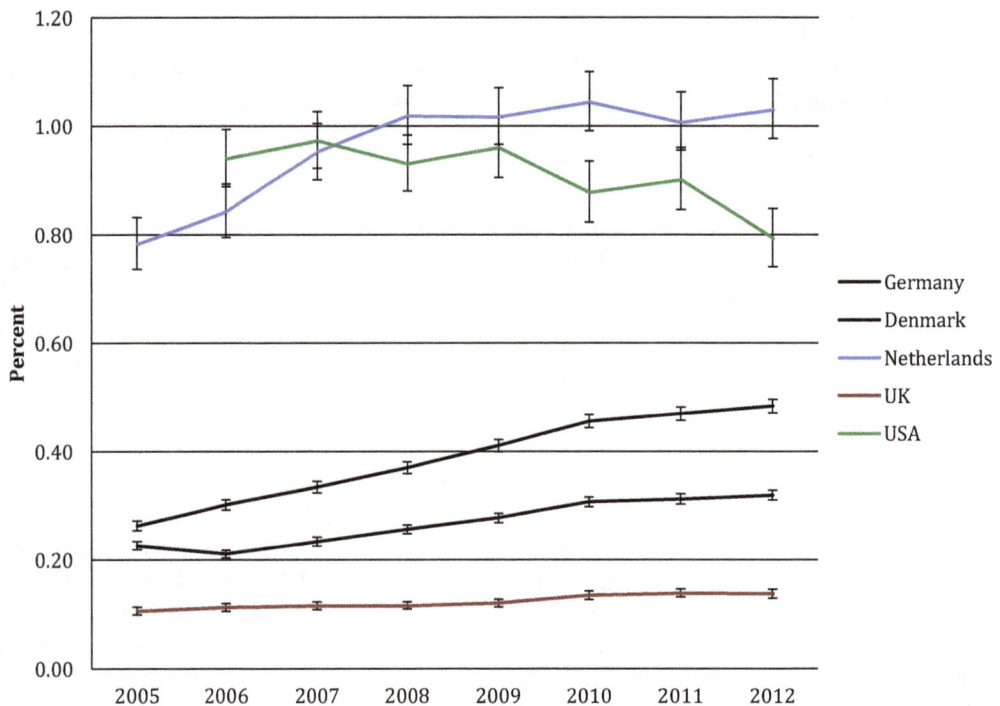

Fig. 1 Annual percent prevalence of antipsychotic drug use in children and adolescents (0–19 years) in cohorts from five countries, 2005/6–2012 (with 95% confidence intervals)

Table 1 Annual percent prevalence of antipsychotic drug use in cohorts from five countries between 2005/6–2012 among children and adolescents in 4 age group

	2005	2006	2007	2008	2009	2010	2011	2012	Difference 2005–2012
Denmark									
0–4 years	0.00 [0.00–0.01]	0.00 [0.00–0.01]	0.00 [0.00–0.01]	0.00 [0.00–0.01]	0.00 [0.00–0.01]	0.00 [0.00–0.01]	0.00 [0.00–0.01]	0.00 [0.00–0.00]	N/A
5–9 years	0.07 [0.06–0.08]	0.08 [0.07–0.09]	0.09 [0.08–0.10]	0.10 [0.09–0.11]	0.12 [0.11–0.13]	0.12 [0.11–0.14]	0.11 [0.10–0.13]	0.10 [0.09–0.12]	44.9%
10–14 years	0.26 [0.24–0.28]	0.27 [0.26–0.29]	0.33 [0.31–0.35]	0.34 [0.32–0.37]	0.39 [0.36–0.41]	0.40 [0.38–0.43]	0.40 [0.38–0.42]	0.42 [0.39–0.44]	61.5%
15–19 years	0.77 [0.73–0.80]	0.88 [0.85–0.92]	0.94 [0.90–0.97]	1.03 [0.99–1.06]	1.11 [1.08–1.15]	1.24 [1.21–1.28]	1.30 [1.26–1.34]	1.33 [1.29–1.37]	74.3%
Total	0.26 [0.25–0.27]	0.30 [0.29–0.31]	0.33 [0.32–0.35]	0.37 [0.36–0.38]	0.41 [0.40–0.42]	0.46 [0.44–0.47]	0.47 [0.46–0.48]	0.48 [0.47–0.50]	83.9%
Germany									
0–4 years	0.15 [0.14–0.16]	0.04 [0.03–0.05]	0.02 [0.02–0.03]	0.02 [0.02–0.03]	0.02 [0.02–0.03]	0.02 [0.01–0.02]	0.02 [0.01–0.02]	0.01 [0.01–0.02]	N/A
5–9 years	0.13 [0.12–0.15]	0.13 [0.12–0.14]	0.15 [0.14–0.17]	0.17 [0.15–0.18]	0.18 [0.16–0.19]	0.17 [0.16–0.19]	0.17 [0.16–0.18]	0.17 [0.16–0.18]	25.7%
10–14 years	0.24 [0.23–0.26]	0.27 [0.25–0.28]	0.31 [0.29–0.33]	0.34 [0.32–0.36]	0.37 [0.35–0.39]	0.42 [0.40–0.44]	0.42 [0.41–0.45]	0.43 [0.41–0.45]	76.8%
15–19 years	0.34 [0.33–0.36]	0.34 [0.33–0.36]	0.37 [0.35–0.39]	0.41 [0.39–0.43]	0.44 [0.42–0.46]	0.51 [0.49–0.54]	0.51 [0.52–0.56]	0.54 [0.52–0.56]	57.4%
Total	0.23 [0.22–0.23]	0.21 [0.20–0.22]	0.23 [0.23–0.24]	0.26 [0.25–0.26]	0.28 [0.27–0.29]	0.31 [0.30–0.32]	0.31 [0.31–0.33]	0.32 [0.31–0.33]	40.8%
Netherlands									
0–4 years	0.12 [0.09–0.17]	0.08 [0.06–0.12]	0.09 [0.07–0.13]	0.09 [0.07–0.13]	0.06 [0.04–0.10]	0.09 [0.06–0.13]	0.06 [0.04–0.09]	0.07 [0.05–0.11]	N/A
5–9 years	0.80 [0.71–0.91]	0.87 [0.77–0.98]	1.01 [0.91–1.12]	0.95 [0.85–1.06]	0.97 [0.87–1.08]	0.96 [0.86–1.07]	0.86 [0.77–0.97]	0.84 [0.75–0.95]	5.3%
10–14 years	1.18 [1.06–1.30]	1.32 [1.20–1.45]	1.56 [1.43–1.70]	1.65 [1.51–1.79]	1.68 [1.55–1.83]	1.69 [1.55–1.83]	1.67 [1.53–1.81]	1.59 [1.47–1.73]	35.5%
15–19 years	1.04 [0.94–1.16]	1.12 [1.02–1.24]	1.15 [1.04–1.26]	1.35 [1.24–1.47]	1.44 [1.33–1.57]	1.37 [1.26–1.49]	1.34 [1.23–1.47]	1.47 [1.35–1.60]	40.8%
Total	0.78 [0.74–0.83]	0.84 [0.80–0.89]	0.95 [0.90–1.01]	1.02 [0.97–1.07]	1.02 [0.97–1.07]	1.04 [0.99–1.10]	1.01 [0.96–1.06]	1.03 [0.98–1.09]	31.7%
UK									
0–4 years	0.00 [0.00–0.01]	0.00 [0.00–0.01]	0.00 [0.00–0.00]	0.00 [0.00–0.00]	0.00 [0.00–0.00]	0.00 [0.00–0.01]	0.00 [0.00–0.00]	0.00 [0.00–0.01]	N/A
5–9 years	0.03 [0.03–0.04]	0.03 [0.03–0.04]	0.04 [0.03–0.05]	0.04 [0.03–0.05]	0.04 [0.03–0.05]	0.05 [0.04–0.06]	0.04 [0.03–0.05]	0.03 [0.02–0.04]	− 16.7%
10–14 years	0.12 [0.11–0.14]	0.13 [0.12–0.15]	0.13 [0.12–0.14]	0.14 [0.12–0.15]	0.14 [0.13–0.16]	0.14 [0.13–0.16]	0.15 [0.13–0.16]	0.16 [0.14–0.17]	27.5%
15–19 years	0.25 [0.23–0.28]	0.27 [0.25–0.29]	0.28 [0.26–0.30]	0.26 [0.24–0.28]	0.26 [0.25–0.29]	0.31 [0.29–0.33]	0.33 [0.31–0.35]	0.31 [0.28–0.33]	20.5%
Total	0.11 [0.10–0.11]	0.11 [0.11–0.12]	0.12 [0.11–0.12]	0.12 [0.11–0.12]	0.12 [0.11–0.13]	0.13 [0.13–0.14]	0.14 [0.13–0.15]	0.14 [0.13–0.15]	29.3%
USA									
0–4 years	N/A	0.16 [0.13–0.19]	0.12 [0.10–0.15]	0.10 [0.08–0.13]	0.07 [0.05–0.09]	0.05 [0.03–0.07]	0.04 [0.03–0.07]	0.02 [0.01–0.04]	N/A
5–9 years	N/A	1.31 [1.18–1.47]	1.39 [1.25–1.54]	1.17 [1.04–1.31]	1.04 [0.92–1.18]	0.82 [0.71–0.94]	0.69 [0.59–0.81]	0.56 [0.47–0.66]	− 57.5%
10–14 years	N/A	2.53 [2.33–2.75]	2.59 [2.39–2.82]	2.50 [2.29–2.72]	2.50 [2.29–2.73]	2.23 [2.03–2.44]	2.31 [2.11–2.53]	1.91 [1.73–2.10]	− 24.6%
15–19 years	N/A	2.41 [2.14–2.71]	2.75 [2.47–3.06]	2.87 [2.59–3.19]	3.07 [2.77–3.41]	2.80 [2.50–3.13]	2.69 [2.41–3.01]	2.53 [2.26–2.83]	5.0%

Table 1 continued

	2005	2006	2007	2008	2009	2010	2011	2012	Difference 2005–2012
Total	N/A	0.94 [0.89–0.99]	0.97 [0.92–1.03]	0.93 [0.88–0.98]	0.96 [0.91–1.02]	0.88 [0.82–0.94]	0.90 [0.85–0.96]	0.79 [0.74–0.85]	− 15.6%

Numbers in brackets = 95% confidence interval

For the USA, only data from 2006 to 2012 were available

Table 2 Percent prevalence of antipsychotic drug use in 2005/6 and 2012 in 0–19 year-olds in cohorts from 5 countries, divided by gender

	2005 (USA:2006)	M/F ratio	2012	M/F ratio
Denmark				
F	0.22 [0.21–0.23]	1.39	0.40 [0.39–0.42]	1.38
M	0.31 [0.29–0.32]		0.56 [0.54–0.58]	
Germany				
F	0.16 [0.15–0.17]	1.85	0.19 [0.18–0.20]	2.28
M	0.29 [0.28–0.30]		0.44 [0.43–0.46]	
Netherlands				
F	0.37 [0.33–0.42]	3.18	0.51 [0.46–0.57]	2.87
M	1.19 [1.11–1.27]		1.54 [1.45–1.63]	
United Kingdom				
F	0.07 [0.06–0.08]	2.15	0.09 [0.08–0.10]	1.88
M	0.14 [0.13–0.16]		0.18 [0.17–0.19]	
USA (2006)[a]				
F	0.55 [0.50–0.61]	2.39	0.52 [0.46–0.59]	1.95
M	1.32 [1.24–1.40]		1.05 [0.97–1.14]	

Numbers in brackets = 95% confidence interval

For the USA, only data from 2006 to 2012 were available

M male; F Female

[a] Based on 2006

of drugs used, both in 2006 (98.5% of all prescriptions) and in 2012 (98.3%). In 2005/6 and 2012, risperidone was the most frequently used AP in all countries' cohorts, with the exception of Denmark, where in 2012 quetiapine ranked first. Use of aripiprazole, a relatively new drug that was approved by the FDA for irritability in autistic children in 2009, increased clearly: While in 2005/6 aripiprazole was only in Denmark and the US data among the top-5 prescribed AP, in 2012 it was in all countries among the five most frequently used AP (Table 3).

Discussion

We observed large differences between samples from 5 countries in the prevalence of AP use, with AP use being highest in the US cohort and lowest in the UK cohort. Since 2007, AP use in the Netherlands' cohort has surpassed use in the US cohort. Also time trends varied significantly: In the Netherlands' data, AP use stabilized

from 2008 to 2012. In the US cohort, the prevalence of AP use stabilized and decreased towards 2012. All other countries showed a trend for increased use. In most countries' data, AP use was greatest in 15–19 year-olds. We observed a strong and in most countries increasing preference for SGA, relative to FGA.

There are several possible explanations for the differences in AP use in youth cohorts from different countries: The attitude of prescribers towards psychotropic drugs and antipsychotic drugs and differences in health systems can be a factor that influences AP prescription rates [31]. For example: the attitude of physicians that SGA should be used to treat aggressive behavior can contribute to higher AP prescription rates [32] and the acceptance of psychiatric medication for children by the general public may be a factor [33]. Several studies indicate a broadening of indications, for example in ADHD and other disruptive behaviour disorders [13, 16, 34, 35].

Higher use of AP drugs can be associated with a stronger representation of medical disciplines in the care for youth with behavioral and psychiatric disorders or with an increasing use of mental health care [36]. Gaps in the mental health care system, e.g. lack of social care for the afore-mentioned patient group, may also lead to higher AP prescriptions [37]. It has been demonstrated that longer duration of treatment—and not only more new users—is a relevant factor in the increase in prevalence [14, 38, 39]. The decrease in use in the US confirms recent findings from the US [35] and could be influenced by measures to constrain AP use in youth. For example, recommendations for a more rigorous monitoring of side effects of AP, e.g.: [40, 41] have appeared. In the US, awareness programs targeting clinicians and the public were developed [42] and a system for prior authorization of antipsychotic prescribing for Medicaid insured youth [43] is implemented in 31 states.

We cannot fully explain the higher AP use in the Netherlands (which parallels the Netherlands position in international ADHD medication use [20]) despite the fact that regulatory approval is harmonized across European countries. In the Netherlands, treatment with AP has been included in some guidance statements, but not as a first line treatment option [44]. This finding may reflect a period of emphasis on the biomedical model in Dutch

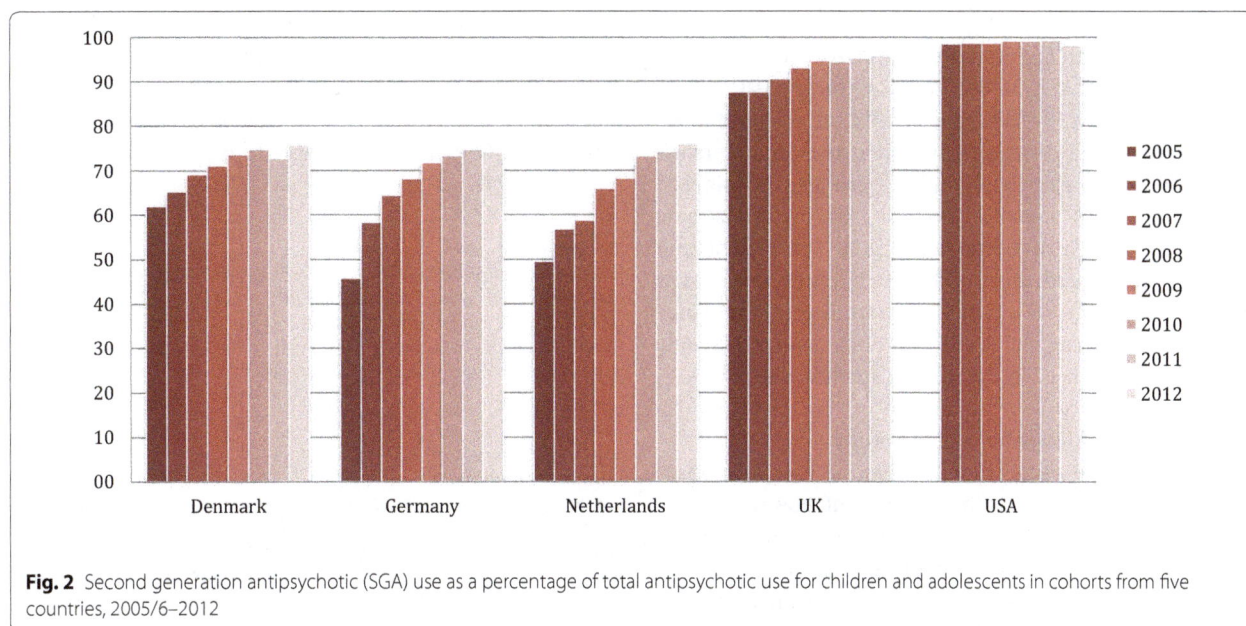

Fig. 2 Second generation antipsychotic (SGA) use as a percentage of total antipsychotic use for children and adolescents in cohorts from five countries, 2005/6–2012

Table 3 The five most commonly used antipsychotic drugs for children and adolescents in cohorts from five countries, 2005/6 vs 2012

Rank	Denmark				Germany				Netherlands				UK				USA			
	2005	%	2012	%	2005	%	2012	%	2005	%	2012	%	2005	%	2012	%	2006¶	%	2012	%
1	RIS	31.9	QUE	24.1	RIS	30.6	RIS	49.6	RIS	57.8	RIS	51.7	RIS	58.2	RIS	53.8	RIS	57.1	RIS	53.1
2	CHP	24.0	RIS	22.0	PIP	20.4	PIP	16.5	PIP	21.4	QUE	14.4	OLA	14.3	ARI	14.1	ARI	30.2	ARI	31.4
3	OLA	9.8	CHP	21.9	TIA	11.9	QUE	9.5	QUE	6.2	PIP	11.7	HAL	5.4	QUE	14.1	QUE	17.9	QUE	16.9
4	QUE	9.1	ARI	19.0	PMZ	6.7	TIA	6.0	OLA	4.9	ARI	11.0	CPZ	5.3	OLA	11.7	OLA	8.1	ZIP	5.5
5	ARI	4.2	OLA	7.0	OLA	5.8	ARI	4.5	PMZ	3.4	OLA	6.0	QUE	3.9	HAL	1.8	ZIP	4.7	OLA	4.3

For the USA, only data from 2006 to 2012 were available

ARI aripiprazole, *CHP* chlorprotixene, *CPZ* chlorpromazine, *HAL* haloperidol, *OLA* olanzapine, *PIP* pipamperone, *PMZ* promazine, *QUE* quetiapine, *RIS* risperidone, *TIA* tiapride, *ZIP* ziprasidone

Child and Adolescent Mental Health care. However, the strongest increase in the use of antipsychotics in youth predates the current period under study and unfolded in the period 1995–2005 [14]. It will be worthwhile to observe trends in the Netherlands from 2015 onwards, since important changes have been implemented since 2015 in the position of Child and Adolescent Mental Health care [45], with as one of the objectives a reduction in the use of psychopharmacological drugs in children.

In contrast, the low prescription rates found in the UK cohort may be related to the nature of the UK data, covering only prescriptions issued in primary care. So prescriptions by specialists are not taken into account. Another reason may be that the NICE guideline for ADHD [46] advices against use of antipsychotics in ADHD and the NICE guideline for antisocial behavior and conduct disorders [47] advices against medication

as routine management for children with this condition—which stands in contrast to some other countries' guidelines.

The greatest AP use in 15–19 year-olds in 4 of the 5 countries replicates findings by other authors where AP use increased towards early adolescence [13]. This is an age-group where behavioral problems tend to peak [48] and where severe mood disorders and psychotic disorders emerge. Another factor may be reluctance in prescribers towards prescribing for younger patients. The highest use in 10–14 year-olds that was found in the Netherlands may be explained by more use in behavioral disorders and by less reluctance towards prescribing in younger patients.

One explanation for the strong trend towards the use of SGA—which constitutes an exceptional growth in comparison to older studies (in 2000, in Germany only

5% of AP were SGA, [49])—may be that the literature about AP in youth is dominated by SGA focused papers, although the actual evidence base for efficacy is weak for most indications [50]. This may possibly an effect of more investment in the development and registration process of newer drugs. Previously, SGA were also considered more safe due to a smaller risk for extrapyramidal side effects [51] and tardive dyskinesia [52]. The insight that SGA are associated with different, but not necessarily smaller risks than FGA [53] is of more recent date since most reports about metabolic and endocrinological side effects have appeared in the last decade [40, 54–58].

Limitations, and implications of this study

This study is one of the first to describe use of antipsychotics in youth cohorts from different countries. The diversity of the underlying databases is a limitation as the underlying populations differ and this will certainly influence the rates that we found: The Danish cohort is nationwide, the US cohort comprises CHIP insured patients from one state, the Netherlands cohort covers a region of the country, the German cohort comprises patients from one large insurance company, while the UK cohort covers prescriptions from primary care. So, between-country comparisons should be made with caution. We were not able to control for co-medication, prescribing physician specialty (GPs vs. specialists) or socio-economic status, factors which influence AP use [51, 59]. Our data sources lack information that could improve the perspective on AP use, such as underlying indication, ethnic background, foster care status, duration of pharmacotherapy, adherence, symptom severity and symptom duration. We did not consider medication for hospitalized children. But the number of hospitalized youth may be small, compared to outpatients [60], and usually medication is continued in the outpatient setting after discharge from hospital.

In this vein, future studies will benefit from the use of harmonized databases, information about diagnosis (e.g. [61]) and use of other treatments, concurrent or sequential, thus giving more insight on indications and unmet needs in care across populations [59]. Data about incidence and duration of AP use is relevant, since longer exposure to the metabolic and endocrinological side effects of AP poses higher risks for health.

The implications of this study are that guidelines and practice parameters for AP use drugs need closer scrutiny. For those drugs where efficacy has been demonstrated in RCTs of limited duration, there is a pressing need for longer lasting observational and discontinuation studies to determine the risks and benefits of long-term use [62–64]. Close monitoring of use of psychopharmacological agents over time and across countries may

sensitize to national discrepancies in mental health care, differences in use of psychopharmacological treatment and populations with special needs or risks. For this purpose, a fixed multinational set of databases, gauged against each other, is an essential tool.

Abbreviations
AP: antipsychotics; FGA: first generation antipsychotic drugs; SGA: second generation antipsychotic drugs; UK: United Kingdom; USA/US: United States of America; ARI: aripiprazole; CHP: chlorprotixene; CPZ: chlorpromazine; HAL: haloperidol; OLA: olanzapine; PIP: pipamperone; PMZ: promazine; QUE: quetiapine; RIS: risperidone; TIA: tiapride; ZIP: ziprasidone.

Authors' contributions
LJK and CJB conceptualized and designed the study. LJK drafted the initial manuscript, undertook the statistical analysis. CJB, LA, MB GG, FH, CCMS, LPW, IP, JMZ acquired, analysed and interpreted data, revised the manuscript critically. All authors mentioned above agree to be accountable for all aspects of the work. All authors read and approved the final manuscript.

Author details
[1] Department of Psychiatry, University of Groningen, University Medical Center Groningen, Groningen, The Netherlands. [2] Freelance Researcher, Marburg, Germany. [3] Life Science Team, IP & Technology, Bech-Bruun Law Firm, Copenhagen, Denmark. [4] Department of Pharmaceutical Health Services Research, University of Maryland, Baltimore, MD, USA. [5] Division of Health Long-term Care and Pensions, University of Bremen, SOCIUM Research Center on Inequality and Social Policy, Bremen, Germany. [6] Department of Health Services Research, Carl von Ossietzky University, Oldenburg, Germany. [7] Department of Primary Care and Population Health, University College London, London, UK. [8] University of Groningen, Pharmacotherapy, Epidemiology & Economics, Groningen, The Netherlands. [9] Population, Policy and Practice, University College London Great Ormond Street Institute of Child Health, London, UK.

Acknowledgements
The authors wish to acknowledge all people and organisations that are instrumental in collecting and processing the datasets that make studies like this possible.

Competing interests
Financial: The authors have no financial relationships relevant to this article to disclose. Non-financial: LJK has received lecture fees from Eli-Lilly, Janssen-Cilag and Shire and has served as a study physician in clinical trials of Eli-Lilly. CJB has received lecture fees from Actelion, Novartis, and Ferring as well as payment from BARMER GEK and from AOK for writing book chapters. He has served as a study physician in clinical trials for Shire and Novartis. GG and FH are active on behalf of a number of statutory health-insurance companies (BARMER GEK, DAK, TK, and various corporate health-insurance funds) in the setting of contracts for third-party payment. LA has received travelling grants from Pfizer and Swedish Orphan BioVitrum. CCMS, LPW, IP, JMZ and MB declare no conflict of interest.

Ethics approval and consent to participate

United Kingdom: The study was approved by the CSD Medical Research Scientific Review Committee in February 2015 (reference number 14–086). The scheme for THIN to obtain and provide anonymous patient data to researchers was approved by the National Health Service South-East Multicentre Research Ethics Committee in 2002. *USA:* The study related to the USA cohort was reviewed and approved by the Institutional Review Board of the University of Maryland, Baltimore. *Denmark, Germany and the Netherlands:* According to the respective national regulations, an ethics review was not necessary for this study.

Funding

No funding was secured for this study.

References

1. Verdoux H, Tournier M, Begaud B. Antipsychotic prescribing trends: a review of pharmaco-epidemiological studies. Acta Psychiatr Scand. 2010;121(1):4–10.
2. Malone RP, Sheikh R, Zito JM. Novel antipsychotic medications in the treatment of children and adolescents. Psychiatr Serv. 1999;50(2):171–4.
3. Glazer WM. Extrapyramidal side effects, tardive dyskinesia, and the concept of atypicality. J Clin Psychiatry. 2000;61(Suppl 3):16–21.
4. Stafford MR, Mayo-Wilson E, Loucas CE, James A, Hollis C, Birchwood M, Kendall T. Efficacy and safety of pharmacological and psychological interventions for the treatment of psychosis and schizophrenia in children, adolescents and young adults: a systematic review and meta-analysis. PLoS ONE. 2015;10(2):e0117166.
5. Liu HY, Potter MP, Woodworth KY, Yorks DM, Petty CR, Wozniak JR, Faraone SV, Biederman J. Pharmacologic treatments for pediatric bipolar disorder: a review and meta-analysis. J Am Acad Child Adolesc Psychiatry. 2011;50(8):749–62.
6. Troost PW, Lahuis BE, Steenhuis MP, Ketelaars CE, Buitelaar JK, van Engeland H, Scahill L, Minderaa RB, Hoekstra PJ. Long-term effects of risperidone in children with autism spectrum disorders: a placebo discontinuation study. J Am Acad Child Adolesc Psychiatry. 2005;44(11):1137–44.
7. Hollis C, Pennant M, Cuenca J, Glazebrook C, Kendall T, Whittington C, Stockton S, Larsson L, Bunton P, Dobson S, Groom M, Hedderly T, Heyman I, Jackson GM, Jackson S, Murphy T, Rickards H, Robertson M, Stern J. Clinical effectiveness and patient perspectives of different treatment strategies for tics in children and adolescents with Tourette syndrome: a systematic review and qualitative analysis. Health Technol Assess. 2016;20(4):1–450.
8. Pringsheim T, Hirsch L, Gardner D, Gorman DA. The pharmacological management of oppositional behaviour, conduct problems, and aggression in children and adolescents with attention-deficit hyperactivity disorder, oppositional defiant disorder, and conduct disorder: a systematic review and meta-analysis. Part 2: antipsychotics and traditional mood stabilizers. Can J Psychiatry. 2015;60(2):52–61.
9. Loy JH, Merry SN, Hetrick SE, Stasiak K. Atypical antipsychotics for disruptive behaviour disorders in children and youths. Cochrane Database Syst Rev. 2012;9:CD008559.
10. de Bildt A, Mulder EJ, Scheers T, Minderaa RB, Tobi H. Pervasive developmental disorder, behavior problems, and psychotropic drug use in children and adolescents with mental retardation. Pediatrics. 2006;118(6):e1860–6.
11. Ben Amor L. Antipsychotics in pediatric and adolescent patients: a review of comparative safety data. J Affect Disord. 2012;138(Suppl):S22–30.
12. Olfson M. Epidemiologic and clinical perspectives on antipsychotic treatment of children and adolescents. Can J Psychiatry. 2012;57(12):715–6.
13. Olfson M, King M, Schoenbaum M. Treatment of young people with antipsychotic medications in the United States. JAMA Psychiatry. 2015;72(9):867–74.
14. Kalverdijk LJ, Tobi H, van den Berg PB, Buiskool J, Wagenaar L, Minderaa RB, de Jong-van den Berg LT. Use of antipsychotic drugs among Dutch youths between 1997 and 2005. Psychiatr Serv. 2008;59(5):554–60.
15. Patten SB, Waheed W, Bresee L. A review of pharmacoepidemiologic studies of antipsychotic use in children and adolescents. Can J Psychiatry. 2012;57(12):717–21.
16. Bachmann CJ, Lempp T, Glaeske G, Hoffmann F. Antipsychotic prescription in children and adolescents: an analysis of data from a German statutory health insurance company from 2005 to 2012. Dtsch Arztebl Int. 2014;111(3):25–34.
17. Burcu M, Zito JM, Ibe A, Safer DJ. Atypical antipsychotic use among medicaid-insured children and adolescents: duration, safety, and monitoring implications. J Child Adolesc Psychopharmacol. 2014;24(3):112–9.
18. Zito JM, Tobi H, de Jong-van den Berg LT, Fegert JM, Safer DJ, Janhsen K, Hansen DG, Gardner JF, Glaeske G. Antidepressant prevalence for youths: a multi-national comparison. Pharmacoepidemiol Drug Saf. 2006;15(11):793–8.
19. Bachmann CJ, Aagaard L, Burcu M, Glaeske G, Kalverdijk LJ, Petersen I, Schuiling-Veninga CC, Wijlaars L, Zito JM, Hoffmann F. Trends and patterns of antidepressant use in children and adolescents from five western countries, 2005–2012. Eur Neuropsychopharmacol. 2016;26(3):411–9.
20. Bachmann. CJ, Wijlaars L, Kalverdijk LJ, Burcu M, Glaeske G, Petersen I, Schuiling-Veninga CM, Hoffmann F, Zito JM. Trends in ADHD medication use in children and adolescents in five Western countries, 2005–2012. 2016 **(Under review)**.
21. Hoffmann F, Bachmann CJ. Differences in sociodemographic characteristics, health, and health service use of children and adolescents according to their health insurance funds. Bundesgesundheitsblatt Gesundheitsforschung Gesundheitsschutz. 2014;57(4):455–63.
22. Visser ST, Schuiling-Veninga CC, Bos JH, de Jong-van den Berg LT, Postma MJ. The population-based prescription database IADB.nl: its development, usefulness in outcomes research and challenges. Expert Rev Pharmacoecon Outcomes Res. 2013;13(3):285–92.
23. Blak BT, Thompson M, Dattani H, Bourke A. Generalisability of The Health Improvement Network (THIN) database: demographics, chronic disease prevalence and mortality rates. Inform Prim Care. 2011;19(4):251–5.
24. Horsfall L, Walters K, Petersen I. Identifying periods of acceptable computer usage in primary care research databases. Pharmacoepidemiol Drug Saf. 2013;22(1):64–9.
25. Maguire A, Blak BT, Thompson M. The importance of defining periods of complete mortality reporting for research using automated data from primary care. Pharmacoepidemiol Drug Saf. 2009;18(1):76–83.
26. Health and social care information centre. The prescribing compliance a review of the proportion of prescriptions dispensed. http://www.hscic.gov.uk/home. 2011. Accessed 02 Jan 2017.
27. http://kff.org/health-reform/state-indicator/medicaid-and-chip-income-eligibility-limits-for-children-as-a-percent-of-the-federal-poverty-level/. Accessed 02 Jan 2017.
28. Byck GR. A comparison of the socioeconomic and health status characteristics of uninsured, state children's health insurance program-eligible children in the united states with those of other groups of insured children: implications for policy. Pediatrics. 2000;106(1 Pt 1):14–21.
29. World Health Organization: (2016) ATC/DDD index. http://www.whocc.no/atc_ddd_index/. Accessed 05 Jan 2017.
30. Tobi H, van den Berg PB, de Jong-van den Berg LT. Small proportions: what to report for confidence intervals? Pharmacoepidemiol Drug Saf. 2005;14(4):239–47.
31. Schomerus G, Matschinger H, Baumeister SE, Mojtabai R, Angermeyer MC. Public attitudes towards psychiatric medication: a comparison between United States and Germany. World Psychiatry. 2014;13(3):320–1.
32. Rodday AM, Parsons SK, Correll CU, Robb AS, Zima BT, Saunders TS, Leslie LK. Child and adolescent psychiatrists' attitudes and practices prescribing second generation antipsychotics. J Child Adolesc Psychopharmacol. 2014;24(2):90–3.
33. McLeod JD, Pescosolido BA, Takeuchi DT, White TF. Public attitudes toward the use of psychiatric medications for children. J Health Soc Behav. 2004;45(1):53–67.
34. Penfold RB, Stewart C, Hunkeler EM, Madden JM, Cummings JR, Owen-Smith AA, Rossom RC, Lu CY, Lynch FL, Waitzfelder BE, Coleman KJ, Ahmedani BK, Beck AL, Zeber JE, Simon GE. Use of antipsychotic medications in pediatric populations: what do the data say? Curr Psychiatry Rep. 2013;15(12):426.

35. Crystal S, Mackie T, Fenton MC, Amin S, Neese-Todd S, Olfson M, Bilder S. Rapid growth of antipsychotic Prescriptions for children who Are publicly insured has ceased but concerns remain. Health Aff (Millwood). 2016;35(6):974–82.

36. Steinhausen HC. Recent international trends in psychotropic medication prescriptions for children and adolescents. Eur Child Adolesc Psychiatry. 2015;24(6):635–40.

37. Murphy AL, Gardner DM, Kisely S, Cooke CA, Kutcher SP, Hughes J. System struggles and substitutes: a qualitative study of general practitioner and psychiatrist experiences of prescribing antipsychotics to children and adolescents. Clin Child Psychol Psychiatry. 2015;21:1–15.

38. Abbas S, Ihle P, Adler JB, Engel S, Gunster C, Linder R, Lehmkuhl G, Schubert I. Psychopharmacological Prescriptions in Children and Adolescents in Germany. Dtsch Arztebl Int. 2016;113(22–23):396–403.

39. Rani F, Murray ML, Byrne PJ, Wong IC. Epidemiologic features of antipsychotic prescribing to children and adolescents in primary care in the United Kingdom. Pediatrics. 2008;121(5):1002–9.

40. Correll CU, Carlson HE. Endocrine and metabolic adverse effects of psychotropic medications in children and adolescents. J Am Acad Child Adolesc Psychiatry. 2006;45(7):771–91.

41. Cahn W, Ramlal D, Bruggeman R, de Haan L, Scheepers FE, van Soest MM, Assies J, Slooff CJ. Prevention and treatment of somatic complications arising from the use of antipsychotics. Tijdschr Psychiatr. 2008;50(9):579–91.

42. ABIM Foundation American Psychiatric Association (2015). Five things physicians and patients should question. http://www.choosingwisely.org/clinicianlists/american-psychiatric-association-antipsychotics-in-children-or-adolescents/. Accessed 27 Jan 2017.

43. Schmid I, Burcu M, Zito JM. Medicaid prior authorization policies for pediatric use of antipsychotic medications. JAMA. 2015;313(9):966–8.

44. Kenniscentrum (2017) Landelijk Kenniscentrum Kinder- en Jeugpsychiatrie. http://www.kenniscentrum-kjp.nl/en/home. Accessed 05 Jan 2017.

45. Hilverdink P, Daamen W, Vink C. Children and youth support and care in the Netherlands. Neth Youth Inst. (www.nji.nl/english); 2015:8.

46. NICE. Attention deficit hyperactivity disorder: diagnosis and management. Clinical guideline [CG72]. 2008. https://www.nice.org.uk/guidance/cg72. Accessed 01 Aug 2017.

47. NICE. Antisocial behaviour and conduct disorders in children and young people: recognition and treatment. [CG158]. 2013. https://www.nice.org.uk/guidance/cg158. Accessed 01 Sept 2017.

48. Moffitt TE. Adolescence-limited and life-course-persistent antisocial behavior: a developmental taxonomy. Psychol Rev. 1993;100(4):674–701.

49. Zito JM, Safer DJ, de Jong-van den Berg LT, Janhsen K, Fegert JM, Gardner JF, Glaeske G, Valluri SC. A three-country comparison of psychotropic medication prevalence in youth. Child Adolesc Psychiatry Ment Health. 2008;2(1):26.

50. Pringsheim T, Gorman D. Second-generation antipsychotics for the treatment of disruptive behaviour disorders in children: a systematic review. Can J Psychiatry. 2012;57(12):722–7.

51. Correll CU. Antipsychotic use in children and adolescents: minimizing adverse effects to maximize outcomes. J Am Acad Child Adolesc Psychiatry. 2008;47(1):9–20.

52. Correll CU, Leucht S, Kane JM. Lower risk for tardive dyskinesia associated with second-generation antipsychotics: a systematic review of 1-year studies. Am J Psychiatry. 2004;161(3):414–25.

53. Leucht S, Corves C, Arbter D, Engel RR, Li C, Davis JM. Second-generation versus first-generation antipsychotic drugs for schizophrenia: a meta-analysis. Lancet. 2009;373(9657):31–41.

54. Correll CU, Lencz T, Malhotra AK. Antipsychotic drugs and obesity. Trends Mol Med. 2011;17(2):97–107.

55. Andrade SE, Lo JC, Roblin D, Fouayzi H, Connor DF, Penfold RB, Chandra M, Reed G, Gurwitz JH. Antipsychotic medication use among children and risk of diabetes mellitus. Pediatrics. 2011;128(6):1135–41.

56. Bobo WV, Cooper WO, Stein CM, Olfson M, Graham D, Daugherty J, Fuchs DC, Ray WA. Antipsychotics and the risk of type 2 diabetes mellitus in children and youth. JAMA Psychiatry. 2013;70(10):1067–75.

57. Correll CU, Manu P, Olshanskiy V, Napolitano B, Kane JM, Malhotra AK. Cardiometabolic risk of second-generation antipsychotic medications during first-time use in children and adolescents. JAMA. 2009;302(16):1765–73.

58. Roke Y, Buitelaar JK, Boot AM, Tenback D, van Harten PN. Risk of hyperprolactinemia and sexual side effects in males 10–20 years old diagnosed with autism spectrum disorders or disruptive behavior disorder and treated with risperidone. J Child Adolesc Psychopharmacol. 2012;22(6):432–9.

59. Sikirica V, Pliszka SR, Betts KA, Hodgkins P, Samuelson T, Xie J, Erder H, Dammerman R, Robertson B, Wu EQ. Comparative treatment patterns, resource utilization, and costs in stimulant-treated children with ADHD who require subsequent pharmacotherapy with atypical antipsychotics versus non-antipsychotics. J Manag Care Pharm. 2012;18(9):676–89.

60. Graaf Md, Schouten D, Konijn C. De Nederlandse jeugdzorg in cijfers 1998–2002. NIZW Jeugd. 2005.

61. Nesvag R, Hartz I, Bramness JG, Hjellvik V, Handal M, Skurtveit S. Mental disorder diagnoses among children and adolescents who use antipsychotic drugs. Eur Neuropsychopharmacol. 2016;26(9):1412–8.

62. Rani FA, Byrne PJ, Murray ML, Carter P, Wong IC. Paediatric atypical antipsychotic monitoring safety (PAMS) study: pilot study in children and adolescents in secondary- and tertiary-care settings. Drug Saf. 2009;32(4):325–33.

63. Glennon J, Purper-Ouakil D, Bakker M, Zuddas A, Hoekstra P, Schulze U, Castro-Fornieles J, Santosh PJ, Arango C, Kolch M, Coghill D, Flamarique I, Penzol MJ, Wan M, Murray M, Wong IC, Danckaerts M, Bonnot O, Falissard B, Masi G, Fegert JM, Vicari S, Carucci S, Dittmann RW, Buitelaar JK, PERS Consortium. Paediatric European Risperidone Studies (PERS): context, rationale, objectives, strategy, and challenges. Eur Child Adolesc Psychiatry. 2014;23(12):1149–60.

64. Persico AM, Arango C, Buitelaar JK, Correll CU, Glennon JC, Hoekstra PJ, Moreno C, Vitiello B, Vorstman J, Zuddas A, European Child and Adolescent Clinical Psychopharmacology Network. Unmet needs in paediatric psychopharmacology: present scenario and future perspectives. Eur Neuropsychopharmacol. 2015;25(10):1513–31.

4

The relationships between gender, psychopathic traits and self-reported delinquency: a comparison between a general population sample and a high-risk sample for juvenile delinquency

L. E. W. Leenarts[1][*][†], C. Dölitzsch[2][†], T. Pérez[1], K. Schmeck[1], J. M. Fegert[2] and M. Schmid[1]

Abstract

Background: Studies have shown that youths with high psychopathic traits have an earlier onset of delinquent behavior, have higher levels of delinquent behavior, and show higher rates of recidivism than youths with low psychopathic traits. Furthermore, psychopathic traits have received much attention as a robust indicator for delinquent and aggressive behavior in both boys and girls. However, there is a notable lack of research on gender differences in the relationship between psychopathic traits and delinquent behavior. In addition, most of the studies on psychopathic traits and delinquent behavior were conducted in high-risk samples. Therefore, the first objective of the current study was to investigate the relationship between psychopathic traits and specific forms of self-reported delinquency in a high-risk sample for juvenile delinquency as well as in a general population sample. The second objective was to examine the influence of gender on this relationship. Finally, we investigated whether the moderating effect of gender was comparable in the high-risk sample for juvenile delinquency and the general population sample.

Methods: Participants were 1220 adolescents of the German-speaking part of Switzerland (N = 351 high-risk sample, N = 869 general population sample) who were between 13 and 21 years of age. The Youth Psychopathic traits Inventory (YPI) was used to assess psychopathic traits. To assess the lifetime prevalence of the adolescents' delinquent behavior, 15 items derived from a self-report delinquency instrument were used. Logistic regression analyses were used to examine the relationship between gender, psychopathic traits and self-reported delinquency across both samples.

Results: Our results demonstrated that psychopathic traits are related to non-violent and violent offenses. We found no moderating effect of gender and therefore we could not detect differences in the moderating effect of gender between the samples. However, there was a moderating effect of sample for the relationship between the callous and unemotional YPI scale and non-violent offenses. In addition, the regression weights of gender and sample were, for non-violent offenses, reduced to non-significance when adding the interaction terms.

Conclusions: Psychopathic traits were found to be present in a wide range of youths (i.e., high-risk as well as general population sample, young children as well as adolescents, boys as well as girls) and were related to delinquent

*Correspondence: laura.leenarts@upkbs.ch
[†]L. E. W. Leenarts and C. Dölitzsch contributed equally to this work
[1] Forschungsabteilung, Kinder- und Jugendpsychiatrische Klinik, Universitäre Psychiatrische Kliniken (UPK), Schanzenstrasse 13, 4056 Basel, Switzerland
Full list of author information is available at the end of the article

behavior. The influence of age and YPI scales on self-reported delinquency was more robust than the influence of gender and sample. Therefore, screening for psychopathic traits among young children with psychosocial adjustment problems seems relevant for developing effective intervention strategies.

Background

In recent years there has been an increasing interest in the manifestation and assessment of psychopathic traits in children and adolescents [1–3]. Studies have shown that youths with high psychopathic traits have an earlier onset of delinquent behavior, have higher levels of delinquent behavior, and show higher rates of recidivism than youths with low psychopathic traits [4, 5]. Furthermore, in conduct-problem youths, it has been found that the presence of psychopathic traits was related to a more severe pattern of antisocial behavior than when these traits were not present [4]. For example, as found in a study by Lindberg et al. [6] adolescent male homicide offenders scoring high on psychopathic traits, more frequently used excessive violence in their crimes. These findings are in agreement with many previous reports showing that juvenile offenders with psychopathic traits form a special subgroup [4]. Recognizing their characteristics would facilitate effective intervention efforts. However, up till now the vast majority of research on psychopathic traits and delinquent behavior has focused on high-risk samples for juvenile delinquency [7]. While, when defining effective intervention efforts, it is important to test whether the predictive value of psychopathic traits on delinquent behavior is confined only to the most antisocial youths or whether the relationship between psychopathic traits and delinquent characteristics is similar for juvenile justice and non-juvenile justice youths [7].

The few studies focusing on psychopathic traits in non-juvenile justice youths demonstrate that psychopathic traits are highly associated with delinquent behavior. For example, Oshukova et al. [8] found that in a community sample, in both boys and girls, psychopathic traits were highly correlated with rule-breaking and aggressive behavior. In addition, the correlation between psychopathic traits and rule-breaking behavior was significantly higher in boys than in girls. The relationship between psychopathic traits and delinquency among adolescents in residential care (i.e., residing non-juvenile justice youths) is unknown, as studies in these settings are scarce. However, a Dutch study on adolescents in residential care [9] identified that youths scoring high on all three YPI scales scored higher on externalizing problem behavior compared to youths with average scores on the YPI scales. In addition, Schmid et al. [10] reported that youths with psychopathic traits are two to three times more likely to drop out of residential care (i.e., unscheduled termination of measurement by the institution, juvenile or other involved people; e.g., expulsion from the institution because of aggressive behavior towards professionals or other juveniles in the institution, little cooperation from the family of the juvenile, no educational opportunities).

There is a controversial discussion about differences between boys and girls in the manifestation of psychopathic traits and its relation to delinquent behavior. Psychopathic traits are believed to exist in both boys and girls [11, 12]. In addition, in both boys and girls elevated psychopathic traits are related to a higher likelihood of delinquent behavior [4]. However, a number of studies have demonstrated that the relationship between psychopathic traits and delinquent behavior is different for boys and girls (e.g., [4, 7]). For example, the results of a meta-analysis by Asscher et al. [4] showed that the effect size of psychopathy on delinquent behavior was larger in adolescent female samples than in adolescent male samples. An explanation for this finding may be that the relatively small group of girls showing psychopathic traits is a highly disturbed and burdened group, showing high levels of delinquent behavior. Whereas Penney and Moretti [13] found that the relationship, in a high-risk sample, between psychopathic features, aggression and antisocial behavior was equivalent for boys and girls. Generally speaking, psychopathic traits have received much attention as a robust indicator for delinquent and aggressive behavior in both boys and girls. However, there is a notable lack of research on gender differences in the relationship between psychopathic traits and delinquent behavior [13]. In addition, as previously mentioned, most of the studies on psychopathic traits and delinquent behavior were conducted in high-risk samples.

Consequently, the first objective of the current study was to investigate the relationship between psychopathic traits and specific forms of self-reported delinquency in a high-risk sample for juvenile delinquency as well as in a general population sample. As different combinations of elevated scores on psychopathic traits may lead to different types of juvenile delinquency [9], with for example a higher score on all three YPI scales predicting the probability for having committed violent offenses and a higher score on only one scale of the YPI predicting the probability for having committed non-violent offenses, we categorized the self-reported delinquency in two types of offenses (i.e., violent offenses and non-violent offenses).[1] Furthermore, given the controversial discussion about the role of gender in the relationship between psychopathic traits and specific forms of self-reported delinquency; the second objective was to examine the influence of gender on this relationship. Finally, we investigated whether the moderating effect of gender was comparable in the high-risk sample for juvenile delinquency and the general population sample. Gaining greater understanding of associations between psychopathic traits and delinquent behavior in a high-risk sample for juvenile delinquency as well as in a general population sample is essential for developing effective intervention strategies.

Methods
Procedure
The current study was part of the larger *Swiss study for clarification and goal-attainment in youth welfare and juvenile justice institutions*, involving the standardized monitoring and evaluation of mental health problems of youths in welfare and juvenile justice institutions in Switzerland [14]. At the same time, the Youth Psychopathic traits Inventory (YPI) and the self-reported delinquency questionnaire were applied to a school sample [15], to obtain data from the general population for purposes of comparison.

The high-risk sample for juvenile delinquency was recruited from 38 welfare and juvenile justice institutions from the German speaking part of Switzerland. Adolescents between 13 and 21 years of age who were admitted to one of the 38 facilities between 2007 and 2011 were asked to participate; with the exception of those who had a placement shorter than 1 month and those who, due to language problems, were not able to complete the assessment tools. Adolescents and their primary caregivers were individually approached by trained staff of the institution who explained the aims and nature of the study. Following Swiss legislation, active informed consent was collected and, if the adolescent was younger than age 18, parental/primary caregiver informed consent was obtained as well. The study was reviewed by the Ethics Review Committees of Basel, Lausanne (Switzerland) and Ulm (Germany). It is important to note that in Switzerland, youths can be placed in welfare and juvenile justice institutions because of: delinquent behavior (*criminal law measure*), youth welfare reasons (*civil law measure*,

e.g., maltreatment, parental psychopathology, prostitution and drug abuse) or *other reasons* (e.g., their own or parents' choice). These three groups currently reside in the same facilities. An analysis by Dölitzsch et al. [16] showed that youths who are placed in youth welfare and juvenile justice institutions because of youth welfare or other reasons, have a high-risk of delinquent behavior: 83.4% reported to have committed at least one offense.

The general population sample was recruited from 18 public schools in the German-speaking part of Switzerland. Schools were selected to cover all curricula and to cover urban as well as rural areas. Youths were included in the study if they were between 13 and 21 years of age and were able to complete the German assessment tools. Assessment took place during a 1-h class. Active informed consent was collected and for minors, parental/ primary caregiver informed consent was collected. Participants had a chance to get free movie tickets. The study was reviewed by the Ethics Review Committee of Basel.

Participants
For the current study, data from 1220 adolescents of the German-speaking part of Switzerland (N = 351 high-risk sample, N = 869 general population sample) who were between 13 and 21 years of age and completed both the YPI [17] and a self-reported delinquency questionnaire [18] were analyzed. Adolescents' ages, from the high-risk sample, ranged from 13 to 21 years (mean = 16.2, SD = 1.8). Among the 242 (68.9%) boys and 109 (31.1%) girls, 26.6% were placed in the facility under a *criminal law measure*, 55.0% under a *civil law measure* and 18.4% because of *other reasons*. Most adolescents (79.5%) were born in Switzerland and 20.5% was born in other countries. More than one third of the mothers (37.7%) and one fifth (20.2%) of the fathers of youths in the high-risk sample had only finished primary or secondary school. The adolescents' ages, from the general population sample, ranged from 13 to 21 years (mean = 17.3, SD = 1.3). Among the 497 (57.2%) boys and 372 (42.8%) girls, 86.7% was born in Switzerland and 13.3% was born in other countries. One fourth of the mothers (25%) and 15.3% of the fathers of youths in the general population sample had only finished primary or secondary school.

Assessment
Demographics
Background information (i.e., age, gender and country of birth) for the high-risk sample was extracted by local staff from personal records. Youths from the general population sample answered questions about their personal background in a questionnaire.

---

[1] The current study focuses on self-reported delinquency, the term delinquency is used as a more general category which is categorized in violent offenses and non-violent offenses.

YPI

The German [Schmeck, Hinrichs & Fegert, 2005, unpublished questionnaire] version of the YPI [17] was used to assess psychopathic traits. The YPI is a self-report questionnaire which consists of 50 items that combine into 10 scales. These scales map onto three domains: grandiose-manipulative (including the subscales dishonest charm, grandiosity, lying and manipulation), callous and unemotional (including the subscales callousness, unemotionality and remorselessness), and impulsive-irresponsible (including the subscales impulsiveness, thrill-seeking and irresponsibility). The respondent rates the questions on a Likert-type four-point rating scale ranging from 1 = does not apply at all to 4 = applies very well. Earlier research on this questionnaire in juvenile justice and non-juvenile justice samples displayed satisfactory psychometric properties [15, 17]. In the current study, Cronbach's alpha coefficients of the scales ranged from 0.82 to 0.90.

Self-reported delinquency

To assess the lifetime prevalence of the adolescents' delinquent behavior, 15 items derived from a validated instrument [18] were used. The items assess three forms of delinquent behavior, namely: vandalism (3 items), property offenses (8 items) and violent offenses (4 items). Vandalism expresses damage to or the destruction of public or private property, caused by a person who is not its owner. Property offenses refers to the taking of property, and does not involve (threat of) force against a victim or damage to or destruction of the property. Violent offenses refers to crimes in which an offender uses or threatens force upon a victim. This entails both crimes in which the violent act is the objective as well as crimes in which violence is the means to an end. Adolescents were asked anonymously, if they had ever committed the designated delinquent behavior, how old they were when they first committed the behavior and how often they had committed the behavior. For the analyses, the three forms of self-reported delinquency were categorized into two variables: violent offenses versus non-violent offenses (i.e., vandalism and property offenses).

Statistics

First, we generated descriptive statistics (using Statistical Package for Social Science, SPSS, 21) for the study variables and compared YPI scores, and self-reported delinquency across the two samples via t-test and Chi square analyses.

Next, we conducted logistic regression analyses, for each YPI scale separately, that regressed violent offenses and non-violent offenses on age, YPI scale, gender and sample. In the second block all the two-way interactions were included in the analyses (excluding interactions

with age). To test for the potential moderating effect of gender, we checked whether the interaction terms contributed significantly to the regression equation. In the third and final block the three-way interaction between gender, sample and YPI scale was included, to investigate whether the moderating effect of gender was comparable in the high-risk sample and the general population sample.

Results

Comparisons across samples

YPI means were compared across the high-risk sample and the general population sample. Youths from the high-risk sample scored significantly higher than youths from the general population sample on all the YPI scales: grandiose-manipulative [10.58 versus 9.38; $t(587) = 7.06$, $p < 0.001$], callous and unemotional [11.01 versus 9.84; $t(1218) = 7.77$, $p < 0.001$], and impulsive-irresponsible [12.92 versus 11.36; $t(577) = 9.33$, $p < 0.001$]. Considering self-reported delinquency; youths from the high-risk sample were more likely than youths from the general population sample to report non-violent offenses [84.3% versus 61.4%; $\chi^2(1) = 60.18$, $p < 0.001$], and violent offenses [60.1% versus 26.2%; $\chi^2(1) = 124.56$, $p < 0.001$].

Logistic regression non-violent offenses

Table 1 presents the models predicting non-violent offenses. First, we considered the YPI grandiose-manipulative scale for non-violent offenses (Table 1, Model 1); the first block significantly predicted non-violent offenses [$\chi^2(4) = 177.17$, $p < 0.001$; Nagelkerke $R^2 = 0.19$]. A significant main effect emerged for age, the YPI grandiose-manipulative scale, gender and sample. The second block revealed no improvement in explained variance compared to the first block [$\chi^2(3) = 3.13$, $p = 0.372$; Nagelkerke $R^2 = 0.19$]. The contributions of age and the YPI grandiose-manipulative scale remained essentially unchanged, while the main effects of gender and sample were reduced to non-significance. The two-way interaction terms did not significantly contribute to the regression equation. The third block, which also included the three-way interaction term, yielded similar results as the second block [$\chi^2(1) = 1.39$, $p = 0.238$; Nagelkerke $R^2 = 0.19$]. The only significant contributors to the equation were age and the YPI grandiose-manipulative scale.

Next, we considered the YPI callous and unemotional scale for non-violent offenses (Table 1, Model 2); the first block significantly predicted non-violent offenses [$\chi^2(4) = 140.25$, $p < 0.001$; Nagelkerke $R^2 = 0.15$]. Again, a significant main effect emerged for age, the YPI callous and unemotional scale, gender and sample. Adding all the two-way interactions to the model significantly improved model fit [$\chi^2(3) = 9.18$, $p = 0.027$; Nagelkerke $R^2 = 0.16$].

Table 1 Logistic regression non-violent offenses

	Model 1 (grandiose-manipulative)			Model 2 (callous and unemotional)			Model 3 (impulsive-irresponsible)		
	B	SE B	Exp (B)	B	SE B	Exp (B)	B	SE B	Exp (B)
Block 1									
Age	0.14	0.05	1.15**	0.14	0.05	1.15**	0.14	0.05	1.15**
YPI scale	0.24	0.03	1.28***	0.20	0.03	1.22***	0.42	0.03	1.53***
Gender (boys = 1, girls = 0)	0.43	0.14	1.53**	0.31	0.14	1.36*	0.50	0.14	1.64***
Sample (high-risk = 1, general = 0)	1.16	0.18	3.20***	1.18	0.18	3.27***	0.97	0.19	2.63***
Block 2									
Age	0.14	0.05	1.15**	0.14	0.05	1.15**	0.14	0.05	1.15**
YPI scale	0.26	0.05	1.30***	0.09	0.05	1.10	0.44	0.06	1.55***
Gender	0.97	0.57	2.64	− 0.56	0.66	0.57	0.90	0.78	2.45
Sample	1.01	0.68	2.74	− 0.27	0.84	0.76	1.03	0.92	2.81
YPI × gender	− 0.05	0.06	0.95	0.11	0.07	1.11	− 0.03	0.07	0.97
YPI × sample	0.05	0.07	1.05	0.19	0.09	1.21*	0.01	0.08	1.01
Gender × sample	− 0.54	0.36	0.58	− 0.63	0.36	0.53	− 0.34	0.37	0.71
Block 3									
Age	0.14	0.05	1.15**	0.14	0.05	1.15**	0.14	0.05	1.15**
YPI scale	0.24	0.05	1.27***	0.10	0.06	1.11	0.44	0.06	1.56***
Gender	0.66	0.63	1.93	− 0.43	0.72	0.65	1.01	0.89	2.74
Sample	− 0.15	1.23	0.86	0.19	1.33	1.21	1.34	1.46	3.81
YPI × gender	− 0.01	0.07	0.99	0.09	0.07	1.10	− 0.04	0.08	0.96
YPI × sample	0.19	0.14	1.21	0.14	0.14	1.15	− 0.02	0.13	0.99
Gender × sample	1.16	1.50	3.20	− 1.39	1.76	0.25	− 0.83	1.86	0.44
YPI × gender × sample	− 0.19	0.17	0.82	0.08	0.18	1.08	0.04	0.16	1.05

B unstandardized regression coefficient, SE B standard error regression coefficient, Exp (B) expected regression coefficient (odds ratio), YPI Youth Psychopathic Traits Inventory

* $p < 0.05$; ** $p < 0.01$; *** $p < 0.001$

Regarding the main effects, only the main effect of age remained significant. In addition, the two-way interaction term sample × YPI callous and unemotional contributed significantly to the regression equation. Meaning that having a higher score on the YPI callous and unemotional scale increased the probability for having committed non-violent offenses for youths from the high-risk sample and not for youths from the general population sample. Adding the three-way interaction did not significantly improve model fit [$\chi^2(1) = 0.20$, $p = 0.658$; Nagelkerke $R^2 = 0.16$]. Age was the only significant contributor to this regression equation.

Finally, we considered the YPI impulsive-irresponsible scale for non-violent offenses (Table 1, Model 3). The first block significantly predicted non-violent offenses [$\chi^2(4) = 299.81$, $p < 0.001$; Nagelkerke $R^2 = 0.30$]. Significant main effects emerged for age, the YPI impulsive-irresponsible scale, gender and sample. The second block revealed no improvement in explained variance compared to the first block [$\chi^2(3) = 1.12$, $p = 0.772$; Nagelkerke $R^2 = 0.31$]. The contributions of age and the

YPI impulsive-irresponsible scale remained essentially unchanged, while the other main effects were reduced to non-significance. None of two-way interactions contributed substantially to the regression equation. Adding the three-way interaction did not improve model fit [$\chi^2(1) = 0.07$, $p = 0.789$; Nagelkerke $R^2 = 0.31$]. Only age and the YPI impulsive-irresponsible scale contributed significantly to this regression equation.

Logistic regression violent offenses

Considering the YPI grandiose-manipulative scale for violent offenses (Table 2, Model 1); the first block significantly predicted violent offenses [$\chi^2(4) = 234.16$, $p < 0.001$; Nagelkerke $R^2 = 0.24$]. A significant main effect emerged for age, the YPI grandiose-manipulative scale, gender and sample. The second block revealed a significant improvement in explained variance compared to the first block [$\chi^2(3) = 9.57$, $p = 0.023$; Nagelkerke $R^2 = 0.25$]. All main effects remained essentially unchanged. In addition, the two-way interaction term gender x sample contributed significantly to the regression equation.

Table 2 Logistic regression violent offenses

	Model 1 (grandiose-manipulative)			Model 2 (callous and unemotional)			Model 3 (impulsive-irresponsible)		
	B	SE B	Exp (B)	B	SE B	Exp (B)	B	SE B	Exp (B)
Block 1									
Age	0.11	0.05	1.12*	0.13	0.05	1.13**	0.11	0.05	1.12*
YPI scale	0.17	0.03	1.18***	0.24	0.03	1.27***	0.23	0.03	1.26***
Gender (boys = 1, girls = 0)	0.86	0.15	2.37***	0.62	0.15	1.86***	0.96	0.15	2.62***
Sample (high-risk = 1, general = 0)	1.41	0.15	4.11***	1.42	0.15	4.14***	1.29	0.16	3.63***
Block 2									
Age	0.12	0.05	1.13**	0.13	0.05	1.14**	0.12	0.05	1.13**
YPI scale	0.23	0.06	1.26***	0.22	0.06	1.25***	0.30	0.06	1.35***
Gender	1.75	0.61	5.78**	0.56	0.71	1.75	2.34	0.76	10.38**
Sample	2.35	0.58	10.49***	2.13	0.68	8.42**	2.02	0.76	7.54**
YPI × gender	− 0.06	0.06	0.94	0.03	0.07	1.03	− 0.09	0.06	0.91
YPI × sample	− 0.04	0.05	0.96	− 0.02	0.07	0.98	− 0.02	0.06	0.98
Gender × sample	− 0.80	0.31	0.45**	− 0.72	0.32	0.49*	− 0.70	0.31	0.50*
Block 3									
Age	0.12	0.05	1.13**	0.13	0.05	1.14**	0.12	0.05	1.13**
YPI scale	0.19	0.07	1.21**	0.25	0.07	1.29***	0.29	0.07	1.34***
Gender	1.33	0.76	3.77	0.97	0.88	2.64	2.23	0.97	9.26*
Sample	1.57	1.04	4.80	2.91	1.20	18.41*	1.82	1.31	6.15
YPI × gender	− 0.02	0.08	0.98	− 0.01	0.09	0.99	− 0.08	0.08	0.92
YPI × sample	0.05	0.11	1.05	− 0.10	0.12	0.90	0.00	0.10	1.00
Gender × sample	0.30	1.25	1.35	− 1.86	1.48	0.16	− 0.41	1.57	0.67
YPI × gender × sample	− 0.11	0.12	0.89	0.11	0.14	1.12	− 0.02	0.12	0.98

B unstandardized regression coefficient, *SE B* standard error regression coefficient, *Exp (B)* expected regression coefficient (odds ratio), *YPI* Youth Psychopathic Traits Inventory

* $p < 0.05$; ** $p < 0.01$; *** $p < 0.001$

Meaning that in the high-risk sample there was no difference between boys and girls in the probability of having committed violent offenses, while in the general population sample boys had a higher probability of having committed violent offenses than girls. In addition, in girls the probability of having committed violent offenses was higher when the girl was from the high-risk sample than when she was from the general population sample. In boys there was no difference between the high-risk sample and the general population sample in the probability of having committed violent offenses. Adding the three-way interaction term did not improve model fit [$\chi^2(1) = 0.84$, $p = 0.360$; Nagelkerke $R^2 = 0.25$]. Only age and the YPI grandiose-manipulative scale contributed significantly to this regression equation.

Next, we considered the YPI callous and unemotional scale for violent offenses (Table 1, Model 2); the first block significantly predicted violent offenses [$\chi^2(4) = 254.85$, $p < 0.001$; Nagelkerke $R^2 = 0.26$]. Again, a significant main effect emerged for age, the YPI callous and unemotional scale, gender and sample. The second

block revealed no improvement in explained variance compared to the first block [$\chi^2(3) = 6.21$, $p = 0.102$; Nagelkerke $R^2 = 0.26$]. Regarding the main effects, all remained the same, except for gender. Gender no longer contributed significantly to the regression equation. Considering the two-way interactions, as in Model 1 for violent offenses gender × sample contributed significantly to the regression equation. Adding the three-way interaction term did not improve model fit [$\chi^2(1) = 0.62$, $p = 0.432$; Nagelkerke $R^2 = 0.26$]. All main effects remained the same. Neither the two-way interactions, nor the three-way interaction contributed significantly to the regression equation.

Finally, we considered the YPI impulsive-irresponsible scale for violent offenses (Table 1, Model 3). The first block significantly predicted violent offenses [$\chi^2(4) = 266.87$, $p < 0.001$; Nagelkerke $R^2 = 0.27$]. Significant main effects emerged for age, the YPI impulsive-irresponsible scale, gender and sample. The second block revealed a significant improvement in explained variance compared to the first block [$\chi^2(3) = 8.61$, $p = 0.035$;

Nagelkerke $R^2 = 0.28$]. A significant main effect emerged for age, the YPI impulsive-irresponsible scale, gender and sample. Considering the two-way interactions, as in Model 1 and 2 for violent offenses gender × sample contributed significantly to the regression analyses. Adding the three-way interaction term did not improve model fit [$\chi^2(1) = 0.04$, $p = 0.849$; Nagelkerke $R^2 = 0.28$]. Only the main effects age, the YPI impulsive-irresponsible scale and gender contributed significantly to this regression equation. Sample no longer contributed significantly to the regression equation. Neither the two-way interactions, nor the three-way interaction contributed significantly to the regression equation.

Discussion

The purpose of the current study was to examine the relationship between psychopathic traits and self-reported non-violent and violent offenses in a high-risk sample for juvenile delinquency as well as in a general population sample and how gender influences this relationship. We also investigated whether the moderating effect of gender was comparable in the high-risk sample for juvenile delinquency and the general population sample. Consistent with previous research [4, 5], our results demonstrated that psychopathic traits are related to non-violent and violent offenses. We found no moderating effect of gender and therefore we could not detect differences in the moderating effect of gender between the samples. However, there was a moderating effect of sample for the relationship between the callous and unemotional YPI scale and non-violent offenses. Youths from the high-risk sample with a higher score on the YPI callous and unemotional scale had a higher probability for having committed non-violent offenses than youths scoring low on this scale. In youths from the general population sample, this was not the case. Because the three-way interaction YPI callous and unemotional scale × gender × sample was not significant, it can be concluded that the moderating effect of sample was comparable for boys and girls. Considering the moderating effect of sample for the relationship between the callous and unemotional YPI scale and non-violent offenses, surprisingly, youths from the high-risk sample with a higher score on the YPI callous and unemotional scale had a higher probability for having committed *non*-violent offenses than youths scoring low on this scale and this was not the case for violent offenses. An explanation for this finding may be found in the fact that higher scores on all three YPI scales predict the probability for having committed violent offenses [9]. This may indicate that youths with a higher score on only one scale of the YPI can be seen as a less 'severe' group of juvenile offenders, committing 'only' non-violent offenses, compared to youths with a higher score on all three YPI scales, committing violent offenses.

The regression weights of gender and sample were, for non-violent offenses, reduced to non-significance when adding the interaction terms. Therefore, it can be concluded that the influence of gender and sample on non-violent offenses was less robust than the influence of age and YPI scales. This finding is in line with earlier research reporting that higher levels of psychopathic traits are associated with higher levels of self-reported delinquency [4] and that the involvement in delinquency increases considerably during adolescence [19]. In addition, the level of offenses such as vandalism (i.e., non-violent offenses), peaks at a younger age (i.e., age 14–15), whereas the level of violent offenses peaks at an older age (i.e., age 16–17 [19]). In our sample however, adolescents were asked if they had *ever* committed the designated delinquent behavior. Consequently, the probability of having committed offenses during lifetime increased the older juveniles of this high-risk sample were.

Several limitations should be considered. First, the cross-sectional design of our study may limit the interpretation of our findings. Second, we relied solely on the participants' self-reported delinquent behavior. As a consequence, under-reporting of delinquent behavior may have occurred. However, analyses have shown that youths from the high-risk sample reported more delinquent behavior than the professional caregivers from their institutions [16]. In addition, psychopathic traits were also measured through self-report only, the socially desirable responding on questions of the YPI may have influenced the scores on the YPI. However, a study by Cauffman et al. [20] demonstrated that self-reported psychopathic traits was a better predictor of self-reported delinquent behavior compared to expert-rated psychopathic traits. Third, the questionnaire for self-reported delinquency included items that assess also mild forms of delinquent behavior (e.g., 'Have you ever sprayed graffiti on places were this was illegal?', 'Have you ever taken something from a supermarket, store or a mall without paying for it?') which may explain the relatively high rates of delinquent behavior in both samples. Lastly, we did not include the level of psychopathology in our study. An extensive body of research has documented that a high proportion of especially youths from the high-risk sample meet criteria for psychopathology [22, 23]. Since psychopathic traits have been found to be related to psychopathology (e.g., [8, 9, 21]) and psychopathology has been found to be related to delinquent behavior in youths (e.g., [22–24]), it is reasonable to suggest that the level of psychopathology influences the relationship between psychopathic traits and specific forms of delinquent behavior, and therefore may have influenced our results.

Despite these limitations the current study leads us to formulate a number of recommendations for future research. The YPI displayed satisfactory psychometric properties in juvenile justice and non-juvenile justice samples [15, 17]. However, a study by Colins et al. [25], demonstrated that YPI scores were not able to predict future offending, which may suggest that the YPI should not yet be used for risk assessment purposes. Therefore, future research should investigate the prognostic usefulness of the YPI. Furthermore, currently the YPI uses the same scoring key for boys and for girls, while the identification of personality traits in juvenile justice youths is influenced by gender variations in symptom expression (boys tend to reveal their feelings on self-report scales less readily than girls [26], it may be reasonable to suggest that the current cut-off scores for boys under-detect certain psychopathic traits. Future research should address whether the current scoring key of the YPI adequately detects psychopathic traits in boys as well as in girls. Moreover, YPI norms (e.g., for different age groups, gender and different samples) should be developed to be able to give meaningful interpretations in individual cases. Lastly, it is crucial that further research includes follow-up data to investigate the long term negative outcomes of youths scoring high on psychopathic traits in, for example, contacts with family, relationships, school/work and living situation.

Conclusion

Overall, the current study contributes to the body of research examining the consequences of psychopathic traits in juveniles. Psychopathic traits are found to be present in a wide range of youths (i.e., high-risk as well as general population sample, young children as well as adolescents, boys as well as girls) and are related to delinquent behavior. This study showed that psychopathic traits are related to non-violent and violent offenses. The influence of age and YPI scales on self-reported delinquency was more robust than the influence of gender and sample. Therefore, based on this study, screening for psychopathic traits among young children with psychosocial adjustment problems seems relevant for developing effective intervention strategies.

Authors' contributions
LL Analysed and interpreted the data, and drafted the manuscript. CD Analysed and interpreted the data, and drafted the manuscript. TP Analysed and interpreted the data, and drafted the manuscript. KS Revised the manuscript critically. JF Revised the manuscript critically. MS Enrolled the study, helped to draft the manuscript and revised the manuscript critically. All authors read and approved the final manuscript.

Author details
[1] Forschungsabteilung, Kinder- und Jugendpsychiatrische Klinik, Universitäre Psychiatrische Kliniken (UPK), Schanzenstrasse 13, 4056 Basel, Switzerland. [2] Klinik für Kinder- und Jugendpsychiatrie/Psychotherapie, Universitätsklinikum Ulm, Steinhövelstrasse 5, 89075 Ulm, Germany.

Acknowledgements
Not applicable.

Competing interests
The authors declare that they have no competing interests.

Funding
The study was funded by the Federal Office of Justice in Switzerland (Bundesamt für Justiz).

References
1. Blair RJ, Leibenluft E, Pine DS. Conduct disorder and callous-unemotional traits in youth. N Engl J Med. 2014;371:2207–16.
2. Cauffman E, Skeem J, Dmitrieva J, Cavanagh C. Comparing the stability of psychopathy scores in adolescents versus adults: how often is "fledgling psychopathy" misdiagnosed? Psychol Public Policy Law. 2016;22:77–91.
3. Vahl P, Colins OF, Lodewijks HPB, Lindauer R, Markus MT, Doreleijers TAH, Vermeiren RR. Psychopathic traits and maltreatment: relations with aggression and mental health problems in detained boys. Int J Law Psychiatry. 2016;46:129–36.
4. Asscher JJ, van Vugt ES, Stams GJJ, Dekovic M, Eichelsheim VI, Yousfi S. The relationship between juvenile psychopathic traits, delinquency and (violent) recidivism: a meta-analysis. J Child Psychol Psychiatry. 2011;52:1134–43.
5. Pechorro P, Goncalves RA, Maroco J, Gama AP, Neves S, Nunes C. Juvenile delinquency and psychopathic traits: an empirical study with Portuguese adolescents. Int J Offender Ther Comp Criminol. 2014;58:174–89.
6. Lindberg N, Laajasalo T, Holi M, Putkonen H, Weizmann-Henelius G, Hakkanen-Nyholm H. Psychopathic traits and offender characteristics—a nationwide consecutive sample of homicidal male adolescents. BMC Psychiatry. 2009;9:11.
7. Frick PJ, Cornell AH, Barry CT, Bodin SD, Dane HE. Callous-unemotional traits and conduct problems in the prediction of conduct problem severity, aggression, and self-report of delinquency. J Abnorm Child Psychol. 2003;31:457–70.
8. Oshukova S, Kaltiala-Heino R, Miettunen J, Marttila R, Tani P, Aronen ET, Marttunen M, Kaivosoja M, Lindberg N. The relationship between self-rated psychopathic traits and psychopathology in a sample of Finnish community youth: exploration of gender differences. J Child Adolesc. 2016;4:7.
9. Nijhof KS, Vermulst A, Scholte RH, van Dam C, Veerman JW, Engels RC. Psychopathic traits of Dutch adolescents in residential care: identifying subgroups. J Abnorm Psychol. 2011;39:59–70.
10. Schmid M, Dölitzsch C, Pérez T, Jenkel N, Schmeck K, Kölch M, Fegert JM. Welche Faktoren beeinflussen Abbrüche in der Heimerziehung—welche Bedeutung haben limitierte prosoziale Fertigkeiten? Kindh Entwickl. 2014;23:161–73.
11. Marsee MA, Silverthorn P, Frick PJ. The association of psychopathic traits with aggression and delinquency in non-referred boys and girls. Behav Sci Law. 2005;23(6):803–17.
12. Sevecke K, Lehmkuhl G, Krischer MK. Examining relations between psychopathology and psychopathy dimensions among adolescent female and male offenders. Eur Child Adolesc Psychiatry. 2009;18:85–95.
13. Penney SR, Moretti MM. The relation of psychopathy to concurrent aggression and antisocial behavior in high-risk adolescent girls and boys. Behav Sci Law. 2007;25:21–41.
14. Schmid M, Kölch M, Fegert JM, Schmeck K, MAZ.-Team: Abschlussbericht Modellversuch Abklärung und Zielerreichung in stationären Massnahmen. 2013. https://www.bj.admin.ch/dam/data/bj/sicherheit/smv/modellversuche/evaluationsberichte/maz-schlussbericht-d.pdf. Accessed 25 May 2017.
15. Stadlin C, Pérez T, Schmeck K, Di Gallo A, Schmid M. Konstruktvalidität und Faktorenstruktur des deutschsprachigen Youth Psychopathic Traits Inventory (YPI) in einer repräsentativen Schulstichprobe. Diagnostica. 2016;62:85–96.
16. Dölitzsch C, Schmid M, Keller F, Besier T, Fegert JM, Schmeck K, Kölch M. Professional caregiver's knowledge of self-reported delinquency in an adolescent sample in Swiss youth welfare and juvenile justice institutions. Int J Law Psychiatry. 2016;47:10–7.

17. Andershed H, Kerr M, Stattin H, Levander S. Psychopathic traits in non-referred youths: initial test of a new assessment tool. In: Blaauw E, Philippa JM, Ferenschild KCMP, van Lodensteijn B, editors. Psychopaths: current international perspectives. The Hague: Elsevier; 2002. p. 131–58.

18. Boers K, Reinecke J, editors. Delinquenz im Jugendalter. Waxmann: Erkenntnisse einer Münsteraner Längsschnittstudie. Münster; 2007.

19. Junger-tas J, Marshall IH, Ribeaud D. Delinquency in an international perspective: The international self-reported delinquency study (ISRD). The Hague: Criminal Justice Press, Kugler Publications; 2003.

20. Cauffman E, Kimonis ER, Dmitrieva J, Monahan KC. A multimethod assessment of juvenile psychopathy: comparing the predictive utility of the PCL:YV, YPI, and NEO PRI. Psychol Assess. 2009;21:528–42.

21. Seals RW, Sharp C, Ha C, Michonski JD. The relationship between the youth psychopathic traits inventory and psychopathology in a U.S. community sample of male youth. J Pers Assess. 2012;94:232–43.

22. Wasserman GA, Mc Reynolds L, Schwalbe CS, Keating JM, Jones SA. Psychiatric disorder, comorbidity, and suicidal behavior in juvenile justice youth. Crim Justice Behav. 2010;37:1361–76.

23. Kataoka SH, Zima BT, Dupre DA, Moreno KA, Yang X, McCracken JT. Mental health problems and service use among female juvenile offenders: their relationship to criminal history. J Am Acad Child Adolesc Psychiatry. 2001;40:549–55.

24. Wasserman GA, McReynolds LS, Ko SJ, Katz LM, Carpenter JR. Gender differences in psychiatric disorders at juvenile probation intake. Am J Public Health. 2005;95:131–7.

25. Colins OF, Fanti KA, Andershed H, Mulder E, Salekin RT, Blokland A, Vermeiren RRJM. Psychometric properties and prognostic usefulness of the Youth Psychopathic Traits Inventory (YPI) as a component of a clinical protocol for detained youth: a multiethnic examination. Psycholl Assess. 2017;9:740–53.

26. Grisso T, Barnum R. Massachusetts Youth Screening Instrument-version 2 (MAYSI-2): User's manual and technical report. Sarasota: Professional Resource Press; 2006.

5

Lifetime and past-year prevalence of children's exposure to violence in 9 Balkan countries: the BECAN study

George Nikolaidis[1]*[iD], Kiki Petroulaki[1], Foteini Zarokosta[1,14], Antonia Tsirigoti[1,15], Altin Hazizaj[2], Enila Cenko[2,16], Jelena Brkic-Smigoc[3], Emir Vajzovic[3], Vaska Stancheva[4], Stefka Chincheva[4], Marina Ajdukovic[5], Miro Rajter[5], Marija Raleva[6], Liljana Trpcevska[6], Maria Roth[7], Imola Antal[7], Veronika Ispanovic[8], Natasha Hanak[8,17], Zeynep Olmezoglu-Sofuoglu[9], Ismail Umit-Bal[9], Donata Bianchi[10], Franziska Meinck[11,12] and Kevin Browne[13]

Abstract

Background: Children's exposure to violence is a major public health issue. The Balkan epidemiological study on Child Abuse and Neglect project aimed to collect internationally comparable data on violence exposures in childhood.

Methods: A three stage stratified random sample of 42,194 school-attending children (response rate: 66.7%) in three grades (aged 11, 13 and 16 years) was drawn from schools in Albania, Bosnia and Herzegovina, Bulgaria, Croatia, Former Yugoslavian Republic of Macedonia (FYROM), Greece, Romania, Serbia and Turkey. Children completed the ICAST-C questionnaire, which measures children's exposure to violence by any perpetrator.

Results: Exposure rates for psychological violence were between 64.6% (FYROM) and 83.2% (Greece) for lifetime and 59.62% (Serbia) and 70.0% (Greece) for past-year prevalence. Physical violence exposure varied between 50.6% (FYROM) and 76.3% (Greece) for lifetime and 42.5% (FYROM) and 51.0% (Bosnia) for past-year prevalence. Sexual violence figures were highest for lifetime prevalence in Bosnia (18.6%) and lowest in FYROM (7.6%). Lifetime contact sexual violence was highest in Bosnia (9.8%) and lowest in Romania (3.6%). Past-year sexual violence and contact sexual violence prevalence was lowest in Romania (5.0 and 2.1%) and highest in Bosnia (13.6 and 7.7% respectively). Self-reported neglect was highest for both past-year and lifetime prevalence in Bosnia (48.0 and 20.3%) and lowest in Romania (22.6 and 16.7%). Experiences of positive parental practices were reported by most participating children in all countries.

Conclusions: Where significant differences in violence exposure by sex were observed, males reported higher exposure to past-year and lifetime sexual violence and females higher exposure to neglect. Children in Balkan countries experience a high burden of violence victimization and national-level programming and child protection policy making is urgently needed to address this.

Keywords: Violence against children, Child abuse and neglect, Child maltreatment, Violence, Epidemiology, Balkans

Background

Violence against children has attracted gradually increasing clinical attention over recent decades. From its first reporting by the American pediatrician Henry Kempe in the 1960s [1] up to its recognition by the World Health Organization as a major public health issue in the late 1990s [2, 3], perspectives on the subject matter have changed drastically. During the last decades, violence against children has experienced increasingly interdisciplinary attention, first predominantly in social policy,

*Correspondence: gnikolaidis@ich-mhsw.gr; geornikolaidis@hotmail.com
[1] Department of Mental Health and Social Welfare, Centre for the Study and Prevention of Child Abuse and Neglect, Institute of Child Health, 7 Fokidos Str., 11526 Athens, Greece
Full list of author information is available at the end of the article

social work, psychology and clinical practice and more recently also in public health. Reasons and causes of the phenomenon's increased visibility over the years should be attributed to the literature on the severe implications of early exposure of children to violence or deprivation. Violence exposure in childhood is associated with negative physical and emotional health outcomes [4] which include anxiety and depression [5–7], suicidal ideation [8–10], substance use [11], dissociation and personality disorders, neurobiological implications [12] as well as with wider psychosocial consequences such as adolescent delinquency, educational shortcomings [13, 14], difficulties in relationships and family roles in adulthood, criminal activity [15] and reproduction of the "circle of violence" [16].

This paper follows the UNICEF definitions of violence against children and uses this interchangeably with the term children's exposure to violence. Physical violence against children includes "all corporal punishment and all other forms of torture, cruel, inhuman or degrading treatment or punishment as well as physical bullying and hazing by adults or other children". Psychological violence includes all "psychological maltreatment, mental abuse, verbal abuse and emotional abuse or neglect". Sexual violence includes "any sexual activities imposed by an adult or child against which the child is entitled to protection by criminal law. [...] Sexual activities are also considered as abuse when committed against a child by any other child if the offender is significantly older than the victim or uses power, threat or other means of pressure". Neglect includes the "failure to meet children's physical and psychological needs, protect them from danger or obtain medical, birth registration or other services when those responsible for their care have the means, knowledge and access to services to do so [17]". Violence against children is thus more broadly defined than child abuse and neglect or child maltreatment.

Violence against children has over the past decade attracted international attention and its prevention and reduction has now been included into the Sustainable Development Goals [18]. There is currently a global interest to multiply efforts and join forces to eradicate children's exposure to all forms of violence and increase awareness of the problem at global and local levels. An increasing number of countries across the globe have prohibited all forms of violence against children [19]. Of the nine countries participating in this study, Greece, Romania, Bulgaria and Croatia had enacted laws prohibiting violence against children in the home and school. Albania and Former Yugoslav Republic Of Macedonia (FYROM) joined them in 2010 and 2013, while Bosnia and Herzegovina, Serbia and Turkey have expressed commitment to law reforms banishing

violence against children in all settings [19]. A recent systematic review found that attitudes condoning corporal punishment and other forms of violence against children decrease drastically in countries with legislation that bans all forms of violence against children, as do prevalence rates [20].

As a result, the necessity for building up a robust evidence base regarding the magnitude of the various types of children's exposure to violence is becoming a necessity for the international scientific community in order to establish trends and changes in violence exposure over the years. One straightforward obstacle to this goal has traditionally been the radical incommensurability of results reported by various researchers around the globe using different tools and measuring fundamentally incompatible concepts of the phenomenon [21]. Moreover, it has been noticed that some of these tools measured subjective perceptions of exposure to violence and therefore suffered from decreased reliability [22].

To tackle such issues, during the last decade, the World Health Organization (WHO) and the International Society for the Prevention of Child Abuse and Neglect (ISPCAN) have initiated a set of recommendations for producing globally compatible and reliable data on measuring children's exposure to violence [23]. This initiative was later supplemented by other similar organizations trying to specify optimum methodological requirements for conducting field research on violence against children [24]. The main characteristics of all such recommendations of international organizations [23, 25] involve applying credible and internationally used tools for inquiring about prevalence and incidence of children's exposure to violence, using questionnaires measuring objective actions and experiences versus subjective perceptions of children's victimization (i.e. asking "how many times have you been beaten, spanked, or smacked" instead of "have you experienced physical violence"). Further recommendations are to follow standardized methodologies of conducting research (e.g. using trained professionals instead of laymen as field researchers, designing strict protocols for research implementation to avoid biased suggestion of researchers' attitudes and prejudices to participant subjects), and conducting field studies in representative randomly selected samples of the respective children's general population in order for results to be a valid estimation of the actual situation in the referred population (in contrast with results deriving from clinical studies) [25].

On these grounds, with the support of the Oak Foundation, ISPCAN collaborated with UNICEF, the UN Secretary General's Study on Violence against Children, the Office of the High Commissioner of Human Rights, and WHO to create the ISPCAN Child Abuse Screening

Tools (ICAST) [26, 27] which allow the systematic collection and comparison of child abuse data concerning children's exposure to violence by any perpetrator.

Within this overall framework the Balkan Epidemiological Child Abuse and Neglect (BECAN) project was undertaken and funded by EU's 7th Framework Program for Research and Innovation (I.D.: 223478/HEALTH/2007) in order to establish past-year and lifetime prevalence of children's exposure to violence in nine countries of the Balkan Peninsula. As there were no empirical data available on children's exposure to violence up to the time of the particular research effort, the aim of this study was to investigate the epidemiology of violence against children in the participating countries for international comparisons and to serve as a baseline rate for future research.

Methods

Research design and sampling

The different steps in the research process are illustrated in Fig. 1.

The BECAN research project was a cross-sectional study of lifetime and past-year prevalence of children's exposure to violence in the following nine countries: Albania, Bosnia and Herzegovina, Bulgaria, Croatia, Former Yugoslavian Republic of FYROM, Greece, Romania, Serbia and Turkey. The study utilized the ICAST-C questionnaire which was developed for use with children

11-years and older. This tool aims at measuring children's self-reported exposure to various types of violence (by all potential perpetrators) and its items are structured in different sub-scales corresponding to children's exposure to physical, psychological and sexual violence and neglect.

A three-stage stratified random sample was drawn from the general school-going population of 11, 13 and 16 year olds in the nine countries. First, official data about the child population and number of schools per region was obtained for the year preceding the study from the respective Offices of Statistics and the Ministries of Education in each country. These data constitute the sampling frame. Within the regions, schools were randomly selected into the sample using random series of numbers generated by a statistician until the number of schools was filled for each stratum. Since classes only partly equate age groups, students in grades reflecting the age clusters 11, 13 and 16 were recruited. All children who were part of that class, present on the day and consented, participated in the research. The vast majority of children in the participating countries attend school to age 18, therefore only school children were recruited for this present study.

The initial targeted sample was 63,250 children. This corresponds to 2–5% of the general population of children according to official figures released by the educational authorities of each country. The percentage varies with respect to the overall size of the population in each

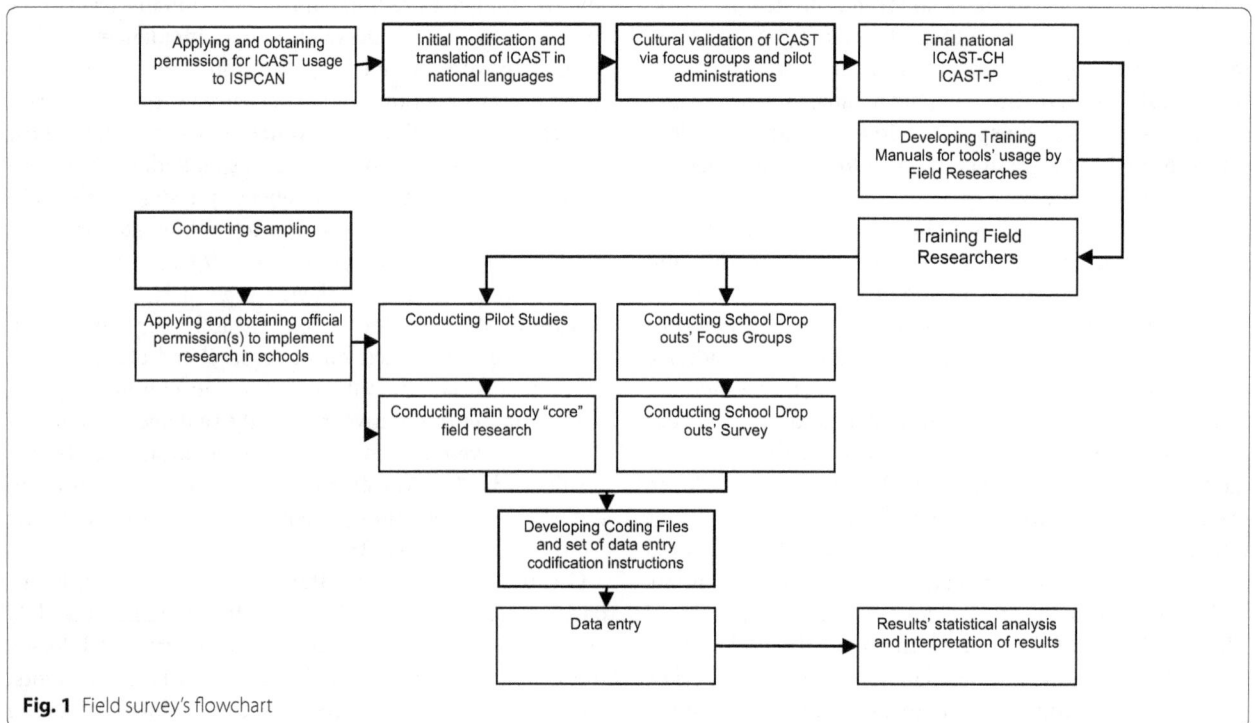

Fig. 1 Field survey's flowchart

country, with smaller percentages in countries with larger populations. However, given the overall sample size and the randomized selection, the sample was regarded as representative of children attending schools in the participating countries.

Measures

Physical, psychological and sexual violence exposure, neglect and positive and non-violent parenting were measured using the ICAST-C, a 38 item self-report measure for children developed by ISPCAN for prevalence studies across diverse contexts [26]. The ICAST measures past-year and lifetime prevalence of physical, psychological and sexual violence by any perpetrator, neglect and positive/non-violent parenting, similar to other instruments which have been used in prevalence studies in other European countries [28]. A limited amount of research is available on the validity and internal consistency of the ICAST-C. The measure showed good internal validity (Cronbrach's alpha greater than 0.70) for the physical violence, psychological violence, sexual violence and neglect sub-scales across countries as diverse as China, Romania, Egypt, India, Russia, Columbia and Iceland in initial validation studies [26, 29, 30].

In accordance with ISPCAN's rules and procedures, the ICAST-C was modified and subsequently translated into the official languages of the participating countries [31]. Modification was undertaken to align items with the parent version which is subject to a separate manuscript. Further, modifications were used to increase ease of reading and understanding by creating separate items for those questions which described multiple violent incidents. Translation was followed by cultural validation, back-translation and the development of a protocol for application of the measure. Small cultural modifications were made to describe specific practices in the different countries, i.e. frightening children with the bogeyman or by evoking evil spirits had to be translated into a locally relevant equivalent. The resulting measure was then subjected to a three round modification process including a consensus panel, 37 focus groups with 392 children and pilot studies in each of the countries (see Table 1 for number of focus groups conducted). These were conducted in rural and urban areas and recruited at last one classroom with pupils aged 11–16 (N = 1861). The focus groups aimed at elucidating whether children in all countries had the same cognitive and cultural understanding of the questions. The pilot studies collected 1331 modified ICAST-C questionnaires (response rate: 71.52%) and found that children in all age groups were able to understand and answer all items. The overall adaptation, piloting and consultation process across the nine countries took approximately 1 year.

The final versions of the modified ICAST-C questionnaires comprised 45 items (children aged 11) and 51 items (adolescents aged > 12) structured in five scales. These measure exposure to psychological (17 items/19 items), physical (15 items/16 items), and sexual violence exposure (5 items/6 items), feelings of neglect (3 items) and reported experiences of nonviolent positive parental practices (5 items/7 items) which were added to the initial ICAST-C questionnaire [32]. For information on the actual phrasing of items please see Additional file 1. Each item inquired about specific violent events in the past year and allowed for the following response options: 'once or twice a year', 'several times a year', 'monthly or every 2 months', 'several times a month', 'once a week or more often', 'not in the past year, but it has happened to me before', 'never in my life' and 'I don't want to answer'. The final order of question items was informed by focus group discussions and expert opinion on the quality of children's responses taking into account their age group and cognitive development [33]. The full questionnaire,

Table 1 Number of focus groups that were conducted and number of children participating in them per country

Country	11 years olds		13 years olds		16 years olds		School dropouts	
	No of FGs	No of children	No of FGs	No of FGs	No of children	No of children	No of FGs	No of children
Albania	1	13	1	1	13	12	–	–
B&H	1	7	2	1	7	26	–	–
Bulgaria	1	14	1	1	14	11	1	6
Croatia	2	19	2	2	19	17	1	9
FYROM	1	16	1	1	16	17	1	4
Greece	1	8	1	1	2	7	–	–
Romania	–	–	2	2	18	36	1	9
Serbia	2	21	1	1	13	14	–	–
Turkey	1	8	1	1	9	7	–	–
Total	10	106	12	11	111	147	4	28

as administered, can be viewed at http://becan.eu/sites/default/files/uploaded_images/EN_ICAST-CH.pdf.

Socio-demographics measured age of child, sex, whether child lives with mother, and urban/rural location of school.

Research protocol

A standard protocol was developed for application of questionnaires to children in classrooms across the nine participating countries. Field researchers had to be certified professionals (psychologists and social workers). They received extensive training in interviewing vulnerable children about sensitive topics. Emphasis in training was placed on confidentiality, privacy and on neutrality during the interview process in order to avoid influencing children's responses [34]. Questionnaires were self-administered in classrooms with interviewers present to answer questions or aid children if they got upset. Children with learning and physical disabilities were interviewed face-to-face. Children in the grade group aged 11 were asked the shorter 45 item version of the modified ICAST-C, children in the grade groups 13 and 16 were asked the longer 51 item version of the modified ICAST-C. Researchers in Turkey were unable to ask the questions about sexual abuse as government permission for this was not granted.

Ethical issues

Permission to conduct the research in the school setting was granted by the educational authorities in each country. All children and their caregivers were informed in advance about the plans to carry out the research and provided consent. In line with in-country legislation, parental consent was either passive or active. However, a wide range of ethical and methodological issues emerged during the set-up of the field research relating to differences in national legislation and authoritative agency responses. These included, among others, the rights of disabled children to participate, the differentiation of oral versus written consent for parents and children and its implications or potential for parental refusal to participate in cases of severe child abuse. To deal with these issues, independent ethical advisory boards were set up in each country to provide supervision and guidance. These were overseen by an international independent ethics advisory board. Further, ad-hoc crisis intervention teams were set up in each country to help with collaborations between the research teams and local community agencies to facilitate referrals following child abuse disclosures where children were considered to be at risk of significant harm.

Data entry and statistical analysis

Data were collected from all nine participating countries and entered into databases by trained professionals. Research teams double checked data entry and data quality on a regular basis. For past-year prevalence, items were dichotomized based on any vs no exposure in the past year on the different abuse sub-scales. For lifetime prevalence, items were dichotomized based on any vs no exposure in the past year or ever. This resulted in past-year prevalence rates for physical, emotional, sexual abuse, contact sexual violence exposure, neglect and positive parenting. Prevalence rates were then calculated using basic descriptive functions of the software package SPSS 18. Sex differences were assessed using χ^2 tests. Internal consistency of the different sub-scales of the ICAST-C measure were calculated using Cronbach's alpha.

Results

Participation rates differed between countries and school grades. Overall, 63,250 pupils were invited to participate in the survey. Of these 42,194 filled in a questionnaire resulting in a 66.7% response rate. Reasons for non-response included non-attendance at school on the day the survey was carried out, parental consent not obtained and child consent not obtained. Country-specific national participation rates ranged from 45.8% in FYROM to 82.7% in Turkey although a direct comparison is difficult between countries due to differences related to gaining parental consent (active–passive–none), enrolment numbers in school and actual student attendance throughout the school year. Participation rates by grade group and by country are presented in Table 2, in which the sample sizes are also presented. Socio-demographic characteristics of participants and their parents and location of school are described in Table 3.

Internal consistency of the ICAST

Internal consistency of the various ICAST sub-scales was measured by calculating Cronbach's alpha and is reported in Table 4. Internal consistency of the psychological violence sub-scale was good with Cronbach's alpha ranging from 0.80 to 0.96. Internal consistency for physical violence was good to excellent with Cronbach's alpha ranging from 0.81 to 0.99. Internal consistency of the sexual violence subscale was adequate to good with Cronbach's alpha ranging from 0.71 to 0.86. Internal consistency of the contact sexual violence sub-scale was poor to adequate ranging from 0.41 to 0.76. Internal consistency of the neglect sub-scale was poor to good with Cronbach's alpha ranging from 0.60 to 0.87. Internal consistency of the positive and non-violent parenting subscale was poor to good with Cronbach's alpha ranging from 0.35 to 0.81.

Table 2 Description of schoolchildren's sample and response rates by grade group and country

Country	Grade group									Total		
	11-year olds			13-year olds			16-year olds					
	N[1]	n[2]	R.R[3]	N[1]	n[2]	R.R[3]	N[1]	n[2]	R.R[3]	N[1]	n[2]	R.R[3]
Albania	1652	1186	71.79	1667	1204	72.23	1125	937	83.29	4444	3327	74.86
Bulgaria	1241	662	53.34	1105	685	61.99	1273	693	54.44	3619	2040	56.37
B & H	1333	676	50.71	1340	675	50.37	1501	1287	85.74	4174	2638	63.20
Croatia	1744	1223	70.13	1771	1188	67.08	1492	1233	82.64	5007	3644	72.78
Greece	4401	2771	62.96	5072	3438	67.78	5847	4242	72.55	15,320	10,451	68.22
FYROM	2058	670	32.56	2183	791	36.23	1408	1125	79.90	5649	2586	45.78
Romania	3471	1976	56.93	2709	1849	68.25	2190	2130	97.26	8370	5955	71.15
Serbia	2131	908	42.61	2623	1400	53.37	2811	1719	61.15	7565	4027	53.23
Turkey	2913	2500	85.82	3162	2564	81.09	3027	2462	81.33	9102	7526	82.69
Total	20,944	12,572	60.03	21,632	13,794	63.77	20,674	15,828	76.56	63,250	42,194	66.71

[1] N: number of children registered to schools that were included in the sample

[2] n: number of children who accepted to participate by filling in the ICAST-C questionnaire

[3] R.R.: response rate (percentage of the children who accepted to participate, out of the total number of invited school children in the selected school)

Table 3 Socio-demographic characteristics of the sample and location of schools

Country	School characteristics	Child characteristics			Parental characteristics
	In rural area	Age	Female	Lives with mother	Married
	% (n)	Mean (SD)	% (n)	% (n)	% (n)
Albania	46.0% (1530)	13.10 (2.05)	54.2% (1802)	96.5% (3212)	94.8% (3153)
Bulgaria	29.0% (592)	13.48 (2.04)	51.5% (1049)	88.8% (1812)	74.5% (1519)
B & H	36.5% (932)	14.26 (2.19)	53.1% (1400)	94.0% (2479)	86.5% (2282)
Croatia	27.5% (967)	13.59 (2.13)	51.1% (1863)	95.8% (3491)	84.9% (3094)
Greece	16.1% (1682)	13.78 (1.85)	52.4% (5480)	97.0% (10,137)	83.8% (8758)
FYROM	13.6% (226)	13.90 (2.17)	58.2% (967)	96.1% (1597)	87.7% (1458)
Romania	43.7% (2602)	13.73 (2.19)	55.5% (3305)	90.2% (5374)	81.0% (4825)
Serbia	35.8% (1441)	14.26 (2.12)	48.6% (1959)	94.9% (3821)	81.6% (3287)
Turkey	13.1% (983)	13.45 (2.14)	49.2% (3703)	93.6% (7046)	89.1% (6709)

Table 4 Internal consistencies (Cronbach's alpha) of scales of exposure to psychological, physical and sexual violence, neglect and positive/non-violent parenting scales, by country

Country	Form of children's exposure (scales of the ICAST-C[R.])					
	Psychological violence	Physical violence	Sexual violence	Contact sexual violence	Feeling of neglect	Positive and non violent parenting
Albania	0.806	0.900	0.819	0.666	0.705	0.354
B & H	0.865	0.897	0.793	0.557	0.748	0.760
Bulgaria	0.816	0.796	0.705	0.411	0.753	0.672
Croatia	0.895	0.920	0.858	0.764	0.756	0.807
FYROM	0.827	0.852	0.772	0.624	0.712	0.705
Greece	0.830	0.892	0.828	0.645	0.601	0.723
Romania	0.833	0.887	0.840	0.715	0.734	0.672
Serbia	0.840	0.890	0.850	0.652	0.653	0.737
Turkey	0.963	0.992	N/A	N/A	0.873	0.732

N/A not available

Table 5 Lifetime prevalence of schoolchildren's exposure to violent behaviors by form of violence experienced, by country

Country	Form of children's exposure (scales of the ICAST-C[R].)											
	Psychological violence		Physical violence		Sexual violence		Contact sexual violence		Feeling of neglect		Positive and non violent parenting	
	% (n)	95% C.I.	% (n)	95% C.I.	% (n)	95% C.I.	% (n)	95% C.I.	% (n)	95% C.I.	% (n)	95% C.I.
Albania	68.62 (2283)	67.04–70.20	59.44 (1977)	57.77–61.11	11.11 (369)	10.04–12.18	4.85 (161)	4.12–5.59	25.73 (854)	24.24–27.22	94.59 (3146)	93.82–95.36
B & H	72.51 (1912)	70.80–69.47	67.68 (1782)	65.89–69.47	18.68 (491)	17.19–20.17	9.75 (256)	8.61–10.88	39.63 (1042)	37.77–41.50	95.94 (2528)	95.19–96.69
Bulgaria	69.51 (1418)	67.51–71.51	62.21 (1269)	60.10–64.31	8.58 (175)	7.36–9.79	4.90 (100)	3.97–5.84	23.68 (483)	21.83–25.52	92.21 (1881)	91.04–93.37
Croatia	73.04 (2661)	71.60–74.49	66.73 (2425)	65.20–68.26	10.18 (369)	9.20–11.17	4.50 (163)	3.83–5.18	35.30 (1281)	33.74–36.85	97.23 (3539)	96.69–97.76
FYROM	64.58 (8691)	62.74–66.42	50.66 (7962)	48.73–52.59	7.60 (1645)	6.58–8.63	3.80 (787)	3.06–4.55	27.47 (3871)	25.74–29.19	83.87 (10,258)	82.45–85.29
Greece	83.16 (1670)	82.44–83.88	76.37 (1307)	75.56–77.19	15.86 (194)	15.16–16.57	7.60 (96)	7.08–8.11	37.20 (707)	36.27–38.13	98.18 (2168)	97.93–98.44
Romania	76.67 (4564)	75.59–77.74	66.94 (2974)	65.74–68.13	7.90 (467)	7.21–8.58	3.56 (210)	3.09–4.03	22.59 (1388)	21.52–23.65	95.97 (5710)	95.47–96.47
Serbia	68.44 (2756)	67.00–69.87	69.18 (2779)	67.75–70.61	8.49 (340)	7.62–9.35	4.90 (196)	4.23–5.57	28.83 (1157)	27.43–30.23	97.34 (3917)	96.84–97.84
Turkey	70.58 (5311)	69.55–71.61	58.38 (4384)	57.27–59.50	N/A[a]		N/A[a]		42.62 (3194)	41.50–43.73	93.91 (7060)	93.37–94.45

[a] Not available

Table 6 Past-year prevalence of schoolchildren's exposure to violent behaviors by form of violence experienced, by country

Country	Form of children's exposure (scales of the ICAST-C^R.)											
	Psychological violence		Physical violence		Sexual violence		Contact sexual violence		Feeling of neglect		Positive and non violent parenting	
	% (n)	95% C.I.	% (n)	95% C.I.	% (n)	95% C.I.	% (n)	95% C.I.	% (n)	95% C.I.	% (n)	95% C.I.
Albania	61.71 (2053)	60.06–63.36	48.41 (1610)	46.71–50.10	9.12 (303)	8.14–10.10	4.07 (135)	3.40–4.74	21.84 (725)	20.44–23.25	92.96 (3092)	92.10–93.83
B & H	64.05 (1689)	62.22–65.88	51.01 (1343)	49.10–52.92	13.62 (358)	12.31–14.93	7.65 (201)	6.64–8.67	33.21 (873)	31.41–35.01	94.27 (2484)	93.38–95.16
Bulgaria	62.01 (1265)	59.90–64.12	48.48 (989)	46.31–50.65	7.50 (153)	6.36–8.64	4.36 (89)	3.48–5.25	19.90 (406)	18.17–21.63	90.15 (1839)	88.85–91.44
Croatia	65.69 (2393)	64.15–67.23	45.54 (1655)	43.92–47.16	7.20 (261)	6.36–8.04	3.26 (118)	2.68–3.84	28.63 (1039)	27.16–30.10	96.18 (3501)	95.56–96.80
FYROM	60.21 (7318)	58.32–62.10	42.40 (4939)	40.50–44.31	6.39 (989)	5.44–7.34	3.37 (461)	2.66–4.07	24.90 (2748)	23.23–26.57	83.02 (10,052)	81.57–84.46
Greece	70.02 (1557)	69.14–70.90	47.38 (1094)	46.42–48.33	9.54 (163)	8.97–10.10	4.45 (85)	4.05–4.85	26.41 (641)	25.56–27.25	96.21 (2146)	95.84–96.58
Romania	65.90 (3923)	64.70–67.10	44.65 (2651)	43.39–45.92	4.99 (295)	4.43–5.54	2.09 (123)	1.72–2.45	16.66 (987)	15.71–17.61	93.19 (5545)	92.55–93.83
Serbia	59.62 (2401)	58.11–61.14	46.48 (1867)	44.94–48.02	6.24 (250)	5.49–6.99	3.70 (148)	3.11–4.28	22.85 (917)	21.55–24.15	94.58 (3806)	93.88–95.28
Turkey	62.82 (4727)	61.73–63.91	46.06 (3459)	44.94–47.19	N/A[a]		N/A[a]		37.55 (2814)	36.45–38.64	90.74 (6822)	90.09–91.40

[a] Not available

Lifetime and past-year prevalence rates of violence exposure by country

Aggregated results for lifetime and past-year prevalence are presented in Tables 5 and 6. Lifetime prevalence for physical violence ranged from 50.6% (FYROM) to 76.4% (Greece), while past year prevalence ranged from 42.5% (FYROM) to 51.0% (Bosnia). Lifetime prevalence for psychological violence ranged from 64.6% (FYROM) to 83.2% (Greece), while past-year prevalence ranged from 59.6% (Serbia) to 70.0% (Greece). Lifetime prevalence of sexual violence ranged from 7.9% (Romania) to 18.6% (Bosnia), while past-year prevalence ranged from 5.0% (Romania) to 14.6% (Bosnia). Lifetime prevalence of contact sexual violence ranged from 3.6% (Romania) to 9.8% (Bosnia), while past-year prevalence ranged from 2.1% (Bosnia) to 7.7% (Bosnia). Lifetime prevalence of feelings of neglect ranged from 22.6% (Romania) to 42.6% (Turkey), while past-year prevalence ranged from 16.7% (Romania) to 37.6% (Turkey). Lifetime prevalence of positive and non-violent parenting ranged from 83.9% (FYROM) to 98.2% (Greece), while past-year prevalence ranged from 83.0% (FYROM) to 96.2% (Greece).

Lifetime differences in violence exposure by sex

Differences between males and females in relation to lifetime violence exposure were examined. No differences were observed in relation to lifetime psychological violence exposure between males and females across countries (see Table 7). For lifetime physical violence exposure, no differences could be observed between sexes across countries except for Turkey, where males reported higher prevalence of physical violence than females (60.6% vs 56.1%). For lifetime sexual violence exposure, no differences were observed between sexes amongst the majority of countries except for Albania, where males reported higher lifetime sexual violence exposure than females (14.5% vs 8.2%) and FYROM, where this was also the case (9.6% vs 6.0%). For lifetime contact sexual violence exposure, differences between males and females could be observed with higher lifetime prevalence among males in Albania (8.1% vs 2.1%), Bosnia (12.3% vs 7.7%), FYROM (5.5% vs 2.5%) and Serbia (6.0% vs 3.8%). For lifetime experiences of feelings of neglect, differences between males and females could be observed with higher lifetime prevalence among females in Albania (30.7% vs 19.8%), Bosnia (47.5% vs 30.8%), Croatia (40.6% vs 29.8%), FYROM (31.0% vs 23.1%), Greece (42.8% vs 31.0%), Romania (26.6% vs 17.6%), Serbia (34.6% vs 23.4%) and Turkey (48.1% vs 37.3%). No differences between sexes were observed for lifetime positive and non-violent parenting (Table 7).

Past-year differences in violence exposure by sex

Differences between males and females in relation to past-year violence exposure were examined. In relation to past-year prevalence, no significant differences were observed in relation to psychological violence exposure apart from in Serbia with females reporting higher exposure (63.3% vs 56.2%). For past-year prevalence of physical violence, differences between males and females were observed with higher levels of exposure for males in Romania (47.7% vs 42.3%) and Turkey (48.5% vs 43.6%). For past-year sexual violence, higher levels of exposure were observed for males in Albania (12.9% vs 6.0%), FYROM (8.3% vs 4.9%) and Serbia (7.5% vs 5.0%). For past-year contact sexual violence, higher levels of exposure were observed for males in Albania (7.3% vs 1.4%), Bosnia (10.0% vs 5.7%), FYROM (4.8% vs 2.3%), Greece (5.5% vs 3.5%), Romania (2.9% vs 1.5%) and Serbia (4.8% vs 2.5%). For past-year exposure to feelings of neglect, higher levels of exposure were observed for females in Albania (26.7 vs 16.1%), Bosnia (40.5% vs 25.0%), Croatia (33.7% vs 23.3%), FYROM (28.75 vs 20.1), Greece (30.9% vs 21.5%), Romania (19.4 vs 13.1%), Serbia (27.7% vs 18.3%) and Turkey (43.1% vs 32.1%). No differences between sexes were observed for past-year positive and non-violent parenting (Table 8).

Discussion

This paper provides data on psychological, physical and sexual violence exposure, feelings of neglect and positive parenting from the Balkan Epidemiological Study of Child Abuse and Neglect (BECAN). It is the first study to examine past-year and lifetime prevalence in multiple countries in the region and the first to use cross-country comparable methodology to do so. The BECAN study used the ICAST-C measure to investigate prevalence of violence exposure in nationally representative samples of 11, 13 and 16 year olds in nine Balkan countries. The ICAST-C is a non-proprietary child violence exposure screening tool that has been designed for use in international research on the prevalence of violence against children and showed good internal consistency in this sample.

Investigating the international epidemiology of children's violence exposure is important, not only for developing monitoring systems in the participating countries, but also for sensitizing and mobilizing communities to engage in child protection efforts. The results presented in this study provide an insight to the magnitude of the phenomenon of children's exposure to violence in countries with no prior quantitative research data [35–37]. Moreover, data presented here also provide a baseline measurement for future research and can be used for the evaluation of large-scale social policies on

Table 7 Lifetime-prevalence of schoolchildren's exposure to violent behaviors by form of violence experienced and by child's sex, per country

Country	Sex	Form of children's exposure (scales of the ICAST-C^R)											
		Psychological violence		Physical violence		Sexual violence		Contact sexual violence		Feeling of neglect		Positive and non violent parenting	
		% (n)	95% C.I.	% (n)	95% C.I.	% (n)	95% C.I.	% (n)	95% C.I.	% (n)	95% C.I.	% (n)	95% C.I.
Albania	Female	70.09 (1263)	67.97–72.20	60.65 (1093)	58.40–62.91	8.22 (148)	6.95–9.49	2.06 (37)	1.40–2.72	30.74* (553)	28.61–32.87	95.23 (1716)	94.24–96.21
	Male	66.93 (1018)	64.57–69.29	58.16 (884)	55.68–60.64	14.50* (220)	12.73–16.27	8.11 (123)	6.74–9.49	19.79 (300)	17.78–21.79	93.95 (1428)	92.75–95.15
B & H	Female	73.36 (1027)	71.04–75.67	67.43 (944)	64.97–69.88	17.93 (251)	15.92–19.94	7.65 (107)	6.26–9.04	47.50* (665)	44.88–50.12	96.57 (1352)	95.62–97.52
	Male	71.67 (878)	69.15–74.20	68.25 (834)	65.64–70.86	19.47 (237)	17.25–21.70	12.25 (149)	10.41–14.10	30.79 (375)	28.20–33.38	95.42 (1167)	94.25–96.59
Bulgaria	Female	68.83 (722)	66.02–71.63	59.87 (628)	56.90–62.83	7.91 (83)	6.28–9.55	4.29 (45)	3.06–5.52	25.93 (272)	23.28–28.58	92.56 (971)	90.98–94.15
	Male	70.23 (696)	67.39–73.08	64.58 (641)	61.71–67.66	9.28 (92)	7.48–11.09	5.55 (55)	4.12–6.98	21.29 (211)	18.74–23.84	91.83 (910)	90.12–93.53
Croatia	Female	73.54 (1370)	71.53–75.54	66.38 (1236)	64.23–68.53	11.96 (222)	10.48–13.44	5.18 (96)	4.17–6.18	40.56* (754)	38.33–42.79	97.91 (1823)	97.26–98.56
	Male	72.53 (1291)	70.45–74.60	67.10 (1189)	64.91–69.29	8.31 (147)	7.03–9.60	3.80 (67)	2.90–4.69	29.77 (527)	27.64–31.90	96.51 (1726)	95.66–97.37
FYROM	Female	63.70 (4590)	61.21–66.18	49.03 (4236)	46.44–51.61	6.01 (907)	4.78–7.24	2.47 (423)	1.66–3.28	30.96* (2343)	28.57–33.36	83.66 (5394)	81.75–85.57
	Male	65.68 (4101)	62.93–68.43	52.71 (3726)	49.82–55.60	9.64* (738)	7.91–11.37	5.50 (364)	4.16–6.84	23.07 (1528)	20.62–25.52	84.13 (4864)	82.02–86.25
Greece	Female	83.76 (916)	82.78–84.74	77.37 (704)	76.26–78.48	16.62 (86)	15.63–17.61	7.76 (35)	7.05–8.47	42.83* (444)	41.52–44.14	98.43 (1203)	98.10–98.76
	Male	82.50 (754)	81.44–83.55	75.27 (603)	74.07–76.47	15.02 (108)	14.03–16.02	7.42 (61)	6.68–8.15	30.96 (263)	29.67–32.25	97.91 (965)	97.51–98.30
Romania	Female	76.91 (2542)	75.48–78.35	65.57 (2163)	63.94–67.19	7.90 (260)	6.98–8.82	3.01 (99)	2.43–3.60	26.56* (876)	25.05–28.07	96.43 (3187)	95.80–97.06
	Male	76.51 (2003)	74.88–78.18	68.79 (1794)	67.01–70.57	7.91 (205)	6.87–8.95	4.26 (110)	3.48–5.04	17.57 (456)	16.10–19.03	95.37 (2949)	94.57–96.18
Serbia	Female	71.31 (1397)	69.31–73.31	68.57 (1342)	66.52–70.63	7.53 (147)	6.36–8.70	3.79 (74)	2.95–4.64	34.56* (676)	32.45–36.67	97.96 (1919)	97.33–98.58
	Male	65.72 (1359)	63.67–67.76	69.76 (1437)	67.77–71.74	9.39 (193)	8.13–10.65	5.95 (122)	4.92–6.97	23.38 (481)	21.55–25.21	96.76 (1998)	95.99–97.52
Turkey	Female	70.89 (2625)	69.43–72.35	56.12 (2077)	54.52–57.72	N/A^a		N/A^a		48.12* (1780)	46.51–49.73	94.65 (3502)	93.92–95.37
	Male	70.28 (2686)	68.83–71.73	60.58* (2307)	59.03–62.14	N/A^a		N/A^a		37.25 (1414)	35.71–38.79	93.19 (3558)	92.39–93.99

^{a} Not available

* Significant at p < 0.05

Table 8 Past-year prevalence of schoolchildren's exposure to violent behaviors by form of violence experienced and by child's sex per country

| Country | Sex | Form of children's exposure (scales of the ICAST-C[R].) | | | | | | | | | | | |
| | | Psychological violence | | Physical violence | | Sexual violence | | Contact sexual violence | | Feeling of neglect | | Positive and non violent parenting | |
		% (n)	95% C.I.	% (n)	95% C.I.	% (n)	95% C.I.	% (n)	95% C.I.	% (n)	95% C.I.	% (n)	95% C.I.
Albania	Female	63.37 (1142)	61.15–65.60	48.83 (880)	46.53–51.14	6.00 (108)	4.90–7.10	1.39* (25)	0.85–1.93	26.68* (480)	24.64–28.73	93.40 (1683)	82.25–94.54
	Male	59.83 (901)	57.37–62.29	48.03 (730)	45.51–50.54	12.85* (195)	11.17–14.54	7.26 (110)	5.95–8.56	16.09 (244)	14.25–17.94	92.57 (1407)	91.25–93.88
B & H	Female	65.93 (923)	63.45–68.41	49.79 (697)	47.17–52.40	12.43 (174)	10.70–14.16	5.65* (79)	4.44–6.86	40.50* (567)	37.93–43.07	95.50 (1338)	94.41–96.59
	Male	62.04 (760)	59.32–64.76	52.62 (643)	49.82–55.42	15.04 (183)	13.03–17.05	10.03 (122)	8.34–11.72	25.04 (305)	22.61–27.47	93.13 (1139)	91.71–94.55
Bulgaria	Female	61.77 (648)	58.83–64.71	47.28 (496)	44.26–50.30	6.96 (73)	5.42–8.50	3.72 (39)	2.57–4.86	22.21 (233)	19.70–24.73	90.75 (952)	89.00–92.51
	Male	62.66 (621)	59.65–65.68	49.75 (493)	46.63–52.86	8.07 (80)	6.38–9.77	5.05 (50)	3.68–6.41	17.46 (173)	15.09–19.82	89.51 (887)	87.60–91.41
Croatia	Female	66.40 (1237)	64.25–68.54	44.58 (830)	42.32–46.83	8.03 (149)	6.79–9.26	3.34 (62)	2.52–4.16	33.67* (626)	31.53–35.82	96.78 (1802)	95.98–97.58
	Male	64.94 (1156)	62.73–67.16	46.56 (825)	44.24–48.88	6.33 (122)	5.20–7.47	3.17 (56)	2.36–3.99	23.33 (413)	21.36–25.30	95.56 (1699)	94.60–96.51
FYROM	Female	59.81 (3833)	57.27–62.34	40.18 (2550)	37.65–42.72	4.89* (484)	3.77–6.01	2.26* (191)	1.49–3.04	28.73* (1689)	26.39–31.07	82.82 (5293)	80.87–84.77
	Male	60.71 (3485)	57.89–63.54	45.19 (2389)	42.31–48.08	8.30 (505)	6.69–9.92	4.78 (270)	3.52–6.03	20.09 (1059)	17.76–22.41	83.26 (4759)	81.10–85.42
Greece	Female	69.95 (860)	68.73–71.16	46.58 (577)	45.25–47.90	8.87 (70)	8.11–9.62	3.50* (32)	3.01–3.99	30.88* (412)	29.65–32.10	96.59 (1191)	96.11–97.07
	Male	70.11 (697)	68.83–71.38	48.26 (517)	46.87–49.65	10.28 (93)	9.43–11.13	5.50 (53)	4.86–6.14	21.45 (229)	20.31–22.60	95.79 (955)	95.23–96.35
Romania	Female	66.02 (2182)	64.41–67.64	42.29* (1395)	40.60–43.97	4.65 (153)	3.93–5.37	1.46* (48)	1.05–1.87	19.44* (641)	18.09–20.79	93.59 (3093)	92.75–94.42
	Male	65.93 (1726)	64.11–67.74	47.70 (1244)	45.78–49.62	5.40 (140)	4.53–6.27	2.86 (74)	2.22–3.51	13.10 (340)	11.80–14.39	92.77 (2426)	91.78–93.76
Serbia	Female	63.25* (1239)	61.11–65.38	45.94 (899)	43.73–48.15	4.92* (96)	3.96–5.88	2.51* (49)	1.82–3.21	27.66* (541)	25.68–29.64	95.05 (1862)	94.09–96.01
	Male	56.19 (1162)	54.05–58.33	46.99 (968)	44.84–49.15	7.49 (154)	6.36–8.63	4.82 (99)	3.90–5.75	18.28 (376)	16.61–19.95	94.14 (1944)	93.13–95.15
Turkey	Female	63.06 (2335)	61.50–64.61	43.61* (1614)	42.01–45.21	N/A[a]		N/A[a]		43.09* (1594)	41.50–44.69	91.73 (3394)	90.84–92.62
	Male	62.59 (2392)	61.05–64.12	48.45 (1845)	46.86–50.04	N/A[a]		N/A[a]		32.14 (122)	30.65–33.62	89.79 (2418)	88.82–90.75

[a] Not available

* Significant at p < 0.05

child protection. Overall, the findings of this research documented in quantitative terms a considerable rate of children's exposure to various harmful practices in the participating countries.

Psychological violence

Rates of exposure to psychological violence were found to be high with the vast majority of children reporting past-year and lifetime exposure. Children's self-reported exposure to psychological violence ranged from 64.6 to 83.2% for lifetime and 58.3 to 70.0% for past-year exposure. As with other studies from the region, except for Serbia where girls reported higher levels of exposure to past-year psychological violence, no significant differences in exposure between males and females could be observed [38]. However, lifetime prevalence rates in this study far exceeded the estimated European prevalence 29.2%, established by a recent meta-analysis which included six European studies [38]. A recent study in Romania using the Adverse Childhood Experiences Questionnaire in 15-year old students found a lifetime prevalence of 39.7% for psychological violence which is higher than the European mean but lower than the 77% found by this present study [39]. Further research is needed to establish the underlying drivers of these high rates of psychological violence in the region.

Physical violence

Rates of physical violence exposure were found to be high with almost every second child reporting past-year exposure and more than every second child reporting lifetime victimization. Equivalent percentages of children's self-reports for exposure to physical violence range from 50.7 to 76.4% for lifetime and 42.4 to 51.0% for past-year victimization. As with other studies from the region, apart from in two countries, no significant differences in physical violence exposure between males and females could be observed [40]. However, lifetime prevalence rates for physical violence exposure in this study far exceeded the European estimate of 22.9% established by a recent meta-analysis which included 19 European studies [40]. A recent study in Romania found a lifetime prevalence of 32.2% for physical violence among 15-year olds which is considerably lower than the 67% found by this present study [39]. Further research is needed to establish the underlying drivers of these high rates of physical violence in the region.

Sexual violence

Rates of sexual violence exposure were found to range from one in twelve to one in six children for lifetime exposure and between one in twenty and one in ten children for past-year prevalence. Equivalent percentages of children's self-reported exposure to contact sexual violence ranged from 2.1 to 7.7% for the last year and 3.5 to 9.8% across the lifespan. While exposure to sexual violence is typically more often associated with female victimization [41] in this study self-reported experiences of boys were found to exceed or equal girls' self-reported exposures. In particular, boys in Albania, Bosnia and Herzegovina, FYROM, Greece, Romania and Serbia reported higher levels of contact sexual violence exposure compared to girls. This is contrary to findings from a recent meta-analysis of 39 publications which established lifetime prevalence of childhood sexual victimization in Europe as 13.5% for females and 5.6% for males, therefore finding lower prevalence of sexual victimization in boys [42]. The global prevalence estimates of sexual abuse in childhood in this meta-analysis also established higher risk for sexual victimization among girls. Recent research from Saudi Arabia and South Africa finds equal exposures for sexual victimization between boys and girls [43, 44]. Why boys report equal or increased exposure to sexual violence than girls in some regions of the world is unclear. Further research, is required to investigate the reasons for these elevated rates of sexual abuse victimization among boys in the participating countries.

Neglect

Rates of subjective feeling of neglect were found to range from one in four to one in two children for lifetime exposure and between one in six and one in three children for past-year prevalence. Equivalent percentages of children's self-reports for neglect experiences range from 16.7 to 37.5% for the last year and 22.6 to 42.6% across the lifespan. Rates of feeling neglected were reported significantly more by female children across almost all countries. A recent meta-analysis of 16 studies on emotional neglect could not establish a prevalence rate for Europe as it could not find any studies from the region [45]. However, the overall lifetime global prevalence estimate for emotional neglect was 18.4% which is lower than the estimates in this study. Further this meta-analysis found no difference in lifetime prevalence between boys and girls. Why girls report equal or increased exposure to neglect than boys is unclear although it may be related to the way in which the questions were framed as they did not ask about specific incidents but a general feeling of being uncared for. Further research is required to investigate the reasons for these elevated rates of neglect among girls in the participating countries.

Positive discipline

Over 90% of participants reported exposure to positive and non-violent parenting. This is in stark contrast to the high numbers of violence exposure also reported in this study. One possible explanation for this phenomenon could be that caregivers make use of a range of disciplinary methods which may include harsh and physical punishment but can also include positive discipline techniques. Another possible explanation is that violence was perpetrated by a range of people in the child's network such as peers, teachers and other relatives rather than just by the caregivers. It is also possible that despite thorough piloting, the questions on positive discipline were not precise enough for participants to understand them correctly. It is likely, that a combination of all three occurred. Further research is required to investigate the performance of the positive and non-violent parenting sub-scale in this sample.

Overall, prevalence of past-year and lifetime violence exposure varied across countries while few statistically significant differences in violence exposure were detected between boys and girls. The most noteworthy difference is that in sexual violence exposure which was more commonly reported by boys.

This study found much higher prevalence rates across all measured violence exposures compared to statistics released by the World Health Organization in 2016. This may be due to differences in design and the use of a more comprehensive questionnaire for the measurement of children's exposure to violence which covered multiple domains and a vast array of violent incidents. It may also be due to differences in participant's ages with younger children generally more likely to be exposed to physical violence and neglect while older children are more likely to be exposed to psychological and sexual violence [46].

Limitations

Since the current study is a large-scale, international, cross-sectional study some common limitations in interpreting results have to acknowledged. First, this study utilized a child self-report measure which may be prone to recall and social desirability bias of responders. However, self-report by children is more reliable than parental report or agency records [47] and research has shown a tendency to under-report abusive experiences in studies using retrospective recall rather than over-report these [48]. Further, care was taken to ensure privacy and confidentiality throughout the research phase to reduce social desirability bias. Second, minor differences in implementation of the research protocol occurred across the different country sites. However, utmost care was taken to follow the protocol as closely as possible and to deviate only out of legal or practical necessity. Third, response-rates showed large variations across countries but no data could be collected with regards to the non-responding students and there is therefore the potential that this study excludes children that are most vulnerable

to violence exposure. Recruitment rates did not differ according to consent procedure used (active vs passive) and neither did disclosure rates of violence exposure. Fourth, although utmost care was taken with the translation of the ICAST-C, there may be slight variations in phrasing across the multiple countries and languages in this study. Sixth, this study only included children enrolled in schools and thus might exclude children who are very vulnerable and out of school. However, pilot studies in the participating countries found that the vast majority of children in the target age groups were enrolled in schools due to mandatory education requirements up to age 18. Seventh, since participating countries have different age distribution of their child population, the samples were drawn using different proportions of 11-, 13- and 16-year old children according to the proportion of this population in the respective country. This should be taken into account particularly when interpreting age aggregated prevalence rates and is one of the reasons why this study does not conduct analyses to compare prevalence rates of violence exposure across the various countries. However, it should also be noted that despite geographical proximity, participating countries have substantial differences in a number of characteristics which are expected to influence prevailing behaviors in societies. Furthermore, it should be also taken into account that some of the participating countries experienced war or civil unrest less than a decade prior to conducting the surveys. This can influence societies' prevailing behaviors and perspectives which could have influenced results in a number of different ways (from actual differences in prevalence of violence against children to differences in responding to such a survey). Finally, this study did not adjust for multiple comparisons based on Rothman's suggestion that this will lead to fewer errors of interpretation when the data under evaluation are actual observations [49].

Conclusions

Research on children's exposure to violence has an increased social utility function over and above providing epidemiological evidence which can help predict the burden of mental health. Providing a robust evidence base for the understanding of the phenomenon of children's victimization can ultimately facilitate effective social and child protection policy design and implementation. From this angle, current evidence indicates new targets for social policies and awareness raising interventions that could tackle currently invisible aspects of the phenomenon of children's exposure to violence. In this context, this particular study generated a first quantitative measurement of the magnitude of the problem in the participant countries and served as a tool for awareness raising among professional communities and policy makers. It created a space for further research not just to verify its findings, but also for shedding more light on all aspects of children's victimization which include medical, mental, psycho-social and human rights challenges for modern societies.

Authors' contributions
GN conceptualised the study together with KP, FZ, AT, AH, EC, JBS, EV, VS, SC, MA, MR, MR, LT, MR, IA, VI, NH, ZOS, IUB, DB and KB. GN, KP, AT, AH, EC, JBS, EV, VS, SC, MA, MR, MR, LT, MR, IA, VI, NH, ZOS and IUB contributed in specification of the study in detail, developed the fieldwork and led data collection in their respective countries. GN, KP and FZ conducted the statistical analyses with assistance from all authors regarding each country's results. GN initially drafted the manuscript. KP, FZ, AT, AH, EC, JBS, EV, VS, SC, MA, MR, MR, LT, MR, IA, VI, NH, ZOS, IUB, DB, KB and FM contributed to the writing and interpretation of the analyses. All authors read and approved the final manuscript.

Author details
[1] Department of Mental Health and Social Welfare, Centre for the Study and Prevention of Child Abuse and Neglect, Institute of Child Health, 7 Fokidos Str., 11526 Athens, Greece. [2] Children's Human Rights Centre of Albania, Tirana, Albania. [3] Faculty of Political Sciences, University of Sarajevo, Sarajevo, Bosnia and Herzegovina. [4] Department of Medical Social Sciences, South-West University "N. Rilski", Blagoevgrad, Bulgaria. [5] Department of Social Work, Faculty of Law, University of Zagreb, Zagreb, Croatia. [6] University Clinic of Psychiatry, University of Skopje, Skopje, Former Yugoslav Republic of Macedonia. [7] Social Work Department, Faculty of Sociology and Social Work, Babes-Bolyai University, Cluj-Napoca, Romania. [8] Faculty for Special Education and Rehabilitation, University of Belgrade, Belgrade, Serbia. [9] Association of Emergency Ambulance Physicians, İzmir, Turkey. [10] Instituto degli Innocenti, Florence, Italy. [11] Centre for Evidence-Based Interventions, University of Oxford, Oxford, UK. [12] School of Behavioural Sciences, North-West University, Vanderbeijlpark, South Africa. [13] Centre for Forensic and Family Psychology (Division of Psychiatry and Applied Psychology), School of Medicine, University of Nottingham, Nottingham, UK. [14] Present Address: Department of Applied Mathematics and Computer Science, Technical University of Denmark, Copenhagen, Denmark. [15] Present Address: "The Smile of the Child", Athens, Greece. [16] Present Address: Humanities and Social Sciences Department, University of New York Tirana, Tirana, Albania. [17] Present Address: AWO Clearinghaus for Unaccompanied Minor Refugees, Dortmund, North Rhine-Westphalia, Germany.

Acknowledgements
This paper is part of the BECAN project that was funded by the EU's 7th Framework Program for Research and Innovation (ID: 223478/HEALTH/CALL 2007-B), coordinated by the Institute of Child Health (GR) and included the following participating organizations: Children's Human Rights Centre of Albania (AL), South-West University "N. Rilski" (BG), University of Sarajevo (BH), University of Zagreb (HR), University of Skopje (MK), Babes-Bolyai University (RO), University of Belgrade (RS), Association of Emergency Ambulance Physicians (TK) and Istituto degli Innocenti (IT).

Competing interests
The authors declare that they have no competing interests.

Ethics approval and consent to participate
The project was subjected to assessment and was granted approval during its submission to the European Commission FP7 program's ethical committee. In the implementation phase of the project, permission to conduct the research in the school setting was granted by the educational authorities in each country. All children and their caregivers were informed in advance about the plans to carry out the research and provided consent. In line with in-country legislation, parental consent was either passive or active. However, a wide range of ethical and methodological issues emerged during the set-up of the field research relating to differences in national legislation and authoritative agency responses. These included, among others, the rights of disabled children to participate, the differentiation of oral versus written consent for parents and children and its implications or potential for parental refusal to participate in cases of severe child abuse. To deal with these issues, independent ethical advisory boards were set up in each country to provide supervision and guidance. These were overseen by an international independent ethics advisory board with experts on conducting research on children's violence exposure monitoring the implementation of the project in all participant countries. Further, ad-hoc crisis intervention teams were set up in each country to help with collaborations between the research teams and local community agencies to facilitate referrals following child abuse disclosures where children were considered to be at risk of significant harm. Monitoring of the research implementation was recorded in three national Ethics Reviews drafted per country by the national advisory boards on ethical issues and three Ethics Reviews drafted by the international advisory board on ethical issues concerning the implementation of the entire research project all of which were published during the project's lifespan. All official permissions and boards' reviews as well as standard parental consent and child ascent forms used are available on reasonable request.

Funding
The research leading to this manuscript was funded by the European Research Council under the EU's 7th Framework Programme for Research and Innovation (ID: 223478/HEALTH/CALL 2007-B). FM received writing support from the Economic and Social Research Council in the UK (ES/N017447/1).

References
1. Kempe CH, Silverman FN, Steele BF, Droegemueller W, Silver HK. The battered-child syndrome. JAMA J Am Med Assoc. 1962;181:17.
2. World Health Assembly. Prevention of violence. Geneva: WHO; 1997.
3. World Health Organziation. Report of the consultation on child abuse prevention. Geneva: WHO; 1999.
4. Norman RE, Byambaa M, De R, Butchart A, Scott J, Vos T. The long-term health consequences of child physical abuse, emotional abuse, and neglect: a systematic review and meta-analysis. PLoS Med. 2012;9:e1001349.
5. Carr CP, Martins CMS, Stingel AM, Lemgruber VB, Juruena MF. The role of early life stress in adult psychiatric disorders. J Nerv Ment Dis. 2013;201:1007–20.
6. Young JC, Widom CS. Long-term effects of child abuse and neglect on emotion processing in adulthood. Child Abuse Negl. 2014;38:1369–81.
7. Lindert J, von Ehrenstein OS, Grashow R, Gal G, Braehler E, Weisskopf MG. Sexual and physical abuse in childhood is associated with depression and anxiety over the life course: systematic review and meta-analysis. Int J Public Health. 2014;59:359–72.
8. Dube S, Anda R, Felittti D, Chapman D, Williamson W. Childhood abuse, household dysfunction, and the risk of attempted suicide throughout the lifespan. JAMA J Am Med Assoc. 2001;286:3089–96.
9. Harford TC, Yi H, Grant BF. Associations between childhood abuse and interpersonal aggression and suicide attempt among US adults in a national study. Child Abuse Negl. 2014;38:1389–98.
10. Liu J, Fang Y, Gong J, Cui X, Meng T, Xiao B, et al. Associations between suicidal behavior and childhood abuse and neglect: a meta-analysis. J Affect Disord. 2017;220:147–55.

11. Proctor LJ, Lewis T, Roesch S, Thompson R, Litrownik AJ, English D, et al. Child maltreatment and age of alcohol and marijuana initiation in high-risk youth. Addict Behav. 2017;75:64–9.

12. Nemeroff CB. Paradise lost: the neurobiological and clinical consequences of child abuse and neglect. Neuron. 2016;89:892–909.

13. Fergusson DM, McLeod GFH, Horwood LJ. Childhood sexual abuse and adult developmental outcomes: findings from a 30-year longitudinal study in New Zealand. Child Abuse Negl. 2013;37:664–74.

14. Boden JM, Horwood LJ, Fergusson DM. Exposure to childhood sexual and physical abuse and subsequent educational achievement outcomes. Child Abuse Negl. 2007;31:1101–14.

15. Debowska A, Boduszek D. Child abuse and neglect profiles and their psychosocial consequences in a large sample of incarcerated males. Child Abuse Negl. 2017;65:266–77.

16. Bartlett J, Kotake C, Fauth R, Easterbrooks A. Intergenerational transmission of child abuse and neglect: do maltreatment type, perpetrator, and substantiation status matter? Child Abuse Negl. 2017;63:84–94.

17. UNICEF. Hidden in plain sight: a statistical analysis of violence against children. Report. New York; 2014.

18. United Nations. Sustainable development goals. 2014. http://www.sustainabledevelopment.un.org/sdgs. Accessed 5 Dec 2016.

19. Global initiative to end all corporal punishment of children. Progress towards prohibiting all corporal punishment in Europe and Central Asia. London; 2017. http://www.endcorporalpunishment.org/. Retrieved at 21 Dec 2017.

20. Zolotor AJ, Puzia ME. Bans against corporal punishment: a systematic review of the laws, changes in attitudes and behaviours. Child Abuse Rev. 2010;19:229–47.

21. Putnam FW. Ten-year research update review: child sexual abuse. J Am Acad Child Adolesc Psychiatry. 2003;42:269–78.

22. Amaya-Jackson L, Socolar R, Hunter W, Runyan D, Colindres R. Directly questioning children and adolescents about maltreatment: a review of survey measures used. J Interpers Violence. 2000;15:725–59.

23. Butchart A, Phinney Harvey A, Kahane T, Mian M, Fuerniss T. Preventing child maltreatment: a guide to taking action and generating evidence. Geneva: World Health Organization; 2006.

24. Bianchi D, Ruggiero R. Guidelines on data collection and monitoring systems on child abuse. Florence: ChildOnEurope; 2009.

25. Meinck F, Steinert JI, Sethi D, Gilbert R, Bellis M, Mikton C, et al. Measuring and monitoring national prevalence of child maltreatment: a practical handbook. Copenhagen: World Health Organization Regional Office for Europe; 2016.

26. Zolotor AJ, Runyan DK, Dunne MP, Jain D, Péturs HR, Ramirez C, et al. ISPCAN Child Abuse Screening Tool Children's Version (ICAST-C): instrument development and multi-national pilot testing. Child Abuse Negl. 2009;33:833–41.

27. Runyan DK, Dunne MP, Zolotor AJ, Madrid B, Jain D, Gerbaka B, et al. The development and piloting of the ISPCAN Child Abuse Screening Tool—Parent version (ICAST-P). Child Abuse Negl. 2009;33:826–32.

28. Radford L, Corral S, Bradley C, Fisher HL. The prevalence and impact of child maltreatment and other types of victimization in the UK: findings from a population survey of caregivers, children and young people and young adults. Child Abuse Negl. 2013;37:801–13.

29. Iovu M. The potential of ISPCAN Child Abuse Screening Tool Children's Version (ICAST-CH) for mapping child maltreatment experiences. In: Dulama E, Valcan T, Ciocian M, editors. Perspect. asupra Probl. din Domen. Educ. - Cercet. si Apl. Cluj-Napoca: Presa Universitara Clujeana; 2012. p. 7–22.

30. Chang H-Y, Lin C-L, Chang Y-T, Tsai M-C, Feng J-Y. Psychometric testing of the Chinese version of ISPCAN Child Abuse Screening Tools Children's Home Version (ICAST-CH-C). Child Youth Serv Rev. 2013;35:2135–9.

31. Runyan D, Brandspigel S, Zolotor A, Dunne M. Manual for Administration: The ISPCAN Child Aubse Screening Tool (ICAST). Aurora: International Society for the Prevention of Child Abuse and Neglect; 2015.

32. Petroulaki K, Tsirigoti A, Nikolaidis G. Training manual and guidelines for researchers for the modified ICAST-CH and ICAST-P Questionnaires. Athens: BECAN Consortium; 2010.

33. Borgers N, de Leeuw E, Hoax J. Children as responders to survey research: cognitive development and response quality. Bull Methodol Sociol. 2000;66:60–6.

34. Petroulaki K, Tsirigoti A, Zarokosta F, Nikolaidis G. Epidemiological survey on child abuse and neglect in 9 Balkan Countries. Athens: BECAN Consortium; 2013.

35. Petroulaki K, Tsirigoti A, Zarokosta F, Nikolaidis G. Epidemiological characteristics of minors' exposure to experiences of violence in Greece: the BECAN study. Psychiatriki. 2013;24:262–71.

36. Ajdukovic M, Susac N, Rajter M. Gender and age differences in prevalence and incidence of child sexual abuse in Croatia. Croat Med J. 2013;54:469–79.

37. Sofuoğlu Z, Oral R, Aydın F, Cankardeş S, Kandemirci B, Koç F, et al. Epidemiological study of negative childhood experiences in three provinces of Turkey. Turk Pediatr Ars Turk Pediatr Assoc. 2014;49:47–56.

38. Stoltenborgh M, Bakermans-Kranenburg MJ, Alink LRA, van IJzendoorn MH. The universality of childhood emotional abuse: a meta-analysis of worldwide prevalence. J Aggress Maltreat Trauma. 2012;21:870–90.

39. Meinck F, Cosma AP, Mikton C, Baban A. Psychometric properties of the Adverse Childhood Experiences Abuse Short Form (ACE-ASF) among Romanian high school students. Child Abuse Negl. 2017;72:326–37.

40. Stoltenborgh M, Bakermans-Kranenburg MJ, van Ijzendoorn MH, Alink LRA. Cultural-geographical differences in the occurrence of child physical abuse? A meta-analysis of global prevalence. Int J Psychol TF. 2013;48:81–94.

41. UNICEF. The state of the world's children 2008: women and children—child survival. New York: UNICEF; 2008. p. 2007.

42. Stoltenborgh M, van IJzendoorn MH, Euser EM, Bakermans-Kranenburg MJ. A global perspective on child sexual abuse: meta-analysis of prevalence around the world. Child Maltreat. 2011;16:79–101.

43. Al-Eissa MA, AlBuhairan FS, Qayad M, Saleheen H, Runyan D, Almuneef M. Determining child maltreatment incidence in Saudi Arabia using the ICAST-CH: a pilot study. Child Abuse Negl. 2015;42:174–82.

44. Artz L, Burton P, Ward CL, Leoschut L, Phyfer J, Loyd S, et al. Optimus study South Africa: technical report sexual victimisation of children in South Africa. Zurich: UBS Optimus Foundation; 2016.

45. Stoltenborgh M, Bakermans-Kranenburg MJ, van Ijzendoorn MH. The neglect of child neglect: a meta-analytic review of the prevalence of neglect. Soc Psychiatry Psychiatr Epidemiol. 2013;48:345–55.

46. Finkelhor D, Turner H, Ormrod R, Hamby SL. Violence, abuse, and crime exposure in a national sample of children and youth. Pediatrics. 2009;124:1411–23.

47. Johnsona R, Kotch J, Catellier D, Winsor J, Dufort V, Hunter W, et al. Adverse behavioural and emotional outcomes from child abuse and witnessed violence. Child Maltreat. 2002;7:179–86.

48. Hardt J, Rutter M. Validity of adult retrospective reports of adverse childhood experiences: review of the evidence. J Child Psychol Psychiatry. 2004;45:260–73.

49. Rothman KJ. No adjustments are needed for multiple comparisons. Epidemiology. 1990;1:43–6.

6

Low mood in a sample of 5–12 year-old child psychiatric patients: a cross-sectional study

Katri Maasalo[1,2]*⬚, Jaana Wessman[1,2] and Eeva T. Aronen[1,2]

Abstract

Background: Not much is known about low mood and its associates in child psychiatric patients. In this study, we examined the prevalence of low mood, how it associates with disruptive behaviour, and affects clinician-rated global functioning in child psychiatric outpatients.

Methods: The study population consisted of 862 5–12 year-old child psychiatric patients. The study sample was a subsample of all 1251 patients attending a child psychiatric outpatient clinic at Helsinki University Hospital in 2013–2015 formed by excluding 4 year-old and 13 year-old patients and those with missing or incomplete data. The parent-rated Strengths and Difficulties Questionnaire, collected as part of the routine clinical baseline measure, was used as a measure of psychiatric symptoms. The diagnoses were set according to ICD-10 by the clinician in charge after an initial evaluation period. The Children's Global Assessment Scale (CGAS) score set by clinicians provided the measure of the patients' global functioning. All information for the study was collected from hospital registers. Associations between emotional symptoms and conduct problems/hyperactivity scores were examined using ordinal regression in univariate and multivariate models, controlling for age and sex. The independent samples T test was used to compare the CGAS values of patient groups with low/normal mood.

Results: In our sample, 512 children (59.4%) showed low mood. In multivariate ordinal regression analysis, low mood associated with conduct problems (OR 1.93, 95% CI 1.39–2.67), but no association was found between low mood and hyperactivity. Low mood was prevalent among children with oppositional defiant disorder or conduct disorder (51.8%). The global functioning score CGAS was lower among children with parent-reported low mood (52.21) than among children with normal mood (54.62, $p < 0.001$). The same was true in the subgroup of patients with no depression diagnosis (54.85 vs. 52.82, $p = 0.001$).

Conclusions: Low mood is prevalent in child psychiatric outpatients regardless of depression diagnosis and it has a negative effect on global functioning. Low mood and behavioural problems are often associated. It is important to pay attention to low mood in all child psychiatric patients. We recommend prevention measures and low-threshold services for children with low mood.

Keywords: Low mood, Behavioural problems, Global functioning

Background

Among children, the coexistence of psychiatric symptoms across diagnostic categories is a rule rather than an exception [1, 2]. Emotional and behavioural symptoms tend to overlap in population-based samples [2–4], and comorbidity is also common among child psychiatric patients [5, 6]. In order to better "convey the mixed patterns of symptomatology" [1] that are common in child psychiatry, a combination of dimensional and categorical approaches to diagnosis is recommended.

As the evidence of the clinical significance of sub-threshold symptoms has grown, many studies support

*Correspondence: katri.maasalo@hus.fi
[1] University of Helsinki and Helsinki University Hospital, Children's Hospital, Child Psychiatry, Tukholmankatu 8 C 613, 00290 Helsinki, Finland
Full list of author information is available at the end of the article

a dimensional rather than categorical view of disorders, also in depressive disorders [7–9]. Subthreshold symptoms of depression impair quality of life and global functioning, and pose a risk of future psychopathology. There is evidence that recognizing and treating them has clinical significance [7, 8], but further studies in clinical child populations are needed.

In our previous study in a Finnish non-clinical population of 4–12 year-old children, emotional problems were associated with conduct problems and hyperactivity, and our findings emphasized the role of low mood in the associations between emotional and behavioural problems [10]. Persistent sad or low mood is one of the core symptoms of depression according to both the DSM-5 [11] and ICD-10 [12] classification systems, and is also a common symptom of subthreshold depression [13, 14]. Some studies on the clinical characteristics of youth with depression report rates of low mood ranging from 50.0 to 100% [14–18]. One study [15] has compared the prevalence of depressive symptoms in depressed (98.2–100%) and other adolescent psychiatric patients (2.9–4.1%). A recent Danish population-based study found low mood to be as frequent among 8–10 year-old children with subthreshold depression as among those with clinical depression (94.5% vs. 94.3%; diagnoses from DAWBA entered online by mothers and reviewed by physicians), and distinctly less common although still quite prevalent (16.4%) among non-depressed children [13]. In our population-based study of Finnish children [10], low mood was reported by 16% of the children's parents. Low mood was associated with family structure, sleep problems, illness or disability of the child, conduct problems, and hyperactivity. Examining low mood at symptom level and how it associates with behavioural symptoms and disorders in a sample of child psychiatric patients is important, as this knowledge deepens the understanding of the relations between mood and behavioural problems in child patients. This knowledge also has relevance for diagnostic decisions and choices of treatment options.

Children with irritable mood (which counts as a symptom of both depression and mania in children) have been the object of vast interest and several studies, partly in a response to diagnosing children with bipolar disorder [19]. Recently, a new diagnosis of disruptive mood dysregulation disorder (DMDD) has been introduced to the DSM-5 [11]. This new mood diagnosis, and the fact that bipolar disorder remains an inadequately understood disorder in children, calls for studies of co-occurrence of mood and behavioural problems in clinical samples.

We found no earlier literature on studies on comorbidity in clinical populations where the presence of emotional and behavioural symptoms is considered without being restricted into diagnostic categories. Studies on low mood are also scarce—we found no studies that report rates of low mood in child psychiatric patients other than those with depression. Further, no studies were found to examine the associations between low mood and externalising behaviour in child psychiatric patients.

Our aim in this study was to evaluate how emotional symptoms, especially low mood and behavioural problems, coexist in a sample of 5–12 year-old child psychiatric outpatients. More specifically, we wanted to examine how conduct problems/hyperactivity associate with emotional symptoms, the prevalence of low mood in different patient groups, how parents' and the children's reports on mood correspond with each other, how low mood associates with disruptive behaviour, and how low mood affects the clinician-rated global functioning of the child. On the basis of our previous results [10], we hypothesized that emotional problems and low mood would be associated with conduct problems and hyperactivity. We also hypothesized that low mood would more frequently be reported by children than their parents, and that it would have a negative effect on the clinician-rated global functioning of the child.

Methods

Our study population consisted of 862 5–12 year-old child psychiatric patients. We formed the study sample from all the 1251 patients who attended the child psychiatric assessment and acute care unit of Helsinki University Hospital in 2013–2015 by excluding the few 4 year-old and 13 year-old patients and those with missing or incomplete data on parent reported psychiatric symptoms. The final study population did not differ from the initial patient population in respect to age, sex or CGAS values.

The information for the study was collected from hospital registers. Strengths and Difficulties Questionnaire (SDQ-parent form) and Quality of Life measure (17D-child report) were collected as a routine clinical baseline measure of the child's psychiatric symptoms and quality of life at Helsinki University Hospital Child Psychiatry Clinic.

A clinician set the diagnoses according to ICD-10 and assigned the CGAS values after an initial evaluation. The initial evaluation included the information from the referral, a meeting with the child and the parents where the anamnesis was taken by the child psychiatrist, and a brief discussion with the parents alone and with the child alone. The researchers divided the detailed diagnoses (e.g. mild, moderate, severe major depressive disorder) into diagnostic groups (e.g. depressive disorder) by assigning a group to each ICD-10 diagnose code in the data. The CGAS [20] was used as a measure of patients' global functioning, the scale of which ranges from 0 to 100; higher scores indicating better functioning. Our clinic routinely uses this scale which has shown to have moderate inter-rater validity in a naturalistic clinical setting [21].

The SDQ is a brief 25-item instrument for screening the emotional and behavioural problems of children and adolescents [22]. The items are scored 0/1/2 for "not/somewhat/certainly true", except for 5 items (items 7, 11, 14, 21 and 25) that are scored in the opposite direction. The items are categorized into emotional problems, conduct problems, hyperactivity, peer problems, and prosocial subscales, with scores ranging from 0 to 10. A total score of 0–40 is generated by summing the scores of the four first-mentioned subscales [23]. Epidemiological studies [24] have shown the SDQ to be applicable to Finnish children. The SDQ subscores were categorized as "normal", "borderline" or "abnormal" using the cut-off points defined on the official SDQ website [23] (0–3, 4, 5–10 for emotional problems, 0–2, 3, 4–10 for conduct problems, and 0–5, 6, 7–10 for hyperactivity). Of the items screening for emotional problems, "often unhappy, down-hearted or tearful" directly describes mood, while the others describe anxiety symptoms and somatic complaints. We used mood item number 13 as a measure for mood as rated by parents in the sample, and a depression dimension (question 17) from the 17D as a measure for mood as reported by children. The 17D is a 17-dimensional, generic measure of perceived health-related quality of life for pre-adolescents [25]. Question 17 asks the child to choose whether they feel cheerful and happy or a little/quite/very/extremely sad, unhappy or depressed. Reports of feeling at least a little sad, unhappy or depressed were interpreted as current low mood.

Statistical analyses

The "somewhat true" and "certainly true" categories of the emotional items of the SDQ were collapsed into a "somewhat or certainly true" category to retain the setting that was used in our population-based study [10] and to add sensitivity to the parents' reports, since parents often underestimate children's internalizing symptoms [26–29]. The associations between emotional symptoms and conduct problem/hyperactivity scores were examined using ordinal regression in univariate and multivariate models. The kappa statistic (presented in the results) was used to assess the level of agreement between parents and children on mood. The independent samples T test was used to compare the CGAS values of patient groups.

Analyses were carried out using IBM SPSS Statistics 22.

Results

Descriptive statistics

Table 1 presents the characteristics and clinical diagnoses of the study population as well as the distribution of the scores on SDQ subscales and emotional problems subscale items. In the SDQ, boys had higher total difficulties scores as well as higher conduct problems and hyperactivity subscale scores than girls, whereas girls had higher emotional problems scores (p = 0.000–0.004). There was no difference between sexes in peer problems scores. Emotional problems increased with age (p = 0.002), whereas the total problems score, hyperactivity score and conduct score decreased with increasing age (p < 0.001). Age had no effect on peer problems or prosocial scores.

Emotional problems, conduct problems and hyperactivity scores in the SDQ

The partial correlation (controlling for age and sex) between the emotional problems score and the conduct problems score in the parent-rated SDQ was 0.124 (p < 0.001), between the emotional problems score and the hyperactivity score 0.052 (p = 0.129), and between the conduct problems score and the hyperactivity score 0.574 (p < 0.001). Of the children with abnormal conduct problems and/or hyperactivity scores, 42.2% also had an abnormal emotional problems score, and 162 (18.8%) of the patients had only an abnormal emotional problems score, with no conduct problems/hyperactivity. Of the patients, 101 (11.7%) had abnormal scores in all three categories, and 210 patients (24.4%) scored under the cut-off point in all three scales. The smallest patient group was that of children with hyperactivity and emotional problems but no conduct problems (n = 21, 2.4%). See also Fig. 1.

Low mood reported by parents and children

In our sample, 512 children (59.4%) showed low mood (defined as SDQ item 13 "Often unhappy, down-hearted or tearful" being rated somewhat or certainly true by a parent). Of the 428 children who responded to the 17D mood question, 48.8% reported feeling at least a little sad, unhappy or depressed and 62.1% were evaluated to have low mood by their parent. In 166 cases, both the child and the parent reported low mood, and in 119 cases, both the child and the parent reported normal mood. In 23.4% of the cases the parent reported low mood although the child did not, and in 10.0% of the cases the situation was vice versa. The parent and child agreed on the child's mood in 66.6% of the cases, and disagreed in 33.4% of the cases. Cohen's kappa for agreement on mood between parent and child was 0.336 (p < 0.001, 95% CI 0.250–0.422). The majority of the children with parent-reported low mood (58.4%) were boys, as were

Table 1 Descriptive statistics (n = 862)

		Diagnosis, n (%)	
Age in years, mean (SD)	9.1 (2.0)	ODD/CD	224 (26.0)
Range	5–12	Hyperkinetic disorder	152 (17.6)
Interquartile range	4	Other emotional diagnoses	136 (15.8)
Preschool age, n (%)	105 (12.2)	Anxiety disorder	114 (13.2)
School age, n (%)	757 (87.8)	Depression	99 (11.5)
Girls, n (%)	313 (36.3)	Learning disability	70 (8.1)
Boys, n (%)	549 (63.7)	Post-traumatic disorder	61 (7.1)
		Autism spectrum disorder	57 (6.6)
CGAS on arrival (n = 849)		Somatic diagnosis	31 (3.6)
Mean (SD)	53.2 (8.1)	Obsessive compulsive disorder	23 (2.7)
Median	52.0	Eating disorder	23 (2.7)
Range	21–92	Sleeping problem diagnosis	21 (2.4)
Interquartile range	12	Other diagnosis	115 (13.3)
The proportions of SDQ scores	**Normal, n (%)**	**Borderline, n (%)**	**Abnormal, n (%)**
Total difficulties score	306 (35.5)	138 (16.0)	418 (48.5)
Emotional problems score	380 (44.1)	113 (13.1)	369 (42.8)
Conduct problems score	300 (34.8)	137 (15.9)	425 (49.3)
Hyperactivity score	471 (54.6)	75 (8.7)	316 (36.7)
Peer problems score	362 (42.0)	145 (16.8)	355 (41.2)
Prosocial score	547 (63.5)	130 (15.1)	185 (21.5)
The proportions of scores on emotional problems subscale	**Not true, n (%)**	**Somewhat true, n (%)**	**Certainly true, n (%)**
Often complains of headaches, stomach-aches or sickness	364 (42.2)	317 (36.8)	174 (20.2)
Many worries, often seems worried	282 (32.7)	376 (43.6)	202 (23.4)
Often unhappy, down-hearted or tearful	350 (40.6)	364 (42.2)	148 (17.2)
Nervous or clingy in new situations, easily loses confidence	310 (36.0)	327 (37.9)	221 (25.6)
Many fears, easily scared	377 (43.7)	330 (38.3)	153 (17.7)

SD standard deviation, *CGAS* the Children's Global Assessment Scale, *ODD* oppositional defiant disorder, *CD* conduct disorder, *SDQ* the Strengths and Difficulties Questionnaire

those with self-reported low mood (55.0%). As the girls were the minority in the whole sample (36.3%), they were over-represented in these groups, making both self-reported and parent-reported low mood more common among girls (59.1% in girls vs. 42.8% in boys, and 68.1% in girls vs. 54.5% in boys, respectively).

Relationship between mood, conduct problems and hyperactivity

In univariate ordinal regression analysis of emotional symptoms and behavioural problems (controlling for age and sex), low mood, worrying, and somatic complaints were associated with conduct problems. The strongest association was between mood and conduct problems (OR 2.03, 95% CI 1.55–2.66). In multivariate analysis, low mood remained the only associate with conduct problems (OR 1.93, 95% CI 1.39–2.67). No association was found between emotional symptoms and hyperactivity. The results are presented in Table 2.

Table 3 presents the proportions of children with normal/low mood relative to other conditions. Of the children who scored within the abnormal range of the conduct problems score, 64.5% also showed parent-reported low mood, and the same was true for 56.0% of the children who scored within the abnormal range of the hyperactivity score. Of the 251 children (29.1% of the whole sample) who scored within the abnormal range in both conduct problems and hyperactivity scales, 60.6% also showed parent-reported low mood (n = 152, 17.6% of the whole sample). Of the 99 children with a depression diagnosis, 81.8% had low mood (48.5% scoring somewhat true, and 33.3% scoring certainly true) according to their parents. Of the children without depression, 56.5% had low mood. The frequency of low mood was 51.8% among the 224 children diagnosed with ODD/CD, and 39.5% among the 152 children diagnosed with a hyperkinetic disorder, the item "often unhappy, down-hearted or tearful" being rated "certainly true" by 15.6

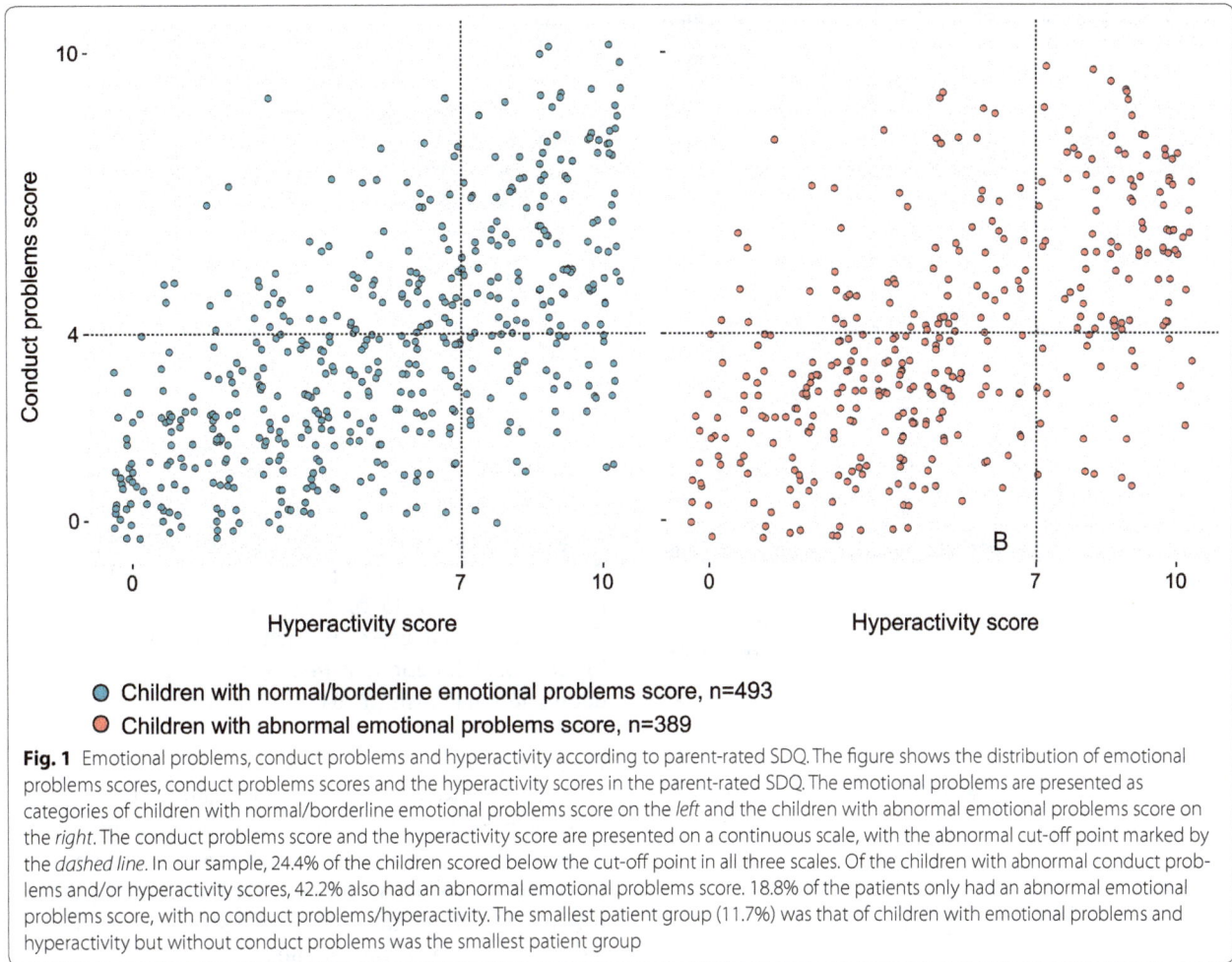

○ Children with normal/borderline emotional problems score, n=493
○ Children with abnormal emotional problems score, n=389

Fig. 1 Emotional problems, conduct problems and hyperactivity according to parent-rated SDQ. The figure shows the distribution of emotional problems scores, conduct problems scores and the hyperactivity scores in the parent-rated SDQ. The emotional problems are presented as categories of children with normal/borderline emotional problems score on the *left* and the children with abnormal emotional problems score on the *right*. The conduct problems score and the hyperactivity score are presented on a continuous scale, with the abnormal cut-off point marked by the *dashed line*. In our sample, 24.4% of the children scored below the cut-off point in all three scales. Of the children with abnormal conduct problems and/or hyperactivity scores, 42.2% also had an abnormal emotional problems score. 18.8% of the patients only had an abnormal emotional problems score, with no conduct problems/hyperactivity. The smallest patient group (11.7%) was that of children with emotional problems and hyperactivity but without conduct problems was the smallest patient group

Table 2 The association of emotional symptoms with conduct problems and hyperactivity in child psychiatric patients (n = 862)

	Conduct problems score		Hyperactive score	
	Univariate	Multivariate	Univariate	Multivariate
	OR (95% CI)	OR (95% CI)	OR (95% CI)	OR (95% CI)
Often unhappy, down-hearted or tearful	2.03 (1.55–2.66)***	1.93 (1.39–2.66)***	0.98 (0.74–1.30)	0.97 (0.70–1.36)
Often complains of headaches, stomach aches or sickness	1.38 (1.05–1.80)*	1.10 (0.83–1.48)	1.10 (0.83–1.45)	1.13 (0.83–1.53)
Many worries, often seems worried	1.50 (1.14–1.98)**	1.12 (0.79–1.59)	0.98 (0.74–1.30)	0.99 (0.69–1.42)
Nervous or clingy in new situations, easily loses confidence	1.21 (0.92–1.58)	1.04 (0.78–1.39)	1.11 (0.84–1.49)	1.16 (0.86–1.58)
Many fears, easily scared	1.19 (0.91–1.54)	0.85 (0.62–1.16)	0.88 (0.67–1.16)	0.82 (0.60–1.14)

Regression analysis examining the problem scores as explained variables and emotional symptoms as predictor variables. The problem scores were categorized as normal, borderline or abnormal (0–2; 3; 4–10 for conduct problems and 0–5; 6; 7–10 for hyperactivity) and the emotional symptoms dichotomized in "not true" and "somewhat/certainly true" (controlling for age and sex)

OR odds ratio, *CI* confidence interval

* p < 0.05, ** p < 0.01, *** p < 0.001

and 7.2% of the children, respectively, and when children with comorbid depression diagnosis were excluded, 14.9 and 6.2% respectively.

Mood and global functioning
The effects of mood on global functioning are presented in Table 4. Global functioning rated by CGAS was lower

Table 3 The prevalence of low mood in different patient groups (whole sample, n = 862)

	Normal mood	Low mood	χ^2	df	p
Whole sample	350 (40.6)	512 (59.4)			
Children with abnormal conduct problems score	151 (35.5)	274 (64.5)	16.849	2	<0.001
Children with borderline conduct problems score	49 (35.8)	88 (64.2)			
Children with normal conduct problems score	150 (50.0)	150 (50.0)			
Children with abnormal hyperactivity score	139 (44.0)	177 (56.0)	2.952	2	0.23
Children with borderline hyperactivity score	32 (42.7)	43 (57.3)			
Children with normal hyperactivity score	179 (38.0)	292 (62.0)			
Children with no depression	332 (43.5)	431 (56.5)			
Children with depression	18 (18.2)	81 (81.8)			
Children with CD/ODD	108 (48.2)	116 (51.8)			
Children with hyperactive disorder	92 (60.5)	60 (39.5)			

ODD oppositional defiant disorder, CD conduct disorder, χ^2 Chi square, df degrees of freedom, p p value

Table 4 The comparison of global functioning between patient groups

	CGAS Mean (SD)
Children with parent-reported low mood (whole sample)	52.21 (7.73)
Children with parent-reported normal mood (whole sample)	54.62 (8.47)***
Children with parent-reported low mood (non-depressed)	52.82 (7.72)
Children with parent-reported normal mood (non-depressed)	54.85 (8.42)**
Children with self-reported low mood	52.36 (7.21)
Children with self-reported normal mood	55.82 (8.49)***
Children with abnormal emotional problems score	52.20 (7.73)
Children with normal or borderline emotional problems score	53.93 (8.83)**
Children with depression	49.25 (7.25)
Children with no depression	53.71 (8.10)***
Children with abnormal hyperactivity score + low mood	51.66 (7.19)
Children with abnormal hyperactivity score + normal mood	53.06 (7.69)
Children with abnormal conduct problems score + low mood	51.60 (7.30)
Children with abnormal conduct problems score + normal mood	52.31 (6.94)
Children with abnormal emotional problems score + low mood	52.08 (7.77)
Children with abnormal emotional problems score + normal mood	53.52 (7.28)

CGAS Children's Global Assessment Scale, SD standard deviation

** p < 0.01, *** p < 0.001, from T test

among children with parent-reported low mood (52.21) than among those with normal mood (54.62, p < 0.001). This effect on global functioning remained when clinically depressed children were excluded from the analysis (52.82 vs. 54.85, p < 0.01). CGAS was also lower in children with self-reported low mood than in those with normal mood (52.36 vs. 55.82 respectively, p < 0.001). Children with a depression diagnosis from a clinician had lower global functioning (49.26) than children with no depression diagnosis (53.64, p < 0.001).

Discussion

In this study, we examined the prevalence of low mood, how the parents' and the children's reports on mood correspond with each other, how low mood associates with behavioural problems, and how low mood affects the clinician-rated global functioning in a sample of 5–12 year-old child psychiatric outpatients.

In our sample, parents reported low mood in 59.4% of the patients. We found no studies that report the prevalence of low mood in child psychiatric patients as such. Instead, studies seem to have examined the clinical characteristics of children and adolescents with depression, and have reported rates of low mood among youths with depression as ranging from 50.0 to 100% [14–18]. Bennet et al. [14] also compared the frequency of depressive symptoms of depressed and other adolescent psychiatric patients. In their clinical control group, low mood was present in 4.1% of the boys and 2.9% of the girls, which is far less than the 56.5% in our sample. This could be due to the different age range of the study participants or to methodological differences. Our sample was younger, and it is possible that with increasing age, symptoms become more specific and better fit the diagnostic categories. In addition, Bennet et al. used the 17-item Depression Rating Scale extracted from the clinician-administered K-SADS interview as a measure of mood, which required at least mild severity, and we used parent/child questionnaires to estimate low mood. Interestingly, Bennet et al. also presented the highest rates available for the frequency of low mood among depressed patients (98.2–100%) and among those with minor depression and dysthymic disorder (100%), which are higher than our rate of low mood in depression (81.8%), suggesting that our definition for low mood was not overly sensitive. Moreover, the rates presented by Bennet et al. are low compared to the study of Wesselhoeft et al. [13], in which 16% of the non-clinical population with no depression or subthreshold depression presented low mood.

To compare the children's and parents' reports of depression, we used a different measure for the children (i.e. not the SDQ), as the 17D response was available for a bigger group of patients (428 vs. 132). To assess the degree of agreement we used Cohen's Kappa, which was 0.336 in this sample. According to widely-used guidelines, values in the range of 0.21–0.4 are considered "fair" agreement, while only values above 0.6 would be considered substantial [30]. Multiple studies have shown that parents' and children's agreement on the child's symptoms is moderate at best [26, 28, 31–33]. In the study of Angold and colleagues [26], 7–25 year-old children and adolescents reported more depressive symptoms than their parents, and agreement was moderate (K = 0.40). Even very low levels of agreement between child and parent regarding the child's feelings of depression have been reported in 6–12 year-old children (0.03 in a community sample and 0.06 in clinical sample) [34]. In our sample, parents recognized the child-reported low mood in about 80% of the children who reported low mood themselves, but 37.6% of the children with parent-reported low mood reported normal mood. In our study, parents reported more low mood than the children, contrary to some earlier statements that children report more internalizing symptoms than their parents [32, 35, 36]. In our study, evaluation of the presence of low mood was made using only one question, and with different measures for children and parents. While the SDQ covers the last 6 months and is a better measure for sustained low mood, the 17D only asks about current feelings, capturing transitory feelings of low mood but missing low mood in children who momentarily are not feeling sad. Parents may also over-report low mood in children because of their own worries or problems [37]. In clinical samples of chronic somatic disorders, adolescents themselves have reported significantly less depression symptoms than their parents [38, 39]. On the other hand it is possible that it is difficult for child psychiatric patients to always recognize their mood symptoms, or to reveal them. Our results and those mentioned above emphasize the importance of asking both the child and the parent about internalizing symptoms, especially in clinical samples.

In a retrospective chart review study on 75 6–17 year-old youths with depression by Breton et al. the reason for consultation in 28% of the youths (and even 59% of the boys 6–12 years old) were behavioural problems [15]. In our previous study of a non-clinical population [10], low mood was the emotional symptom that associated most with conduct problems. We also found this association between low mood and the abnormal conduct problems score in the parent-rated SDQ in the present clinical sample, though it was not as strong as that in the population sample. Of the children with clinician-diagnosed ODD/CD, 7.1% were diagnosed with comorbid depression. Interestingly, more than half of the children with ODD/CD were reported as having low mood, and 14.9% of the children with ODD/CD but without depression rated the "often unhappy, downhearted or tearful" item as certainly true. Non-clinical samples have shown comorbidity rates of 0–45.9% for depression in children with ODD/CD [2] and clinical samples have shown rates of 10.0–50.0% [17, 40, 41]. A similar prevalence has been reported for comorbidity between subthreshold depression and ODD/CD [8, 13]. We found no earlier studies reporting the prevalence of low mood in children with ODD/CD for comparison. Do these children with low mood and conduct problems have a comorbid state of subthreshold depressive disorder and ODD/CD that meets the criteria for a categorical diagnosis (heterotypic comorbidity)? Or are they children with a depressive disorder presented with irritability, thus misconstrued as a conduct disorder (artificial comorbidity)? Do they represent a totally distinct patient group with a disruptive mood dysregulation disorder? More studies are clearly needed on the associations between low and irritable mood and conduct problems in clinical samples to address these questions.

Contrary to our finding in the non-clinical population, we found no association between mood and hyperactivity in parent-rated SDQ. However, over one-third of the children with a diagnosed hyperkinetic disorder had low mood. The reported comorbidity rates of depression in children with ADHD range from 0 to 75% [2, 42, 43]. A recent meta-analysis [44] on the correlations between ADHD and depression reported mixed evidence on the associations of the two disorders. The overall meta-analysis resulted in a moderate association, but there was heterogeneity across studies, and certain subgroup analyses resulted in small or unreliable associations. In a study by Elia et al. [45], minor depression/dysthymia (MDDD) was among the most common comorbidities in youths with ADHD (21.6%). It also found that 10.8% of children with ADHD met the criteria for simultaneous ODD, MDDD and combined type ADHD. Most of these children had irritability as a symptom, and accounted for nearly half of the children with irritability in the whole study population. Irritability is a mood state; it is closely related to low mood but is also an externalizing symptom that makes the child prone to anger and temper outbursts [19, 46]. It seems to predict future depression and anxiety, but not CD or ADHD at follow-up [19].

As recently reviewed by Zisner and Beauchaine [47], shared mechanisms of neural dysfunction in dopaminergic mesolimbic circuits associated with irritability, anhedonia and impulsive behaviour could in part account for the comorbidity patterns between depression and externalizing symptoms.

The finding that almost a quarter (24.4%) of the patients had no abnormal emotional problems, conduct problems or hyperactivity scores in the SDQ is somewhat surprising for patients in a tertiary clinic, but a Chinese study also reported similar findings, in which only half (51% when parent rated and 52% when self rated) of the adolescents scored within the abnormal range of the SDQ total problems score [48]. Our study population most likely also includes a group of children who only have abnormal peer problems scores not examined in this study, so that the number of children with no abnormal scores in any problems subscales of the SDQ is probably at least a little smaller than the 24.4% above. The problems in ADD without hyperactivity, and autism spectrum disorders with mild severity may not fall into SDQ problems categories or may be limited to peer problems. Moreover, as taken into account in the algorithms when predicting psychiatric diagnosis from SDQ, even scores below the abnormal cut-off points are of clinical relevance when combined with symptoms that impact the child's everyday life.

Low mood according to either parent or child lowered the global functioning of the child, implying that recognition of low mood is important. This was true even in children without a depression diagnosis, which is in line with the findings that subthreshold depression affects the quality of life and performance [8]. In addition, children with low mood and either conduct problems or hyperactivity had lower CGAS values than the children with normal mood, but this difference did not reach statistical significance. This can be interpreted to mean that behavioural problems in children with an abnormal hyperactivity or conduct problems score are more relevant in respect to global functioning.

It is important to view these results in the light of certain limitations of this study. As the data were cross-sectional, no conclusions can be made on the longitudinal associations of the co-occurring symptoms or of low mood and global functioning. In addition, we can only state that children with low mood have poorer global functioning than children with normal mood; we cannot claim that low mood is the reason for the decline. It can be speculated that the opposite could also be true: that children feel sad or unhappy if they are unable to function normally. We used diagnoses set by clinicians according

to ICD-10, based on clinical information collected during the initial assessment of the children. The diagnoses for the patients were compiled from medical records. As no structured diagnostic interviews were conducted, some of the co-occurring problems may have remained unnoticed by clinicians, and thus not diagnosed.

According to our results, low mood is a common symptom in children first coming to a child psychiatric clinic—in children with depression as well as with behavioural problems. In clinical practice the importance of careful assessment to define the temporal relationship of different symptoms to determine the principal target of treatment is pointed out. It has also been suggested that by paying attention to depressive symptoms with children with ODD/CD future depression could be prevented [49] as well as depression and other comorbidities in children with ADHD [50].

According to our results, patients with low mood have lower global functioning than patients with normal mood indicating that these children need special attention. The children with significant depressive symptoms have been seen as a potential object of intervention and secondary prevention decreasing the risk for recurrent depression [51].

Conclusion
We conclude that it is important to assess mood in all child psychiatric patients and to pay attention to low mood even in the absence of clinical depression. We recommend prevention measures and low-threshold services for children with low mood.

Abbreviations
ADD: attention-deficit disorder; ADHD: attention-deficit/hyperactivity disorder; CD: conduct disorder; CGAS: The Children's Global Assessment Scale; CI: confidence interval; DAWBA: the Development and Well-Being Assessment; DMDD: disruptive mood dysregulation disorder; DSM-5: the Diagnostic and Statistical Manual of Mental Disorders, 5th edition; ICD-10: International Statistical Classification of Diseases and Related Health Problems, 10th edition; K-SADS: the Kiddie Schedule for Affective Disorders and Schizophrenia; MDDD: minor depression/dysthymia; ODD: oppositional defiant disorder; OR: odds ratio; SDQ: Strengths and Difficulties Questionnaire.

Authors' contributions
All authors participated in the drafting or the revision of the manuscript, and read and approved the final manuscript. In addition, KM participated in the design of the study and performed the statistical analysis. JW gathered the diagnostic groups and participated in forming the sample. EA supervised and led the design of the study. All authors read and approved the final manuscript.

Author details
[1] University of Helsinki and Helsinki University Hospital, Children's Hospital, Child Psychiatry, Tukholmankatu 8 C 613, 00290 Helsinki, Finland. [2] Helsinki Pediatric Research Center, Laboratory of Developmental Psychopathology, Helsinki, Finland.

Competing interests
The authors declare that they have no competing interests.

Funding
This study was supported by grants from non-profit organizations: Finnish Brain Foundation Child Psychiatry Funds and Helsinki University Hospital Research Funds (TYH2013207, TYH2016202).

References

1. Rutter M. Research review: child psychiatric diagnosis and classification: concepts, findings, challenges and potential. J Child Psychol Psychiatry. 2011;52:647–60. doi:10.1111/j.1469-7610.2011.02367.x.

2. Angold A, Costello EJ, Erkanli A. Comorbidity. J Child Psychol Psychiatry. 1999;40:57–87. doi:10.1017/S0021963098003448.

3. Costello EJ, Mustillo S, Erkanli A, Keeler G, Angold A. Prevalence and development of psychiatric disorders in childhood and adolescence. Arch Gen Psychiatry. 2003;60:837–44. doi:10.1001/archpsyc.60.8.837.

4. Wichstrøm L, Berg-Nielsen TS, Angold A, Egger HL, Solheim E, Sveen TH. Prevalence of psychiatric disorders in preschoolers. J Child Psychol Psychiatry. 2012;53:695–705. doi:10.1111/j.1469-7610.2011.02514.x.

5. Staller JA. Diagnostic profiles in outpatient child psychiatry. Am J Orthopsychiatry. 2006;76:98–102. doi:10.1037/0002-9432.76.1.98.

6. Kessler RC, Chiu WT, Demler O, Merikangas KR, Walters EE. Prevalence, severity, and comorbidity of 12-month DSM-IV disorders in the National Comorbidity Survey Replication. Arch Gen Psychiatry. 2005;62:617–27. doi:10.1001/archpsyc.62.6.617.

7. Bertha EA, Balázs J. Subthreshold depression in adolescence: a systematic review. Eur Child Adolesc Psychiatry. 2013;22:589–603. doi:10.1007/s00787-013-0411-0.

8. Wesselhoeft R, Sørensen MJ, Heiervang ER, Bilenberg N. Subthreshold depression in children and adolescents—a systematic review. J Affect Disord. 2013;151:7–22. doi:10.1016/j.jad.2013.06.010.

9. Bjelland I, Lie SA, Dahl AA, Mykletun A, Stordal E, Kraemer HC. A dimensional versus a categorical approach to diagnosis: anxiety and depression in the HUNT 2 study. Int J Methods Psychiatr Res. 2009;18:128–37. doi:10.1002/mpr.284.

10. Maasalo K, Fontell T, Wessman J, Aronen ET. Sleep and behavioural problems associate with low mood in Finnish children aged 4–12 years: an epidemiological study. Child Adolesc Psychiatry Ment Health. 2016;10:37. doi:10.1186/s13034-016-0125-4.

11. American Psychiatric Association. Diagnostic and statistical manual of mental disorders. 5th ed. Arlington: American Psychiatric Association; 2013.

12. World Health Organization. The ICD-10 classification of mental and behavioural disorders: clinical descriptions and diagnostic guidelines. Geneva: World Health Organization; 1992.

13. Wesselhoeft R, Heiervang ER, Kragh-Sørensen P, Juul Sørensen M, Bilenberg N. Major depressive disorder and subthreshold depression in prepubertal children from the Danish National Birth Cohort. Compr Psychiatry. 2016;70:65–76. doi:10.1016/j.comppsych.2016.06.012.

14. Bennett DS, Ambrosini PJ, Kudes D, Metz C, Rabinovich H. Gender differences in adolescent depression: do symptoms differ for boys and girls? J Affect Disord. 2005;89:35–44. doi:10.1016/j.jad.2005.05.020.

15. Breton J-J, Labelle R, Huynh C, Berthiaume C, St-Georges M, Guilé J-M. Clinical characteristics of depressed youths in child psychiatry. J Can Acad Child Adolesc Psychiatry. 2012;21:16–29.

16. Fu-I L, Wang YP. Comparison of demographic and clinical characteristics between children and adolescents with major depressive disorder. Rev Bras Psiquiatr. 2008;30:124–31.

17. Yorbik O, Birmaher B, Axelson D, Williamson DE, Ryan ND. Clinical characteristics of depressive symptoms in children and adolescents with major depressive disorder. J Clin Psychiatry. 2004;65:1654–9 **(quiz 1760)**.

18. Luby JL, Heffelfinger AK, Mrakotsky C, Brown KM, Hessler MJ, Wallis JM, et al. The clinical picture of depression in preschool children. J Am Acad Child Adolesc Psychiatry. 2003;42:340–8. doi:10.1097/00004583-200303000-00015.

19. Vidal-Ribas P, Brotman MA, Valdivieso I, Leibenluft E, Stringaris A. The status of irritability in psychiatry: a conceptual and quantitative review. J Am Acad Child Adolesc Psychiatry. 2016;55:556–70. doi:10.1016/j.jaac.2016.04.014.

20. Shaffer D, Gould MS, Brasic J, Ambrosini P, Fisher P, Bird H, et al. A children's global assessment scale (CGAS). Arch Gen Psychiatry. 1983;40:1228–31. doi:10.1001/archpsyc.1983.01790100074010.

21. Lundh A, Kowalski J, Sundberg CJ, Gumpert C, Landén M. Children's Global Assessment Scale (CGAS) in a naturalistic clinical setting: interrater reliability and comparison with expert ratings. Psychiatry Res. 2010;177:206–10. doi:10.1016/j.psychres.2010.02.006.

22. Goodman R. The Strengths and Difficulties Questionnaire: a research note. J Child Psychol Psychiatry. 1997;38:581–6.

23. Goodman R. Information for researchers and professionals about the Strengths & Difficulties Questionnaires. 2014. http://www.sdqinfo.org. Accessed 3 Apr 2017.

24. Koskelainen M, Sourander A, Kaljonen A. The Strengths and Difficulties Questionnaire among Finnish school-aged children and adolescents. Eur Child Adolesc Psychiatry. 2000;9:277–84.

25. Apajasalo M, Rautonen J, Holmberg C, Sinkkonen J, Aalberg V, Pihko H, et al. Quality of life in pre-adolescence: a 17-dimensional health-related measure (17D). Qual Life Res. 1996;5:532–8.

26. Angold A, Weissman MM, John K, Merikangas KR, Prusoff BA, Wickramaratne P, et al. Parent and child reports of depressive symptoms in children at low and high risk of depression. J Child Psychol Psychiatry. 1987;28:901–15.

27. Herjanic B, Reich W. Development of a structured psychiatric interview for children: agreement between child and parent on individual symptoms. J Abnorm Child Psychol. 1997;25:21–31.

28. Edelbrock C, Costello AJ, Dulcan MK, Conover NC, Kala R. Parent-child agreement on child psychiatric symptoms assessed via structured interview. J Child Psychol Psychiatry. 1986;27:181–90.

29. Cantwell DP, Lewinsohn PM, Rohde P, Seeley JR. Correspondence between adolescent report and parent report of psychiatric diagnostic data. J Am Acad Child Adolesc Psychiatry. 1997;36:610–9. doi:10.1097/00004583-199705000-00011.

30. Landis JR, Koch GG. The measurement of observer agreement for categorical data. Biometrics. 1977;33:159–74. doi:10.2307/2529310.

31. Kazdin AE, French NH, Unis AS, Esveldt-Dawson K. Assessment of childhood depression: correspondence of child and parent ratings. J Am Acad Child Psychiatry. 1983;22:157–64.

32. Moretti MM, Fine S, Haley G, Marriage K. Childhood and adolescent depression: child-report versus parent-report information. J Am Acad Child Psychiatry. 1985;24:298–302.

33. van der Ende J, Verhulst FC, Tiemeier H. Agreement of informants on emotional and behavioral problems from childhood to adulthood. Psychol Assess. 2012;24:293–300. doi:10.1037/a0025500.

34. Mokros HB, Poznanski E, Grossman JA, Freeman LN. A comparison of child and parent ratings of depression for normal and clinically referred children. J Child Psychol Psychiatry. 1987;28:613–24.

35. Reynolds WM, Graves A. Reliability of children's reports of depressive symptomatology. J Abnorm Child Psychol. 1989;17:647–55.

36. Herjanic B, Herjanic M, Brown F, Wheatt T. Are children reliable reporters? J Abnorm Child Psychol. 1975;3:41–8.

37. Pirinen T, Kolho KL, Simola P, Ashorn M, Aronen ET. Parent-adolescent agreement on psychosocial symptoms and somatic complaints among adolescents with inflammatory bowel disease. Acta Paediatr. 2012;101:433–7. doi:10.1111/j.1651-2227.2011.02541.x.

38. Väistö T, Aronen ET, Simola P, Ashorn M, Kolho K-L. Psychosocial symptoms and competence among adolescents with inflammatory bowel disease and their peers. Inflamm Bowel Dis. 2010;16:27–35. doi:10.1002/ibd.21002.

39. Canning EH. Mental disorders in chronically ill children: case identification and parent-child discrepancy. Psychosom Med. 1994;56:104–8.

40. Ezpeleta L, Domènech JM, Angold A. A comparison of pure and comorbid CD/ODD and depression. J Child Psychol Psychiatry. 2006;47:704–12. doi:10.1111/j.1469-7610.2005.01558.x.

41. Boylan K, Vaillancourt T, Boyle M, Szatmari P. Comorbidity of internalizing disorders in children with oppositional defiant disorder. Eur Child Adolesc Psychiatry. 2007;16:484–94. doi:10.1007/s00787-007-0624-1.

42. Biederman J, Newcorn J, Sprich S. Comorbidity of attention deficit hyperactivity disorder with conduct, depressive, anxiety, and other disorders. Am J Psychiatry. 1991;148:564–77. doi:10.1176/ajp.148.5.564.

43. Reale L, Bartoli B, Cartabia M, Zanetti M, Costantino MA, Canevini MP, et al. Comorbidity prevalence and treatment outcome in children and adolescents with ADHD. Eur Child Adolesc Psychiatry. 2017. doi:10.1007/s00787-017-1005-z.

44. Meinzer MC, Pettit JW, Viswesvaran C. The co-occurrence of attention-deficit/hyperactivity disorder and unipolar depression in children and adolescents: a meta-analytic review. Clin Psychol Rev. 2014;34:595–607. doi:10.1016/j.cpr.2014.10.002.

45. Elia J, Ambrosini P, Berrettini W. ADHD characteristics: I. Concurrent co-morbidity patterns in children & adolescents. Child Adolesc Psychiatry Ment Health. 2008;2:15. doi:10.1186/1753-2000-2-15.

46. Stringaris A, Maughan B, Copeland WS, Costello EJ, Angold A. Irritable mood as a symptom of depression in youth: prevalence, developmental, and clinical correlates in the Great Smoky Mountains Study. J Am Acad Child Adolesc Psychiatry. 2013;52:831–40. doi:10.1016/j.jaac.2013.05.017.

47. Zisner A, Beauchaine TP. Neural substrates of trait impulsivity, anhedonia, and irritability: mechanisms of heterotypic comorbidity between externalizing disorders and unipolar depression. Dev Psychopathol. 2016;28:1177–208. doi:10.1017/S0954579416000754.

48. Mellor D, Cheng W, McCabe M, Ling M, Liu Y, Zhao Z, et al. The use of the SDQ with Chinese adolescents in the clinical context. Psychiatry Res. 2016;246:520–6. doi:10.1016/j.psychres.2016.10.034.

49. Lavigne JV, Gouze KR, Bryant FB, Hopkins J. Dimensions of Oppositional Defiant Disorder in young children: heterotypic continuity with anxiety and depression. J Abnorm Child Psychol. 2014;42:937–51. doi:10.1007/s10802-014-9853-1.

50. Jerrell JM, McIntyre RS, Park Y-MM. Risk factors for incident major depressive disorder in children and adolescents with attention-deficit/hyperactivity disorder. Eur Child Adolesc Psychiatry. 2015;24:65–73. doi:10.1007/s00787-014-0541-z.

51. Dietz LJ. Family-based interventions for childhood depression. J Am Acad Child Adolesc Psychiatry. 2017;56:464–5. doi:10.1016/j.jaac.2017.03.019.

7

Association between attempted suicide and academic performance indicators among middle and high school students in Mexico: results from a national survey

Ricardo Orozco[1]*[ID], Corina Benjet[1], Guilherme Borges[1], María Fátima Moneta Arce[2], Diana Fregoso Ito[1], Clara Fleiz[1] and Jorge Ameth Villatoro[1]

Abstract

Background: Students' mental health is associated to academic performance. In high income countries, higher students' grades are related to lower odds of suicidal behaviors, but studies on other indicators of academic performance are more limited, specially in middle income countries.

Methods: Data from 28,519 middle and high school students selected with multistage clustered sampling in the Mexican National Survey of Student's Drug Use. Using a self-administered questionnaire, lifetime suicidal attempt and four indicators of academic performance were assessed: age inconsistency with grade level, not being a student in the last year, perceived academic performance and number of failed courses. Multiple logistic regression models were used to control for sociodemographic and school characteristics.

Results: The lifetime prevalence of attempted suicide was 3.0% for middle school students and 4.2% for high school students. Among middle school students, statistically adjusted significant associations of suicide attempt with academic performance indicators were: not being a student the year before, worse self-perceived performance and a higher number of failed courses; among high school students, predictors were failed courses and self-perceived academic performance, with ORs of 1.65 and 1.96 for the categories of good and fair/poor respectively, compared to those who reported very good performance.

Conclusion: Self-perceived academic performance was the main indicator for suicide in both school levels. Suicide prevention efforts in Mexico's schools should include asking students about the perception they have about their own academic performance.

Keywords: Suicide, Attempted, Academic performance, Epidemiology

Background

According to the Global Burden of Disease Study, suicide is the leading cause of death for children and adolescents from 10 to 19 years of age living in developing countries. Among the 10–14 year old population, suicide has gone from the 14th place in 1990 to the 10th in 2013, increasing 17%; among young people aged 15–19, suicide has remained the second cause of death, but has increased by 18% [1]. In Mexico, completed suicide rates have been constant and steadily increasing, being of particular concern among the young population, increasing rapidly in the group of 15–29 year olds [2]. Population surveys have estimated that one in every 100 Mexican students made a suicide attempt in the previous year [3].

Peer relationships, teachers and families have a significant impact on academic performance, as well as

*Correspondence: ric_oz@imp.edu.mx
[1] Department of Epidemiology and Psychosocial Research, National Institute of Psychiatry (Mexico), Calzada Mexico-Xochimilco No. 101, Col. San Lorenzo Huipulco, 14370 Mexico City, Mexico
Full list of author information is available at the end of the article

on mental health and suicidal behaviors during school years [4]. Previous studies [5] show that mental health is associated with academic performance, as the latter is an important source for the development of identity, the development of social relationships between peers, the improvement of skills such as critical thinking and problem solving, and because it contributes to better opportunities for the future.

Cohort studies with vital statistics in Sweden have estimated that the odds of a serious suicide attempt in students decreased 60% for each point increase in its grading system (range 1–5) [5]. Some cross-sectional studies have reported an association between low grades and statistically significant increases of twice the odds of suicidal ideation and suicidal plan, but not with suicide attempts [6]. Other studies have established a fivefold increased likelihood of a suicide attempt among students with low perceived academic performance compared to those who rated their achievement as above average [7].

Epidemiologic studies in Mexican students have a long tradition [8, 9], mainly through local surveys of students living in Mexico City, but also through national ones. A study in 2000 found that, among 802 females students in Mexico City who had attempted suicide, 5% did it because of poor academic performance [10]. A national study in 2007, which included public schools only (n = 12,424), estimated that the prevalence of attempted suicide among high school students who reported low academic recognition was 12 and 8% among those with high academic recognition with an adjusted Odds Ratio (OR) of 1.04 (0.84–1.30) [11]. However, academic recognition is only one indicator of academic performance, and studies are needed which focus on identifying other indicators which may be associated with suicidal behaviors, to inform how to better implement effective suicide prevention programs in schools. Such policies are needed since the goal of member States of the World Health Organization (WHO)—including developing nations—is to reduce suicide rates by 10% by 2020 [12].

The purpose of this paper is to describe the national prevalence of suicide attempts among Mexican students, their distribution through different population groups and to estimate the magnitude of the association between suicide attempts and four indicators of academic performance, independent of other sociodemographic variables. We analyze a recent, large national epidemiologic survey (n = 28,519) that covered both public and private schools in rural and urban areas. Our hypothesis is that students with worse indicators of academic performance have a higher prevalence of suicide attempts.

Methods
Population and sample
The National Survey of Student's Drug Use (Encuesta Nacional de Consumo de Drogas en Estudiantes—ENCODE) is a national survey of urban and rural schools in Mexico, selected using stratified clustered random sampling. In 2014, ENCODE's target population included middle (12–14 years of age) and high school students (15–17 years of age) from all the country. Strata were formed by school level (middle and high school), state (all 32 Mexican States) and nine cities (Acapulco, Tijuana and Ciudad Juarez, among others) that were of special interest. The sample frame was formed by public and private schools: 34,733 middle and 12,841 high schools, excluding those from towns with more than 60% indigenous population and some specialized schools (e.g. for migrants).

In every school, classrooms were randomly selected by systematic sampling with random start according to the average number of students per class in each level [13]. All students in the classroom answered the questionnaire. It was not possible to conduct the survey in 61 of the selected classrooms due to safety issues in several municipalities. The response rate was 89.4%.

Data were weighted based on selection probabilities and subsequently adjusted for distribution of students by grade within each stratum. The ENCODE sample consists of 114,364 students (57,402 from middle school and 56,962 from high school). Academic performance indicators were asked only to a 25% random subsample. Hence, the sample size used for all analyses was n = 28,519; 14,435 middle school and 14,084 high school students.

Instruments
Data were obtained from a self-administered questionnaire which was standardized, validated and administered in previous surveys [14]. The questionnaire consists of a main section, answered by all participants (sociodemographic information, substance use, antisocial behavior, social environment, among others) and four extra questionnaires that were applied only to a random sample of a quarter of the students each. For this paper we analyzed the sections of sociodemographic characteristics, suicide attempts and academic performance, which were included in one of the random samples.

Main measurements
Lifetime suicide attempt
Based on González-Forteza's "Parasuicide Indicator Data Sheet" (PIDS) [15], students where coded as suicide attempters if they: (1) responded positively to the question: "Have you ever injured, cut, poisoned or harmed yourself in order to take your life?" and, (2) gave valid

answers to follow-up questions about: age at the only (or last) attempt, the motive, method and indicators of seriousness [10] and, (3) confirmed that they tried to "[...] hurt yourself on purpose in order to take your life?".

Academic performance

For the present study, we created four variables of academic performance which have also been used in previous research [16–18]: (1) *age inconsistency with grade level*, students who reported being 2 or more years older than the expected age and year level that they were studying during the survey; (2) *Not being a student in the last year*, students who reported that did not attend school the previous year; (3) *Perceived academic performance*, which was measured with the question: "In general, how do you consider your academic performance in school?" with four possible answers: very good, good, regular and bad; (4) *Number of failed courses*, divided into four categories: none, one, two, and three or more.

Covariates
Sociodemographic characteristics

The sociodemographic characteristics considered included sex, age, having a job most of the previous year and if it was full or part time, speaking an indigenous language, size of the locality where the student has lived most of his/her life (big, medium or small city, small town/rural community), family constellation (living with: both parents, both parents but one is a surrogate, single mother (or surrogate), single father (or surrogate) or others), mother's (or surrogate's) education level and father's (or surrogate's) education level.

School characteristics

The school characteristics considered were the school shift (morning, afternoon and other, such as full time or extra time) and school grade (in Mexico, 7th, 8th and 9th grades are equivalents to the three grades of middle school and 10th, 11th and 12th to the three grades of high school, even though in México middle and high school are divided separately into 3 grades each).

Statistical analyses

The bivariate analysis consisted of frequencies and percentages for contingency tables with categorical variables. Comparisons between categories were conducted using the Chi square Pearson statistic, corrected for by the survey design. Statistical significance was assessed with the *p* value less than 0.05. Multiple logistic regression models were performed, with attempted suicide as the dependent variable, each academic performance as the main independent variable and sociodemographic characteristics and school characteristics as covariates.

In the final models for either middle or high school, only variables with $p < 0.20$ in the bivariate models were entered as covariates. Further pairwise comparisons for significant variables with three or more categories were performed using Stata's *test* command.

All statistical analyses were stratified by school level, in order to estimate associations for students in middle and high school separately. Data were analyzed in Stata version 13.1 [19] using the module for analysis of complex surveys *svy*, which corrects standard errors through the Taylor series method [20], based on the sample design, weighting and clustering of observations.

Results

The analysis of the sociodemographic composition of Mexican students shows slightly more women in high school (51.2%) than in middle school (49.5%) (Table 1). Just over 5% of middle school students were 15 years or older and no young people under 14 attended high school. Approximately two out of ten students worked either full or part time during the previous year, and having a part-time job was reported more frequently by high school students than middle school students ($p < 0.001$). Less high school students spoke an indigenous language and lived most of their lives in small towns or rural areas as compared to their middle school counterparts. 75% of middle school students lived with both parents, decreasing to 72% for high school students. Level of education both for father and mother (or their surrogates) was higher in high school students than in middle school ones. In terms of school characteristics, three quarters of middle schoolers attended at morning shift (78%), as well as 58% of high school students; at both levels the highest proportion of students was concentrated in the 7th and 10th year (41.1% for middle school students and 42.2% for high school students).

The lifetime prevalence of attempted suicide was 3% for middle school students and 4.2% for high school students. In both middle and high school students, the prevalence of attempts in women (5.2 and 6.8%) was higher than in men (1.1 and 1.5%) with a statistically significant difference (Table 2). In relation to other variables, the highest prevalence rates in middle school students were estimated among students who were enrolled in their second or third year. For the variables of academic performance, the only statistically significant difference was observed among middle school students, with a higher proportion of suicide attempts among those who rated their academic performance as fair or poor (3.8%) compared to those who perceived it as good (3.2%) or very good (1.8%), $p = 0.011$.

Table 3 shows the estimates of adjusted ORs from multiple logistic regression models for middle school

Table 1 Sociodemographic and school characteristics of Mexican public and private school students. Mexico, 2014

	Level						X^2	df	p value
	Middle school		High school		Total				
	(n = 14,435)		(n = 14,084)		(n = 28,519)				
	n	%	n	%	n	%			
Sex							31.8	1	0.289
Male	7253	50.5	6990	48.8	14,243	49.9			
Female	7182	49.5	7094	51.2	14,276	50.1			
Age (years)							94,470	8	< 0.001
11	734	5.8	–	–	734	3.6			
12	4463	31.4	–	–	4463	19.4			
13	4874	31.9	–	–	4874	19.7			
14	3515	25.0	414	3.2	3929	16.6			
15	717	4.9	4527	29.5	5244	14.3			
16	93	0.7	4457	33.5	4550	13.2			
17	25	0.2	3292	23.6	3317	9.2			
18	13	0.1	918	6.2	931	2.4			
19–29	1	0.0	476	3.9	477	1.5			
Worked the year before							544.0	2	< 0.001
No	11,422	79.2	10,690	77.6	22,112	78.6			
Yes, part time job	1550	11.7	2266	15.7	3816	13.2			
Yes, full time job	1164	9.1	941	6.7	2105	8.2			
Speaks an indigenous language							401.0	1	0.001
No	13,231	94.2	13,329	96.8	26,560	95.2			
Yes	784	5.8	420	3.2	1204	4.8			
Size of locality							323.0	2	0.182
Big city	3650	24.5	3853	28.1	7503	25.9			
Medium/small city	6450	40.9	6555	42.0	13,005	41.3			
Small town or rural area	4155	34.6	3567	29.9	7722	32.8			
Family structure							140.8	4	0.006
Both parents	10,595	74.5	9954	72.5	20,549	73.8			
Both parents (one surrogate)	899	5.3	767	4.7	1666	5.1			
Mother (or surrogate)	2202	15.1	2477	17.2	4679	15.9			
Father (or surrogate)	325	2.2	328	2.2	653	2.2			
Other	414	2.8	558	3.4	972	3.0			
Mother's (or surrogate's) education level							3059.6	5	< 0.001
Elementary or no education	3590	28.2	3096	22.1	6686	25.9			
Middle school	4523	31.3	4379	30.8	8902	31.1			
High school	2493	17.0	3442	24.5	5935	19.9			
University/college	1428	9.3	1718	12.5	3146	10.5			
Postgraduate studies	1021	6.2	1056	7.8	2077	6.8			
Other	1088	7.9	283	2.2	1371	5.7			
Father's (or surrogate's) education level							3092.5	5	<0.001
Elementary or no education	3439	27.2	2919	20.7	6358	24.7			
Middle school	4170	29.7	3949	29.0	8119	29.5			
High school	2426	16.4	3274	23.8	5700	19.2			
University/college	1508	10.0	1937	14.2	3445	11.7			
Postgraduate studies	1115	6.6	1194	8.4	2309	7.3			
Other	1427	10.0	515	3.8	1942	7.6			

Table 1 continued

	Level						χ^2	df	p value
	Middle school		High school		Total				
	(n = 14,435)		(n = 14,084)		(n = 28,519)				
	n	%	n	%	n	%			
School shift							5271.1	2	< 0.001
Morning	11,038	77.7	8688	58.9	19,726	70.5			
Afternoon	3145	19.3	4156	30.8	7301	23.7			
Other	252	3.1	1240	10.2	1492	5.8			
School year[a]							453.9	2	0.437
First (7th, 10th)	5711	41.1	6542	42.2	12,253	41.5			
Second (8th, 11th)	5471	34.5	3826	29.1	9297	32.4			
Third (9th, 12th)	3253	24.3	3716	28.7	6969	26.0			

Missing Values: Worked last year (486); indigenous language speaker (755); place of residence (289); mother's education (402); father's education (646)

Percentages are weighted, frequencies are unweighted; p value adjusted due to the survey design

[a] 7th, 8th and 9th grades as equivalents to the three grades of middle school and 10th, 11th and 12th for the three grades of high school. In México, middle and high school are divided into 3 grades each

students. Significant predictors of suicide attempt related to academic performance were: not being a student the year before, worse self-perceived performance and having failed three or more courses. Compared to those who perceived themselves to have very good academic performance, those who reported only good performance had almost twice the odds of attempted suicide (OR = 1.86; 95% CI = 1.16–2.99), whereas those who reported having fair or poor performance had 2.35 times the odds (95% CI = 1.56–3.54), controlling for all other variables in the model (sex, age, shift, grade, etc.), further pairwise comparisons did not show significant differences in these two last estimates (p = 0.25). Regarding the number of failed courses, the only statistically significant association was observed between those who reported three or more failed courses compared with those with none, with an OR = 2.41 (95% CI = 1.26–4.60).

Adjusted estimates for high school students are shown in Table 4. After controlling for sociodemographic and school characteristics variables, the statistically significant predictors were having failed two courses compared to none (OR = 1.78; 95% CI = 1.10–2.86) and self-perceived academic performance, with associations of 1.65 (95% CI = 1.08–2.52) and 1.96 (95% CI = 1.25–3.06) for the categories of good and fair/poor respectively, compared to those who reported very good performance. Again, further pairwise comparisons did not reveal significant differences in these two last estimates (p = 0.22).

Discussion

In Mexico, prior estimates of the lifetime prevalence of attempted suicide among students vary from 1.4% of middle school students and 2% of high school students,

[21], up to 9% in high school students [11]. In this paper we estimated a prevalence of 3% in students from middle school and 4.2% for those attending high school. While other national studies have used a single question to identify suicide attempts, in our study we used a battery of questions that increased the instrument's sensitivity to detect young people with a genuine suicide attempt. The results are very similar to those reported by Mexican adolescents in the general population (3.1%) obtained through other instruments like the WHO Composite International Diagnostic Interview [22].

On the other hand, while the prevalence of attempted suicide increases with school year in students attending middle school (probably due to stress related to adjustments to adolescence), as it goes from 1.8 in the 7th year to practically 4 in 8th and 9th grade, among the high school population the prevalence decreased. Because the data comes from a survey, it is possible that school dropout plays a role in the prevalence of attempts, especially in the high school level: in Mexico, only 57% of the population between 15 and 18 attends school [23], with a dropout rate of 15.9% [24]. The latter could be explained because young people with major mental health problems, including suicide, are most likely to leave school at this level, thus, the prevalence diminishes through this selection effect.

Of the four indicators of academic performance we studied, only perceived academic performance was associated to suicide attempt in middle school students in bivariate analysis. After adjustment for potential confounders, self-perceived academic performance was identified as a risk factor for suicide attempt, suggesting a dose–response for both school levels. This is consistent

Table 2 Prevalence of attempted suicide by sociodemographic, school and academic performance variables

	Level											
	Middle school (n = 14,435)						High school (n = 14,084)					
	Sample	Attempts	%	X^2	df	p value	Sample	Attempts	%	X^2	df	p value
Sociodemographic and school												
Sex				803.0	1	< 0.001				963.0	1	< 0.001
Male	7198	75	1.1				6963	119	1.5			
Female	7136	389	5.2				7069	471	6.8			
School shift				16.9	2	0.406				3.9	2	0.805
Morning	10,963	336	3.1				8654	363	4.1			
Afternoon	3121	125	3.3				4141	172	4.5			
Other	250	3	1.5				1237	55	4.3			
School year[a]				220.3	2	< 0.001				31.0	2	0.169
First year (7th, 10th)	5667	100	1.8				6511	295	4.8			
Second year (8th, 11th)	5436	218	4.0				3819	145	3.8			
Third year (9th, 12th)	3231	146	3.9				3702	150	3.9			
Academic performance												
Two years older than expected for grade level				5.6	1	0.357				19.5	1	0.162
No	13,797	452	3.1				12,831	529	4.1			
Yes	537	12	2.3				1201	61	5.4			
Studying previous year				62.0	1	0.085				0.6	1	0.781
Yes	13,557	440	3.0				12,906	549	4.3			
No	478	19	6.2				891	37	4.0			
Perceived academic performance				94.9	2	0.011				49.9	2	0.052
Very good	2997	67	1.8				2082	64	2.8			
Good	6458	216	3.2				7489	308	4.3			
Fair or poor	4606	177	3.8				4305	213	4.7			
Number of failed courses				48.3	3	0.105				28.9	3	0.298
None	11,582	353	3.0				10,266	409	4.1			
1	952	41	3.3				1449	69	4.7			
2	615	30	3.2				838	43	5.9			
3 or more	631	30	5.4				992	55	4.2			

Missing Values: Attempted suicide (153; 101 middle school and 52 high school); studying the previous year (544); self-perceived school performance (512); failed courses (1126)

Percentages are weighted, frequencies are unweighted; p values adjusted due to the survey design

[a] 7th, 8th and 9th grades as equivalents to the three grades of middle school and 10th, 11th and 12th for the three grades of high school. In México, middle and high school are divided into 3 grades each

with other findings reported in both longitudinal and cross-sectional studies [5, 7, 25]. In middle school students, those who did not attend school the previous year had higher odds of suicidal attempt. Regarding the number of failed courses, we found a significantly higher prevalence among middle school students who failed three or more, and in high school students among those with two. Therefore, it would be appropriate to identify students that have a higher number of failed courses in order to screen them for suicidal behaviors. Since the number of failed courses was self-reported, caution must be exerted in the interpretation of this results, since students might conceal that they failed a course or, quite the

contrary, to over-report them by interpreting the question as not doing well.

The fourth indicator that we studied, being 2 years older for their school grade, was not associated with suicidal attempt among this population. Nevertheless, this indicator could be related with other suicidal behaviors such as ideation or suicidal plan, which at the same time are precursors to more serious behaviors [17, 26, 27]. Given that our subjective indicator (perceived academic performance) was consistently more associated with attempts than the objectives ones (like age inconsistency with grade level), it is possible that cognitive distortions resulting from depressive states change student's

Table 3 Association between four school performance indicators and school sociodemographic variables in middle school students

	Two years older than expected for grade level			Studying last year			Perceived academic performance			Number of failed courses		
	(a) No (b) Yes			a) Yes b) No			a) Very good b) Good c) Fair or poor			a) None b) 1 c) 2 d) 3 or more		
	(n = 13,624)			(n = 13,403)			(n = 13,380)			(n = 13,123)		
	OR	95% CI	Sig.	OR	95% CI	Sig.	OR	95% CI	Sig.	OR	95% CI	Sig.
School performance variable												
(a)	1.00	–		1.00	–		1.00	–		1.00	–	
(b)	0.83	(0.31–2.21)		2.75	(1.17–6.50)	*	1.86	(1.16–2.99)	*	1.18	(0.74–1.88)	
(c)	–	–		–	–		2.35	(1.56–3.54)	***	1.12	(0.63–1.98)	
(d)	–	–		–	–		–	–		2.41	(1.26–4.60)	**
Sex												
Male	1.00	–		1.00	–		1.00	–		1.00	–	
Female	5.79	(4.15–8.07)	***	5.74	(4.13–7.98)	***	6.45	(4.56–9.11)	***	6.05	(4.32–8.47)	***
Age (continuous)	1.02	(0.75–1.39)		0.98	(0.78–1.23)		0.98	(0.77–1.23)		0.96	(0.76–1.22)	
Worked last year												
No	1.00	–		1.00	–		1.00	–		1.00	–	
Yes, part-time	2.49	(1.51–4.10)	***	2.34	(1.48–3.71)	***	2.41	(1.43–4.06)	***	2.50	(1.51–4.14)	***
Yes, full-time	1.34	(0.71–2.51)		1.35	(0.71–2.57)		1.37	(0.72–2.59)		1.32	(0.69–2.52)	
Size of locality												
Big city	1.00	–		1.00	–		1.00	–		1.00	–	
City	1.01	(0.72–1.42)		1.01	(0.72–1.42)		1.01	(0.71–1.42)		1.00	(0.71–1.41)	
Small town or hamlet	0.80	(0.50–1.29)		0.78	(0.48–1.26)		0.82	(0.51–1.32)		0.79	(0.48–1.28)	
Family constellation												
Both parents	1.00	–		1.00	–		1.00	–		1.00	–	
Both parents (one surrogate)	1.37	(0.90–2.09)		1.37	(0.90–2.08)		1.32	(0.86–2.03)		1.33	(0.87–2.03)	
Mother (or surrogate)	1.12	(0.75–1.68)		1.09	(0.74–1.61)		1.11	(0.74–1.67)		1.09	(0.73–1.63)	
Father (or surrogate)	2.42	(1.06–5.48)	*	2.44	(1.07–5.58)	*	2.50	(1.08–5.77)	*	2.50	(1.08–5.79)	*
Other	1.88	(1.02–3.45)	*	1.89	(1.02–3.48)	*	1.93	(1.04–3.56)	*	1.83	(0.95–3.51)	
Mother's (or surrogate's) education level												
Elementary or no education	1.00	–		1.00	–		1.00	–		1.00	–	
Middle school	1.25	(0.84–1.86)		1.24	(0.82–1.86)		1.25	(0.84–1.85)		1.25	(0.84–1.86)	
High school	1.37	(0.89–2.10)		1.38	(0.90–2.12)		1.41	(0.91–2.17)		1.35	(0.88–2.09)	
University/college	1.57	(0.97–2.54)		1.57	(0.97–2.54)		1.70	(1.03–2.79)	*	1.53	(0.94–2.49)	
Postgraduate studies	1.50	(0.78–2.87)		1.53	(0.80–2.94)		1.62	(0.84–3.12)		1.52	(0.79–2.91)	
Other	0.61	(0.33–1.13)		0.60	(0.32–1.11)		0.58	(0.30–1.10)		0.55	(0.29–1.06)	
School year[a]												
First year (7th)	1.00	–		1.00	–		1.00	–		1.00	–	
Second year (8th)	2.15	(1.25–3.70)	**	2.42	(1.47–3.96)	***	2.19	(1.36–3.52)	**	2.30	(1.41–3.74)	***
Third year (9th)	2.03	(0.96–4.28)		2.38	(1.30–4.37)	**	2.04	(1.10–3.78)	*	2.29	(1.23–4.28)	**

OR Odds Ratio, *95% CI* 95% Confidence Interval

* p < 0.05; ** p < 0.01; *** p < 0.001

[a] 7th, 8th and 9th grades as equivalents to the three grades of middle school in México

Table 4 Association between the school performance indicators and school sociodemographic variables in high school students

	Two years older than expected for grade level			Studying last year			Perceived academic performance			Number of failed courses		
	(a) No (b) Yes			(a) Yes (b) No			(a) Very good (b) Good (c) Fair or poor			(a) None (b) 1 (c) 2 (d) 3 or more		
	(n = 13,423)			(n = 13,219)			(n = 13,279)			(n = 12,970)		
	aOR	95% CI	Sig.	aOR	95% CI	Sig.	aOR	95% CI	Sig.	aOR	95% CI	Sig.
Academic performance variable												
(a)	1.00	–		1.00	–		1.00	–		1.00	–	
(b)	1.31	(0.64–2.67)		0.84	(0.49–1.44)		1.65	(1.08–2.52)	*	1.36	(0.93–2.00)	
(c)	–	–		–	–		1.96	(1.25–3.06)	**	1.78	(1.10–2.86)	*
(d)	–	–		–	–		–	–		1.40	(0.90–2.18)	
Sex												
Male	1.00	–		1.00	–		1.00	–		1.00	–	
Female	4.86	(3.59–6.58)	***	4.80	(3.54–6.49)	***	5.01	(3.67–6.84)	***	5.25	(3.84–7.19)	***
Age (continuous)	1.04	(0.87–1.24)		1.09	(0.96–1.23)		1.08	(0.97–1.21)		1.08	(0.96–1.21)	
Speaks an indigenous language												
No	1.00	–		1.00	–		1.00	–		1.00	–	
Yes	0.51	(0.24–1.06)		0.52	(0.25–1.09)		0.52	(0.25–1.07)		0.54	(0.26–1.12)	
Family constellation												
Both parents	1.00	–		1.00	–		1.00	–		1.00	–	
Both parents (one surrogate)	1.99	(1.25–3.15)	**	2.00	(1.26–3.18)	**	1.98	(1.24–3.15)	**	1.97	(1.23–3.16)	**
Mother (or surrogate)	1.82	(1.36–2.44)	***	1.84	(1.38–2.47)	***	1.81	(1.35–2.42)	***	1.87	(1.40–2.49)	***
Father (or surrogate)	1.39	(0.61–3.16)		1.44	(0.63–3.28)		1.36	(0.59–3.11)		1.37	(0.59–3.22)	
Other	1.52	(0.92–2.51)		1.47	(0.88–2.48)		1.49	(0.90–2.46)		1.51	(0.89–2.54)	
Father's (or surrogate's) education level												
Elementary or no education	1.00	–		1.00	–		1.00	–		1.00	–	
Middle school	1.30	(0.97–1.76)		1.32	(0.97–1.78)		1.30	(0.96–1.77)		1.34	(1.00–1.80)	
High school	0.94	(0.65–1.36)		0.93	(0.64–1.35)		0.96	(0.66–1.39)		0.98	(0.67–1.41)	
University/college	0.82	(0.53–1.29)		0.82	(0.53–1.28)		0.85	(0.54–1.32)		0.86	(0.55–1.35)	
Postgraduate studies	0.99	(0.63–1.56)		0.98	(0.62–1.55)		1.01	(0.63–1.62)		1.01	(0.64–1.60)	
Other	0.97	(0.54–1.75)		0.92	(0.51–1.67)		1.00	(0.56–1.80)		0.90	(0.49–1.63)	
School year[a]												
First year (10th)	1.00	–		1.00	–		1.00	–		1.00	–	
Second year (11th)	0.75	(0.53–1.05)		0.69	(0.50–0.95)	*	0.71	(0.52–0.96)	*	0.70	(0.51–0.95)	*
Third year (12th)	0.74	(0.47–1.18)		0.66	(0.44–1.00)		0.69	(0.47–1.01)		0.63	(0.42–0.95)	*

aOR Adjusted Odds Ratio, *95% CI* 95% Confidence Interval

* p < 0.05; ** p < 0.01; *** p < 0.001

[a] 10th, 11th and 12th for the three grades of high school in México

perceptions of academic achievement, being this a consequence of poor mental health instead of a real decline of academic performance. Future investigations should research this area.

In middle school students three sociodemographic risk factors were identified in the self-perceived academic performance models: sex, having worked part time and the type of family structure. Women are generally at greater risk of suicidal ideation plan and attempt [28] and in our study being female was the largest predictor of suicide attempt. It is noteworthy that students who are studying and working part-time rather than full-time are at the greatest risk, yet this association has been documented elsewhere [29]. It is likely that families' financial stress is the main driving force that makes middle schoolers to look for a job, putting them at increased burden. Our results suggest that prevention programs in middle schools may screen students for suicidal behaviors, among those who share this burden, or who have left school for a year and came back.

Because this is a cross-sectional study, its main limitation is the impossibility to estimate the incidence of suicide attempts in the student population since the first follow-up year. It is likely that students with mental health problems and suicide attempts abandon school [30], so it is very important to identify and treat currently enrolled students who have these behaviors, since only half of adolescents who reported suicide attempts received mental health care once in a lifetime [22]. Furthermore, with this design we are not able to determine the direction of the association (timing) between our academic performance indicators and suicidal attempts, and it is possible that some mental health problems, such as depression, are risk factors for low academic performance [31].

Another limitation of the study was measuring suicide attempts: despite the use of the PIDS, a scale proved and used throughout the years in Mexico, in this study we incorporate the criterion that students confirm their suicidal action, with the intention of increasing the sensitivity of the measurement of an actual attempt and not only self-harming behavior (deliberate self-harm) [15]. The effect of this criteria could (providing that this effect it is non-differential for dichotomous variables) underestimate the extent of association measures (i.e. OR) [32] so the magnitude of the relationship of suicide attempts with academic performance variables could be even higher than estimated.

Finally, this work does not take into account the role that psychiatric disorders have on suicide attempts, since they are one of its main risk factors. Studies in Mexico [33] indicate that young people with depression have a 16-fold greater risk of suicidal ideas and 5 times higher for suicide attempts compared with those without. Also, because the questionnaire was divided and applied in four different sub-samples, with the sections on academic performance and depression (which also included suicide thoughts) being applied separately, it was not possible to include any of these last measures in the analysis.

Conclusions

Our results show that suicide prevention efforts in México's schools may include assessing adolescents' perception about their own academic performance. This recommendation could be implemented through "gatekeepers" such as teachers and school personnel, who can be trained in suicide prevention and in identifying people at risk in order to direct them to an evaluation and appropriate treatment. Moreover, suicide prevention efforts in the public education system should consider comprehensive interventions at the individual, selective and universal levels, as recommended by the WHO [34] with support from other branches of the government, such as the health and public security sectors, in order to consolidate a national suicide prevention program, with the intention to cover all the way from the adequate registration of suicidal behavior to the adequate reference for treatment of students with suicide attempts.

Abbreviations
ENCODE: Encuesta Nacional de Consumo de Drogas en Estudiantes; WHO: World Health Organization; PIDS: Parasuicide Indicator Data Sheet; OR: odds ratio; CI: confidence interval.

Authors' contributions
RO, CB, GB and JAV were responsible for the study concept and design. DFI, CF and JAV contributed to the acquisition of data. RO, CB, GB, FMA, JAV were involved in the interpretation of the data. RO, CB and FMA were responsible for drafting the manuscript, and all authors were involved in critical revisions of the manuscript. All authors read and approved the final manuscript.

Author details
[1] Department of Epidemiology and Psychosocial Research, National Institute of Psychiatry (Mexico), Calzada Mexico-Xochimilco No. 101, Col. San Lorenzo Huipulco, 14370 Mexico City, Mexico. [2] General Office of Psychiatric Services, Ministry of Health (Mexico), Av. Paseo de la Reforma No. 450 Piso 1, Col. Juárez, 06600 Mexico City, Mexico.

Acknowledgements
Not applicable.

Competing interests
The authors declare that they have no competing interests.

Funding
This work was supported by the Centro Nacional para la Prevención y el Control de las Adicciones (CENADIC México). The founding source did not intervene in the study design; collection, analysis or interpretation of data; the writing of the report nor the decision to submit the manuscript for publication.

References

1. Institute for Health Metrics and Evaluation [IHME]. Institute for Health Metrics and Evaluation GBD 2013. http://vizhub.healthdata.org/gbd-compare/. Accessed 17 Jul 2015.
2. Borges G, Orozco R, Benjet C, Medina-Mora ME. Suicidio y conductas suicidas en México: retrospectiva y situación actual. Salud Publica Mex. 2010;52:292–304.
3. Borges G, Medina-Mora ME, Orozco R, Ouéda C, Villatoro J, Fleiz C. Distribución y determinantes sociodemográficos de la conducta suicida en México. Salud Ment. 2009;32(5):413–25.
4. Björkenstam C, Weitoft GR, Hjern A, Nordström P, Hallqvist J, Ljung R. School grades, parental education and suicide—a national register-based cohort study. J Epidemiol Community Health. 2011;65(1):993–8.
5. Jablonska B, Östberg V, Hjern A, Lindberg LD, Rasmussen F, Modin B. School effects on risk of non-fatal suicidal behaviour: a national multilevel cohort study. Soc Psychiatry Psychiatr Epidemiol. 2014;49(4):609–18.
6. Jiang Y, Perry DK, Hesser JE. Adolescent suicide and health risk behaviors: Rhode Island's 2007 youth risk behavior survey. Am J Prev Med. 2010;38(5):551–5.
7. Richardson AS, Bergen HA, Martin G, Roeger L, Allison S. Perceived academic performance as an indicator of risk of attempted suicide in young adolescents. Arch Suicide Res. 2005;9(2):163–76.
8. Jiménez-Tapia A, González-Forteza C. Veinticinco años de investigación sobre suicidio y psicosociales del Instituto Nacional de Psiquiatría "Ramón de la Fuente". Salud Ment. 2003;26(6):35–46.
9. Mondragón L, Borges G, Gutiérrez R. La medición de la conducta suicida en México: Estimaciones y procedimientos. Salud Ment. 2001;24(6):4–15.
10. González-Forteza C, Villatoro J, Alcántar I, Medina-Mora ME, Fleiz C, Bermúdez P, et al. Prevalencia de intento suicida en estudiantes adolescentes de la cuidad de México:1997 y 2000. Salud Ment. 2002;25(6):1–12.
11. Pérez-Amezcua B, Rivera-Rivera L, Atienzo EE, Castro FD, Leyva-López A, Chávez-Ayala R. Prevalencia y factores asociados a la ideación e intento suicida en adolescentes de educación media superior de la República Mexicana. Salud Publica Mex. 2010;52(4):324–33.
12. World Health Organization [WHO]. Mental health action plan 2013–2020. Geneva: World Health Organization Press; 2013.
13. Comisión Nacional Contra las Adicciones [CONADIC], Instituto Nacional de Psiquiatría Ramón de la Fuente Muñiz [INPRF], Secretaría de Salud [SSA], Secretaria de Educación Pública [SEP]. Encuesta Nacional de Consumo de Drogas en Estudiantes 2014 "Metodología del Estudio". México: INPRFM; 2015.
14. López E, Medina-Mora ME, Villatoro J, Juárez F, Berenzon S. Factores relacionados al consumo de drogas y al rendimiento académico en adolescentes. Psicología Soc México. 1996;6(1):561–7.
15. González-Forteza C, Arana-Quezadas DS, Jiménez-Tapia JA. Problemática suicida en adolescentes y el contexto escolar: Vinculación autogestiva con los servicios de salud mental. Salud Ment. 2008;31(1):23–7.
16. Lugo EKL, Villatoro J, Medina-Mora ME, García FJ. Autopercepción del rendimiento académico en estudiantes mexicanos. Rev Mex Psicol. 1996;13(1):37–47.
17. González-Forteza C, Berenzon S, Tello AM, Facio D, Medina-Mora ME. Ideación suicida y características asociadas en mujeres adolescentes. Salud Publica Mex. 1998;40:430–7.

18. Delgado P, Palos A. Desempeño académico y conductas de riesgo en adolescentes. Revista de educación y desarrollo. 2007;7:5–16.
19. Stata Statistical Sofware. Release 13. College Station: StataCorp LP; 2013.
20. Corp Stata. Stata 13 survey data reference manual. College Station: Stata Press; 2013.
21. Olaiz-Fernández G, Rivera-Dommarco J, Shamah-Levy T, Rojas R, Villalpando-Hernández S, Hernández-Avila M, et al. Encuesta Nacional de Salud y Nutrición 2006. México: INSP; 2006.
22. Borges G, Benjet C, Medina-Mora ME, Orozco R, Familiar I, Nock MK, et al. Service use among Mexico city adolescents with suicidality. J Affect Disord. 2010;120(1):32–9.
23. Instituto Nacional de Estadística y Geografía [INEGI]. Asistencia escolar. http://cuentame.inegi.org.mx/poblacion/asistencia.aspx?tema=P. Accessed 1 Dec 2015.
24. Instituto Nacional para la Evaluación de la Educación [INEE]. Panorama Educativo de México 2010. http://www.inee.edu.mx/bie/mapa_indica/2010/PanoramaEducativoDeMexico/AT/AT02/2010_AT02__d-vinculo.pdf. Accessed 1 Dec 2015.
25. Jablonska B, Lindblad F, Östberg V, Lindberg L, Rasmussen F, Hjern A. A national cohort study of parental socioeconomic status and non-fatal suicidal behaviour-the mediating role of school performance. BMC Public Health. 2012;12(1):1–8.
26. Nock MK, Borges G, Cromet EJ, Alonso J, Angermeyer M, Beautrais A, et al. Cross-national prevalence and risk factors for suicidal ideation, plans and attempts. Brit J Psychiat. 2008;192(2):98–105.
27. Borges G, Benjet C, Medina-Mora ME, Orozco R, Nock MK. Suicide ideation, plan and attempt in the Mexican Adolescent Mental Health Survey. J Am Acad Child Adolesc Psychiatry. 2008;47(1):41–52.
28. Nock MK, Borges G, Ono Y. Suicide. Global perspectives from the WHO World Mental Health Surveys. New York: Cambridge University Press; 2012.
29. Jo SJ, Yim HW, Lee MS, Jeong H, Lee WC. Korean youth risk behavior surveillance survey association between part-time employment and suicide attempts. Asia Pac J Public Health. 2015;27(3):323–34.
30. Maynard BR, Salas-Wright CP, Vaughn MG. High school dropouts in emerging adulthood: substance use, mental health problems, and crime. Community Ment Health J. 2014;51(3):289–99.
31. Quiroga CV, Janosz M, Bisset S, Morin AJS. Early adolescent depression symptoms and school dropout: mediating processes involving self-reported academic competence and achievement. J Educ Psychol. 2013;105(2):552–60.
32. Szklo M, Nieto FJ. Epidemiology: beyond the basics. Gaithersburg: AN Aspen Publication; 1999.
33. Rodríguez C, Román-Pérez R, Valdez EA, Galaviz-Barreras AL. Depresión y comportamiento suicida en estudiantes de educación media superior en Sonora. Salud Ment. 2012;35(1):45–50.
34. Mann JJ, Apter A, Bertolote J, Beautrais A, Currier D, Haas A, et al. Suicide prevention strategies: a systematic review. JAMA. 2005;294(16):2064–74.

8

A longitudinal study of socioeconomic status, family processes, and child adjustment from preschool until early elementary school: the role of social competence

Rikuya Hosokawa[1,2]* and Toshiki Katsura[2]

Abstract

Objective: Using a short-term longitudinal design, this study examined the concurrent and longitudinal relationships among familial socioeconomic status (SES; i.e., family income and maternal and paternal education levels), marital conflict (i.e., constructive and destructive marital conflict), parenting practices (i.e., positive and negative parenting practices), child social competence (i.e., social skills), and child behavioral adjustment (i.e., internalizing and externalizing problems) in a comprehensive model.

Methods: The sample included a total of 1604 preschoolers aged 5 years at Time 1 and first graders aged 6 years at Time 2 (51.5% male). Parents completed a self-reported questionnaire regarding their SES, marital conflict, parenting practices, and their children's behavioral adjustment. Teachers also evaluated the children's social competence.

Results: The path analysis results revealed that Time 1 family income and maternal and paternal education levels were respectively related to Time 1 social skills and Time 2 internalizing and externalizing problems, both directly and indirectly, through their influence on destructive and constructive marital conflict, as well as negative and positive parenting practices. Notably, after controlling for Time 1 behavioral problems as mediating mechanisms in the link between family factors (i.e., SES, marital conflict, and parenting practices) and behavioral adjustment, Time 1 social skills significantly and inversely influenced both the internalization and externalization of problems at Time 2.

Conclusions: The merit of examining SES, marital conflict, and parenting practices as multidimensional constructs is discussed in relation to an understanding of processes and pathways within families that affect child mental health functioning. The results suggest social competence, which is influenced by the multidimensional constructs of family factors, may prove protective in reducing the risk of child maladjustment, especially for children who are socioeconomically disadvantaged.

Keywords: Socioeconomic status, Marital conflict, Parenting practice, Social competence, Behavioral problems, Preschool children

Background

An extensive amount of research has consistently found associations between childhood socioeconomic status (SES) and mental health functioning [1–3], with marital conflict and parenting practices seeming to mediate these associations. SES is a construct that consists of multiple dimensions of social position [4, 5]. Previous related empirical and theoretical research has focused on economic and educational aspects as SES indicators. Family income has been associated with children's developmental outcomes, as have parental educational levels [6–12]. However, despite the many studies conducted in this area, few have simultaneously investigated the influence

*Correspondence: rikuya@med.nagoya-cu.ac.jp
[1] School of Nursing, Nagoya City University, Mizuho-cho, Mizuho-ku, Nagoya 467-8601, Japan
Full list of author information is available at the end of the article

of family income and maternal and paternal education levels as predictors in the relationships between SES, family processes (e.g., marital conflict and parenting practices), and child mental health functioning.

Additionally, despite extensive studies concerning the relationships between SES, family processes, and child mental health functioning, most have only minimally considered the effects of the positive dimensions of marital conflict and parenting practices (e.g., constructive marital conflict and positive parenting practices), rather than the negative dimensions thereof (e.g., destructive marital conflict and negative parenting practices), as mediators in the link between SES and child mental health functioning [7, 13–16]. Moreover, a limitation of previous empirical work concerning these associations (i.e., SES, family processes, and child mental health functioning) is that these studies focused on negative developmental outcomes (e.g., internalizing and externalizing problems) [17, 18]. Further studies examining positive dimensions of child mental health functioning, especially the issue of social competence, are needed. Social competence, which is defined as an individual's ability to act in a socially appropriate manner [19, 20], has received comparatively less attention as a mediator in the link between SES, family processes, and child behavioral adjustment, despite preliminary evidence suggesting it may be an important indicator.

When considering the complex relationships between these variables, it is important to consider independent associations, while controlling for other variables. However, previous studies have primarily examined individual relationships between different types of SES, marital conflict, and parenting practices, as well as child social competence and behavioral adjustment, without considering these associations in a comprehensive model. Therefore, this study examined mediators of the associations between SES and children's functioning in greater detail. Specifically, destructive and constructive marital conflict, negative and positive parenting practices, and child social skills were investigated as mediators in the associations between SES indicators, including family income and parental education levels, and children's internalizing and externalizing behaviors in a unified model. Regarding social skills, we especially focused on the mediating role of social competence in the relationships between family factors (i.e., SES, marital conflict, and parenting attitude) and child behavioral problems, from preschool to the first grade.

Socioeconomic status and child adjustment

Research in the past decade has shown that SES is an important contextual factor that strongly predicts child outcomes [1–3]. Extensive research has shown that SES affects the well-being and development of children, including their internalizing (e.g., anxiety, depression, and withdrawal) and externalizing (e.g., aggression, opposition, and hyperactivity) symptoms, as well as their cognitive and language development [1, 3, 21–27].

It has been well documented that economic problems, such as low income and financial instability, adversely influence inter-parental and parent/child interactions, which in turn are related to a range of harmful outcomes for child development [28]. Studies have shown that economic problems are associated with destructive parental interactions that predict increased domestic problems and lower levels of marital quality. Furthermore, it has also been shown that economic problems place children at an increased risk of exposure to family conflict [7, 29–32]. Economic problems are also predictors of negative parenting, including lack of warmth and involvement, parental harshness, and authoritarian parenting methods [28, 33–36].

The family stress model (FSM), which was proposed by Conger et al., explains the relationships among SES, marital conflict, and parenting style, while also providing solid evidence for the negative effects of family economic problems on both parents and children [15, 37]. The FSM proposes that economic hardship predicts economic pressure, which in turn exacerbates emotional distress (e.g., depression, anxiety, anger, and alienation) for both parents [37]. In turn, parental emotional distress has a direct, negative impact on the parents' relationships with each other, as indicated by conflict. This conflict then spills over into parent/child relationships, in the form of negative parenting, resulting in harsh, uninvolved, and/or inconsistent child-rearing practices; these parenting styles are associated with an increase in negative outcomes for children [29, 37–39].

Educational status and economic aspects are typical quantitative SES indicators [4, 5]. Many previous studies have focused on the educational aspects of SES in the relationship between SES and child development, with parental educational levels being associated with child developmental outcomes [1, 2, 10–12, 25, 26]. However, despite the many studies completed in this area, few have simultaneously investigated the influence of multiple components of SES, including family income, and maternal and paternal education levels, as predictors in the relationships among SES, family processes, and child mental health functioning. In several studies that include both educational and economic aspects of SES indicators, educational status has often either previously been used as a control variable, or it has been combined with income in the construction of an overall index of SES indicators [6, 7]. Furthermore, a limitation of previous empirical work on the FSM is that studies have also focused exclusively on the economic aspect of SES in the relationship between SES and family processes, dedicating little research attention to the educational aspects of SES [28]. It is well known that education is an important predictor of family income across the life course [40]. Therefore, it may be reasonable to expect the influence of educational status on parental interactions and parent/child interactions to be indirect and mediated by economic well-being.

Education is an important component of SES that helps identify a social class or position, and has been linked to individual competence [4]. Higher education is likely to enhance various individual skills for competent functioning, such as problem-solving skills, cognitive skills, and capacity to cope with change. People with higher levels of education tend to be able to solve problems that are more complex and perform jobs with more autonomy and creativity [41–44]. Moreover, educational achievement provides persons with more employment opportunities, enhances their ability to make significant contributions to their fields, and demonstrates significant positive associations with occupational prestige and income [40, 45–47]. Furthermore, according to human capital theory, the education level of an individual's spouse also helps accumulate human capital and has an important impact on economic outcomes [48, 49]. For example, a spouse with a higher education might provide constructive advice and information that can affect career and decision making in the family, such as consumption, fertility, and where to live [50–52]. Additionally, spouses are likely to affect each other through values, attitudes, and other abilities associated with education. Many studies have revealed common findings that the education level of an individual's spouse is positively correlated with the individual's earnings. Especially, numerous studies have suggested that a wife's education affects her husband's earnings [51–56], and vice versa. Additionally, other studies have shown that an individual's earnings are positively correlated with their spouse's education level [53, 57]. This correlation might be due to marital matching, as individuals that are more productive are more likely to marry better-educated individuals.

However, despite the fact that parental education levels strongly interact with income, education levels and economic conditions could have different effects on family processes and child mental health functioning, possibly acting through different pathways. Regarding the relationship between educational level and marital relationship, higher education is likely to help parents to strengthen their communication and analytical skills, allowing for more effective problem solving between parents [44, 50, 58]. Moreover, higher education is also likely to enhance self-control and coping mechanisms

of parents, possibly increasing the positive association between education and psychological well-being [58]. Consequently, parental education levels might positively affect marital relationship through parental psychological well-being [44, 59–61]. A large amount of evidence for the beneficial nature of education on marriage exist, as studies have demonstrated a negative relationship between parental educational levels and marital conflict [62], a positive association between educational attainment and greater marital satisfaction [30, 63], and higher levels of educational attainment are associated with greater marital stability [64, 65].

In addition, previous research has suggested that parental education is the strongest and most important predictor of parenting behavior [66]. Regarding the relationship between educational level and parent/child interactions, higher education is likely to promote the ability to process information, and enable parents to acquire more knowledge and skills about childrearing and child development, allowing parents with higher education to use more effective strategies for childrearing [66–68]. Moreover, as mentioned above, a higher level of education is likely to boost parental psychological well-being, which, in turn, could positively influence parenting style [69–71]. Many studies found that higher maternal education levels are associated with more supportive parenting [72, 73], which is also associated with positive cognitive, behavioral, emotional, and physical child outcomes [74–77]. While few studies have investigated the influence of paternal education levels on fathers' involvement in childrearing, some studies have found paternal education levels to be somewhat associated with parent/child interactions. For example, several studies revealed that fathers with higher educational attainment tend to be more involved, show more positive engagement, and be more accessible to their children than fathers with a lower education level [78–80]. However, other studies have found little association between paternal educational attainment and fathers' involvement, after controlling for factors such as family income and maternal education level [6–9]. As there are conflicting results in the literature regarding the influence of paternal education level on parental involvement, it is possible that parental education levels may influence parenting attitudes directly, or they may do so indirectly through family economic factors or other SES indicators. Given this information, we are unable to form strong expectations regarding the possible pathways of how both maternal and paternal education levels may influence childhood mental health problems.

When considering the complex relationships in the above-mentioned variables, it is important to consider independent associations, while controlling for other SES

74

Psychiatry and Mental Health

variables. However, few previous studies have primarily examined individual relationships between SES, including family income and parental educational levels, interparental interactions, parent/child interactions, and/or child mental health functioning, taking into account associations in a comprehensive model. Therefore, investigations into SES, including family income and parental educational levels, are needed to clarify how each SES indicator flows through the family processes to influence child development. Studying individual markers of SES, including family income and maternal and paternal education, enables us to study the unique and combined contributions of family income and parental education towards family functioning and child adjustment.

Family processes and child adjustment

As mentioned earlier, the FSM has shown that economic hardship predicts greater economic pressure, in turn exacerbating emotional distress among parents, which then negatively affects their relationship with each other, as indicated by parental relationship conflict [29, 39]. This marital conflict spills over into parent/child relationships, which are characterized by more hostile, harsh, emotionally neglectful parenting, and less warmth. These types of relationships are associated with more negative outcomes (e.g., emotional, behavioral, mental, and physical health problems) in childhood and adulthood [7, 15, 16].

The "spillover hypothesis" has been proposed to explain this relationship between marital conflict and child outcomes. According to this hypothesis, the negativity and positivity experienced in the inter-parental relationship transfer to the parent/child relationship, affecting child outcomes [17, 18, 81–83]. The hypothesis further posits that destructive marital conflict, such as verbal and physical aggression, requires excessive energy that makes parents less emotionally available and less sensitive to the needs of their children. The negative interactions "spill over" into the parent/child relationship, resulting in an increase in negative parenting practices, such as poor monitoring, inconsistency, and harsh discipline. In contrast, constructive marital conflict, such as satisfaction, support, and positive interaction, spills over into the parent/child relationship, which is characterized by increased availability to meet children's needs, and results in more positive parenting practices, such as involvement and praise. Moreover, several studies examining the effects of conflict on children's emotional and behavioral outcomes, have also demonstrated ways of categorizing conflict into destructive and constructive marital conflict [84–88]. These studies suggest that destructive marital conflict make children more vulnerable to developing adjustment problems including aggression, conduct disorders, anxiety, and depressive symptomatology.

Conversely, these studies also suggest that constructive marital conflict, including progress towards the resolution of the conflicts and explanations about how conflicts were resolved, is likely to be beneficial to children, helping them learn effective problem-solving and communication skills. Therefore, the findings illustrate the need to examine marital conflict as a multidimensional construct to understand how conflict affects children.

However, despite the extensive research completed in this area, studies have minimally considered the impact of positive dimensions of marital conflict and in turn, parenting practices (positive spillover), rather than negative dimensions (negative spillover), as mediators in the link between SES and child mental health functioning. Previous studies have consistently found that destructive marital conflict fosters negative spillover, resulting in more negative parent/child interactions [18]. Furthermore, a limitation of previous empirical work is that studies have focused exclusively on negative outcomes (e.g., internalizing and externalizing behavioral problems) [17, 18]. Further studies examining a positive association between family factors and child mental health functioning, including positive outcomes, have been called for. Therefore, investigations into positive spillover practices (i.e., constructive marital conflict, positive parenting practices, and positive child outcomes) are needed to clarify how family functioning affects child development in a comprehensive model.

Social competence and child adjustment

School maladjustment is one of the most prevalent and significant health problems threatening children. Previous studies have suggested that one of the factors related to child maladjustment is a child's inability to adjust socially, as a result of a lack of social competence [89]. Social competence has been broadly defined as effectiveness in social interactions [20]. Social skills are discrete abilities that contribute to social competence [19]. Specifically, these skills have been defined as socially acceptable learned behaviors that enable children to interact effectively and avoid unacceptable responses from others [90]. In short, social competence refers to an individual's overall ability to act in a socially appropriate manner [19], whereas social skills refer to specific and distinct behaviors representing social competence [91].

Social skills are some of the most important accomplishments in childhood. Aspects of social skills, such as cooperation, self-control, and assertion, which were clustered by Gresham and Elliott [90], affect social adaptation in later life. Social skills help children initiate positive peer interactions, which help them learn positive behaviors through peer modeling and provide them with resources, such as support and acceptance [92–95].

Conversely, children who fail to develop social skills in early developmental phases often display social problems. Children who persistently exhibit deficits in social skills experience both short- and long-term negative consequences, which may often be precursors to more severe social problems later in life [96, 97]. Children who lack social skills may experience emotional difficulties, and tend to have trouble interacting with their peers, teachers, and families [97–100]. Furthermore, social skill deficits frequently demonstrate a negative association with behavioral adjustment [99–102].

Behavioral adjustment is generally associated with two broad symptom dimensions: internalizing and externalizing behaviors. Internalizing behaviors include worry, anxiety, depression, and somatic complaints; while externalizing behaviors include hyperactivity, inattention, aggression toward peers, and management problems [103–110]. Internalizing and externalizing behaviors consistently influence each other over time, with prior studies showing that internalizing behaviors predict later externalizing behaviors, and vice versa [111–116]. Further, there is evidence of co-morbidity with internalizing and externalizing behaviors later in the life course.

Social competence predicts internalizing and externalizing behaviors across longer periods in childhood, adolescence, and adulthood. Additionally, lower social competence forecasts higher levels of both internalizing and externalizing problems [99–102, 117, 118]. Children who lack social skills have difficulties in expressing themselves and understanding others, such as sending appropriate social messages and responding to their peers, teachers, and families. They have fewer positive interactions and have more trouble interacting with others. Consequently, these individuals are more prone to be disliked and deemed socially incompetent by others [119]. Therefore, children with social skill deficits are at an elevated risk for social isolation, including anxious solitude and peer rejection.

Social isolation is associated with behavioral adjustment. For instance, increased childhood social isolation longitudinally predicts depressive symptoms [120–122]. Therefore, early peer difficulties with social skill deficits are predictive of later maladjustment. The cross-sectional and longitudinal associations between social competence deficits and internalizing symptoms have been well documented from preschool to adolescence [123–125]. Similarly, several studies suggest childhood peer rejection longitudinally predicts externalizing behaviors, including aggression, conduct disorders involving peers, and other under-controlled behaviors during the school-age years and into adolescence [101, 102, 126]. However, several social skill abilities among children that are associated with externalizing behaviors, such as abilities in emotion regulation, verbally expressing emotions, and self-regulation of behavior, generally increase with age [127, 128]. Therefore, as social skills improve with age, the rates of externalizing problems tend to decrease in comparison to internalizing problems [127–129]. Eventually, the failure to develop social skills and successful childhood interpersonal relationships could promote mental health difficulties and both internalizing and externalizing problems over time.

Early childhood is a pivotal period for social development. The transition period from early childhood to elementary school first grade is a pivotal period for social development that leads to school readiness. Previous research has indicated that the preschool years are a sensitive period for the acquisition of social skills and related abilities [130–135]. Preschool-aged children learn and frequently display various prosocial behaviors [136]. Therefore, this period is an important developmental stage during when children are expected to acquire social skills to prepare them for broader social activity. Social skill deficits in early childhood gradually become permanent over time, are related to poor academic performance, and are predictive of social adjustment problems and serious psychopathology in adolescence. Understanding the factors that influence these developmental processes in early childhood may enable the prevention of later socio-emotional difficulties.

There is an extensive body of literature demonstrating that the development of social competence among children is significantly affected by environmental factors in childhood [137–139]. For example, family functioning (e.g., the inter-parental relationship, parent/child interactions) has been shown to predict children's social competence. Positive parenting, such as emotional expressiveness, responsiveness, and support, has been shown to enhance empathy and social functioning in children [140–143], while negative parenting behavior, such as harsh discipline, emotional neglect, or rejecting behavior, is often associated with lower sociability/social competence and increased problem behaviors in children [16, 25, 143].

Many previous studies have also shown that destructive marital conflicts negatively affect social competence [144]. This type of marital conflict may put children at risk of developing adjustment problems, including internalizing and externalizing disorders, due to their inability to control their emotions. Moreover, they may learn through these interactions to solve problems through aggressive behavior [18, 145–147]. Since research has primarily focused on destructive marital conflict, few studies have investigated constructive marital conflict, which may foster social competence. Constructive marital conflict may also aid in the development of problem-solving, coping, and conflict resolution abilities by teaching children how to effectively communicate with others to solve issues [148–150]. Previous studies consistently suggest that destructive conflict increases the risk of adjustment disorders, whereas constructive conflict may positively influence adjustment. Despite the differential effects of destructive and constructive conflict on child development, there is no distinction between these two types of conflict and their implications for social development within the literature. Moreover, even though marital conflict and parenting practices affect social competence [144, 151], few studies have addressed the various ways that this may occur within a comprehensive model.

As mentioned previously, a limitation of empirical work on the FSM is that studies have focused exclusively on negative outcomes, such as internalizing and externalizing problems [7, 15]. This myopic focus leads to a strong need for the examination of positive associations, such as positive developmental outcomes among children (e.g., social competence). The current study highlights the ways that family processes within the FSM promote desirable child outcomes, specifically focusing on the development of social competence.

Various studies have demonstrated the significant effects of family processes on social competence, primarily examining the individual relationships between different types of SES, marital conflict, parenting practices, and child mental health functioning, without considering associations in a comprehensive model. When considering the complex relationships among these variables, it is also important to consider independent associations, while controlling for other variables. For a more detailed exploration of the early protective factors potentially influencing diverse developmental maladjustment, the purpose of this preliminary study was to examine, in greater detail, social competence as a mediator of the relationships between SES, family processes, and children's adjustment.

Present study
Although several studies have demonstrated a significant impact of SES and family processes (i.e., marital conflict and parenting practices) on general adjustment among children, few have considered the relationship between child behavioral problems and SES, including family economic and parental educational levels, negative and positive aspects of marital conflict and parenting practices, and child social competence, in conjunction with one another. Most prior studies including the FSM have focused little attention on the educational domain of SES or the positive aspects of family functioning and child outcomes. When considering the complex relationships between these variables, it is important to consider

independent associations, while controlling for other variables in a comprehensive model. Most studies have examined these complex relationships in a more piecemeal fashion, rarely integrating them into a unified conceptual model. Within the risk and resilience research framework, relational risk or protective factors are thought to make either additive or contingent contributions to adjustment.

Based on the observations above, the aim of this study was to clarify the roles of SES (i.e., family income and maternal and paternal educational levels), marital conflict (i.e., destructive and constructive marital conflict), parenting practices (i.e., negative and positive parenting practices), and child social competence (i.e., social skills) and behavioral problems (i.e. internalizing and externalizing problems), by analyzing these relationships in a comprehensive model. In the present study, we used longitudinal assessments of children's externalizing and internalizing behaviors to evaluate the hypothesis that SES, marital conflict, and parenting practices predict children's social competence, which is then related to later child adjustment. The mediational model in Fig. 1 was tested to estimate the direct effects of Time 1 (T1; participants were 5 years old, in preschool) SES, marital conflict, and parenting practices on Time 2 (T2; participants were 6 years old, in the first grade) behavioral problems, and to examine the indirect effects of T1 variables, through their effects on T1 social competence, on T2 behavioral problems. As a result, our study provides theoretical contributions to the FSM by incorporating additional critical factors (i.e., parental educational levels, positive aspects of family functioning, and positive child outcomes). Investigating the role of social competence as a mediating process in the link between relational risks such as SES and later child adjustment will enable important theoretical contributions to the understanding of processes involved in the development of adaptation among children with higher relational risks, and will provide implications for prevention and intervention efforts.

We hypothesized the following pathways: (1) SES indicators (i.e., family income and maternal and paternal educational levels) are, as predictors, differentially associated with family processes (i.e., marital conflict and parenting practices) and child mental functioning (i.e., social competence and adjustment) through distinct pathways; (2) both negative and positive aspects of family processes will mediate the relationship between SES and child mental health functioning; and (3) social competence in preschool, which is influenced by multidimensional family factors, will reduce the risk of behavioral problems in the first grade.

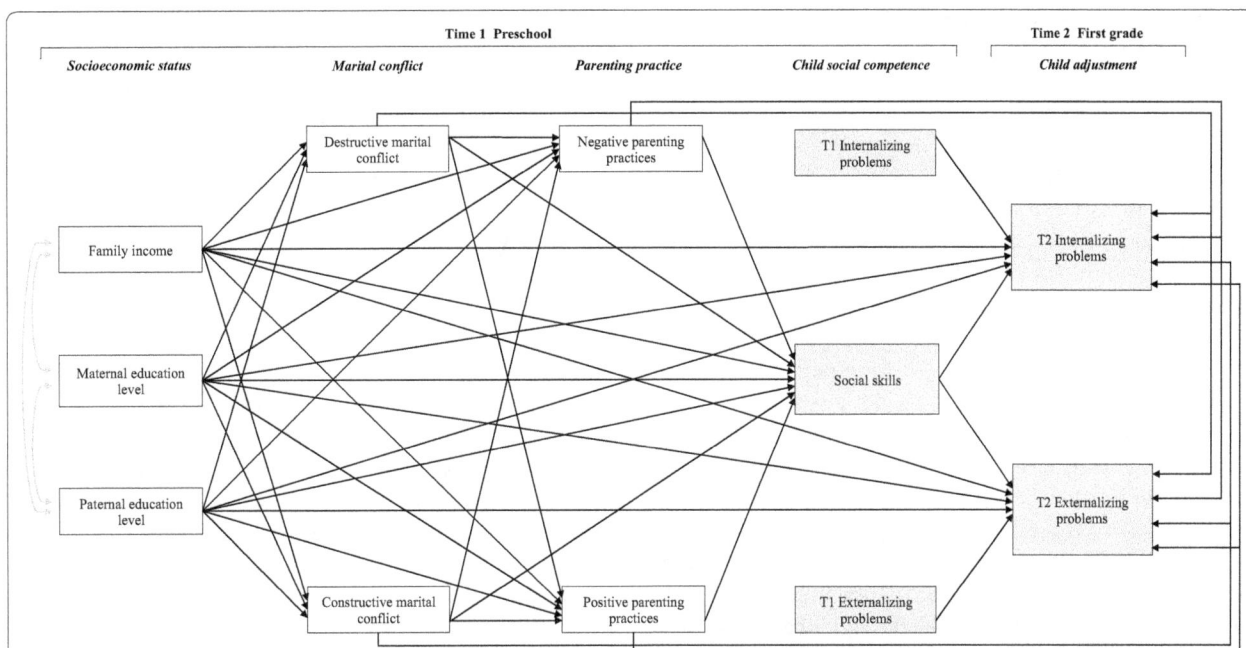

Fig. 1 Hypothesized model. This model includes the hypothesized pathways among socioeconomic status, marital conflict, parenting practices, and children's mental health functioning

Methods

Participants

The current investigation consisted of two waves of data, taken 1 year apart, and was part of a longitudinal study that examined the influence of family factors on child social developmental outcomes. Figure 2 illustrates the

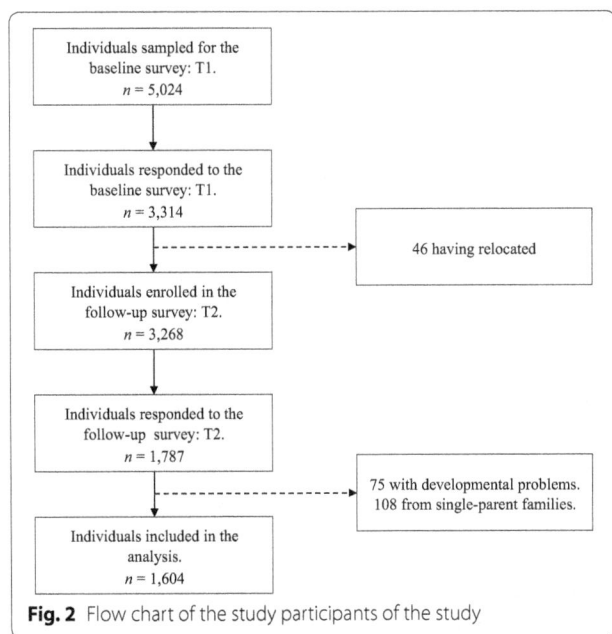

Fig. 2 Flow chart of the study participants of the study

flow chart of participants for this study. At T1 in 2014, participants were 5 years old and in preschool. Self-reported questionnaires were provided to the parents of children ($n = 5024$) enrolled in 52 kindergartens and 78 nursery schools in Nagoya city, which is a major urban area in Japan. A total of 3314 parents completed the questionnaires. At T2 in 2015, participants were 6 years old and in the first grade. Parents returned 1 year (12 months) after T1 to participate in the second wave of data collection. The retention rate from T1 to T2 was 53.9%, resulting in an ultimate sample size of 1787 for the current study.

In the present paper, to clarify the associations between SES accurately, including parents' educational levels, marital relationship, parenting practices, and child developmental outcomes, the following individuals were excluded from analyses: (1) children from single-parent families, (2) children diagnosed with developmental problems, and (3) children whose mothers did not return completed questionnaires. For inclusion in this study, parents did not have to be the target child's biological parent; however, they did need to reside with the child. For both T1 and T2, of the 1787 children, 1604 (89.8%) met the inclusion criteria. The children's data, as provided by the mothers, were analyzed in this study.

At T1, mean age was 6.09 years ($SD = .30$), with 51.5% of the sample being males ($n = 826$) and 48.5% being females ($n = 778$). In total, 48.5% of the sample were children attending kindergarten ($n = 778$), and 51.5% were children attending nursery schools ($n = 826$). The mean ages of the mothers and fathers were 37.41 ($SD = 4.47$) and 39.33 ($SD = 5.44$) years, respectively. SES indicators (i.e., family income and parental education level) are shown in Table 1. The median household income was between ¥ 5,000,000 and ¥ 5,999,999 per year (approximately $ 50,000 and $ 59,999 USD per year). On average, mothers and fathers had completed comparable years of education, at 14.13 years ($SD = 1.75$) and 14.56 years ($SD = 2.25$), respectively.

We compared the T2 non-returning participants with the T2 returning participants on demographic features (i.e., parental age, family income, and parental education level). The mean ages of T2 non-returning participant mothers and fathers were 36.79 ($SD = 4.82$) and 38.92 ($SD = 5.86$) years, respectively. The T2 non-returning participants were comparatively younger parents that returned at T2, according to independent samples t tests ($p < .05$). A Chi square test yielded a significant ($p < .001$) difference between household incomes, with 24.8% of the T2 non-returning participants reporting below ¥ 3,999,999 per year, while only 17.7% of T2 returning participants reported this level. On average, the T2 non-returning participants' mothers and fathers had comparable years of completed education, at 13.72 years ($SD = 1.87$) and 14.01 years ($SD = 2.42$), respectively.

Table 1 Parent and family characteristics of the study sample in percentages ($n = 1604$)

Description	n	%
Annual household income (in millions of yen)		
< 4	284	17.7
4–5	536	33.4
6–7	368	22.9
8–9	185	11.5
10–11	107	6.7
≥ 12	86	5.4
No response	38	2.4
Maternal education level		
Compulsory education (9 years)	35	2.2
Upper secondary school (12 years)	370	23.1
Less than 4 years at college/university (13–15 years)	661	41.2
Over 4 years at college/university (≥ 16 years)	529	33.0
No response	9	.6
Paternal education level		
Compulsory education (9 years)	77	4.8
Upper secondary school (12 years)	382	23.8
Less than 4 years at college/university (13–15 years)	239	14.9
Over 4 years at college/university (≥ 16 years)	895	55.8
No response	11	.7

Additionally, a t-test revealed that the education level of non-returning participants was significantly lower ($p < .001$) than the education level of individuals that did return. Thus, the non-returning participants tended to have relatively lower SES than did returning participants, meaning that there was a lower response rate of individuals with low SES compared to high SES.

Ethics statement
The children's parents and teachers were informed of the study's purpose and procedures, and they were made aware that they were not obligated to participate. The teachers provided their written informed consent, and the parents submitted the same on behalf of their children prior to participating in this research. Ethical approval for this study was obtained from Kyoto University's Ethics Committee in Kyoto, Japan (E2322).

Measures
All the questions used for the self-developed questionnaire were questions translated into Japanese.

Predictors
Socioeconomic status At T1, SES was defined as information about family income levels, as provided by the parents, and parental education. Parents were asked to report their total yearly family income, their education in years, and their completed education levels by choosing one of the following response options: compulsory education (9 years), vocational upper-secondary school/general upper-secondary school (12 years), less than 4 years at college/university (13–15 years; i.e., junior college, vocational school, or professional school), and over 4 years at college/university (≥ 16 years). Each of the SES scores (i.e., yearly family income and years of parental education) were converted to z scores.

Mediators
Marital conflict At T1, the Quality of Co-parental Communication Scale (QCCS), a 10-item self-report questionnaire, was used to assess each parent's feelings or behaviors within the context of the co-parenting relationship [120]. This measure is composed of the following two subscales: Co-parental Conflict (four items relating to conflict, hostility, tension, and disagreements) and Co-parental Support (six items relating to accommodation, helpfulness, and resourcefulness). Items are rated on a 5-point Likert scale ranging from 1 (*Never*) to 5 (*Always*). The Conflict and Support subscales assess parents' perceptions of the co-parenting relationship. The Conflict subscale measures the negative aspect of the co-parenting relationship, with higher conflict scores indicating more co-parental communication conflict [152]. In the current study, we con-

sidered Co-parental Conflict as destructive conflict. Conversely, the Support subscale measures positive aspects of the co-parenting relationship, with higher support scores indicating more supportive co-parental communication [152]. Specifically, the Support subscale measures "general support" including helpfulness, resourcefulness, and cooperation [152], as opposed to the constructive aspects of conflict. However, in the current study, we considered Co-parental Support as constructive marital conflict. The scales have adequate internal consistency and construct validity [152–154]. The internal consistency was .88 and .74 for Conflict and Support scales, respectively [152]. The current study found internal consistencies of .77 and .86 for the Conflict and Support scales, respectively. Each QCCS total score was converted to a z score.

Parenting practice   At T1, the Alabama Parenting Questionnaire (APQ), a 42-item self-report questionnaire, was used to assess various aspects of parenting behavior [155, 156]. The measure is composed of the following five subscales: Poor Monitoring/Supervision, Inconsistent Discipline, Corporal Punishment, Positive Parenting, and Involvement. Items are rated on a 5-point Likert scale ranging from 1 (*Never*) to 5 (*Always*). Participants self-reported their own parenting behavior. The developers have reported that the measure has adequate internal consistency and construct validity [156]. The internal consistency of the subscales ranges from .46 to .80 [156]. In this study, the subscales' internal consistency ranged from .71 to .76.

In this study, we standardized the separate positive and negative parenting composite scores [157]. Scores on the Poor Monitoring/Supervision, Inconsistent Discipline, and Corporal Punishment subscales of the APQ were combined to form a negative parenting composite score, whereas scores on the Positive Parenting and Involvement subscales were combined to form a Positive Parenting composite score. The Negative Parenting composite score was calculated by converting the Poor Monitoring/Supervision, Inconsistent Discipline, and Corporal Punishment subscale scores to z scores and then averaging them, with higher scores indicating more negative parenting. Similarly, the Positive Parenting composite score was calculated using the same method for the Positive Parenting and Involvement subscale scores, with higher scores indicating more positive parenting.

Child social competence   At T1, the Social Skills Questionnaire (SSQ) was used as an index of observer ratings of child social competence. In the current study, the children's teachers evaluated their social skills using this scale. The SSQ is a 24-item measure of children's social competence in relation to "cooperation", "self-control", and

"assertion" [158–160], as factors affecting social adaptation in later life [90]. These clusters of social behaviors can briefly be characterized as follows: Cooperation—behaviors such as helping others, sharing with a peer, and complying with rules such as sharing and obeying; Self-control—behaviors that emerge in conflict situations, such as responding appropriately to (i.e., controlling one's temper) teasing or corrective feedback from an adult; and Assertion—behaviors such as asking others for help/information and responding to others' actions (e.g., responses to peer pressure).

The SSQ has the following three subscales: Cooperation (eight items; e.g., the child helps someone voluntarily), Self-control (eight items; e.g., the child behaves if there is a need), and Assertion (eight items; e.g., the child initiates a conversation with someone). These factors are based upon, and positively correlated with, the Social Skills Rating System (SSRS) [90], which is one of the most widely used social skills scales and was used in the National Institute of Child Health and Human Development (NICHD) study [161, 162]. The SSQ's items are rated on a 3-point scale ranging from 0 (*Not at all*) to 2 (*Often*), yielding total scores for cooperation, self-control, and assertiveness. The SSQ has adequate internal consistency and construct validity; the subscales' internal consistency has previously ranged from .91 to .93 [158], with a range from .84 to 94 in the current study. Furthermore, the present study combined total scores for cooperation, self-control, and assertiveness to form a social skills score, with higher scores indicating better social skills. The social skills score was calculated by converting scores on the Cooperation, Self-control, and Assertion subscales to z scores, and then averaging them.

Criterion variables
Child adjustment   The Strengths and Difficulties Questionnaire (SDQ) is a 25-item measure of parents' perceptions of their children's prosocial and difficult behaviors, and it is designed to assess general internalizing and externalizing emotional and behavioral problems [163]. In this study, children's mothers evaluated their behavioral adjustment using this scale at both T1 and T2. The measure is composed of the following five subscales: Emotional Symptoms, Conduct Problems, Hyperactivity-Inattention, Peer Problems, and Prosocial Behavior. Items were rated on a 3-point Likert scale ranging from 0 (*Not true*) to 2 (*Certainly true*). The scales' internal consistency and construct validity were reported as adequate [164–166].

In this study, the Emotional Symptoms and Peer Problems subscales of the SDQ were combined to form an Internalizing Problems scale (Cronbach's α = .65, .71), while the Conduct Problems and Hyperactivity-Inattention subscales were combined to form an Externalizing

Problem scale (Cronbach's $\alpha = .74, .77$), as suggested by Goodman et al. [167], with higher scores indicating more behavioral problems. Each SDQ total score was converted to a z score.

Procedure

To conduct our study, we asked the kindergartens and nursery schools with 50 or more students, in Nagoya city, to participate. As a result, principals of 130 facilities (52 kindergartens and 78 nursery schools) gave us permission to conduct our survey and meet with participating parents. To recruit families at T1, self-reported questionnaires were distributed at the participating facilities to all parents of 5 year olds ($n = 5024$). Participants received an information sheet and questionnaires on childrearing, in relation to family factors (i.e., SES, family relationships, and parenting style), and child behavioral adjustment (i.e., externalizing and internalizing problems). Participants provided written informed consent and agreed to participate. The parents completed the questionnaires at a single time point and returned these to participating facilities in sealed envelopes to prevent teachers from seeing the questionnaires. Then, the teachers evaluated the children's social skills using the SSQ. All sealed envelopes containing questionnaires and SSQ evaluations were returned to the researcher from the respective principals.

At T2, 12 months later, participants were contacted again when the children were in the first grade. At T1, the researcher obtained the address of participants, and, at T2, the researcher mailed the participants questionnaires on childrearing in relation to family factors and child behavioral adjustment. Participants who completed the questionnaires returned them to the researcher by mail. Access to the data was restricted to the researchers of the current longitudinal study.

Data analyses

First, prior to developing a model of the relationships among SES, parental relationship, parenting practices, and child social competence and adjustment, correlation analyses were utilized to determine the associations among SES (i.e., T1 family income, maternal and paternal levels of education), marital relationship (i.e., T1 destructive and constructive marital conflict), parenting practices (i.e., T1 negative and positive parenting practices), child social competence (i.e., T1 social skills), and child adjustment (i.e., T1 and T2 internalizing and externalizing problems).

Second, path analyses were conducted to estimate direct and indirect paths between SES, parental relationship, parenting practices, and child social competence and adjustment. Structural equation modeling analyses were conducted using full information maximum-likelihood estimation in the presence of missing data. The hypothesized model is presented in Fig. 1. In the models, SES (i.e., T1 family income and parental level of education) was specified as a predictor of the marital relationship (i.e., T1 destructive and constructive marital conflict), parenting practices (i.e., T1 negative and positive parenting practices), child social competence (i.e., T1 social skills), and behavioral adjustment (i.e., T1 and T2 externalizing and internalizing problems). We estimated how family factors (i.e., SES, marital conflict, and parenting) and child social competence in preschool influenced the children's behavioral adjustment in the first grade. The model also included T1 behavioral adjustment as control variables; through controlling for initial levels of maladjustment, the model would appropriately address changes in behavioral adjustment. Based on previous findings in the literature, we expected the effect of T1 SES indicators on T2 behavioral adjustment to be mediated by the T1 parental relationship, parenting practices, and social competence. Moreover, we expected an inverse effect between T1 social competence and T2 adjustment.

To assess fit, we examined the Comparative Fit Index (CFI) [168], the Incremental Fit Index (IFI) [169], and the Root Mean Square Error of Approximation (RMSEA) [170]. Good model fit is reflected in CFI and IFI values above .90 [168, 169]. Regarding the RMSEA, good fit was represented by a value smaller than .05 and reasonable fit was represented by values ranging from .05 to .08 [171]. All the statistical analyses were conducted using SPSS version 23.0 and Amos version 23.0.

Results
Preliminary analyses

SES indicators are shown in Table 1. Other descriptive statistics for all variables measured by the scales (i.e., marital conflict, parenting practices, child social competence, and behavioral adjustment) are presented in Table 2. A correlation matrix of the SES indicators, marital conflict, parenting practices, and child social competence and behavioral adjustment is shown in Table 3. Analyses in study composites showed that all correlations of the study composites were statistically significant. The indicators of SES, marital conflict, parenting practice, and child social competence and behavioral adjustment were interrelated, supporting our hypotheses and previous empirical findings. Each SES variable (i.e., family income and maternal and paternal educational levels) was negatively related to destructive marital conflict, negative parenting, and the children's externalizing and internalizing behavioral problems. Conversely, it was positively related to constructive marital conflict, positive parenting, and children's social skills. In turn, social skills inversely

Table 2 Descriptive statistics for the study variables (n = 1604)

Description	Range	M	SD	Cronbach's α
Marital conflict: Quality of Co-Parental Communication Scale (QCCS)				
Co-parental Conflict	4–20	9.88	3.01	.77
Co-parental Support	6–30	25.16	4.14	.86
Parenting practice: Alabama Parenting Questionnaire (APQ)				
Poor monitoring/supervision	10–50	12.87	2.94	.71
Inconsistent discipline	6–30	14.53	3.77	.73
Corporal punishment	3–15	7.06	2.17	.72
Positive parenting	6–30	22.35	3.49	.76
Involvement	10–50	37.99	5.07	.75
Social competence: Social Skills Questionnaire (SSQ)				
Cooperation	0–16	10.97	4.13	.94
Self-control	0–16	14.18	2.64	.90
Assertion	0–16	14.08	2.37	.84
Child adjustment: Strengths and Difficulties Questionnaire (SDQ)				
T1 internalizing problems	0–20	3.34	2.70	.65
T1 externalizing problems	0–20	5.02	3.21	.74
T2 internalizing problems	0–20	3.88	3.04	.71
T2 externalizing problems	0–20	5.15	3.29	.77

T1: Time 1, preschool; T2: Time 2, first grade

correlated with children's externalizing and internalizing behavioral problems.

Mediational models for SES, marital conflict, parenting practices, child social skills, and child adjustment

Longitudinal models examined the impact of SES, marital conflict, and parenting practices on child social competence and behavioral adjustment (Hypothesized model; Fig. 1). Figure 3 depicts the final path models, and the path diagram specifies both direct and indirect paths linking T1 SES indicators (i.e., family income and maternal and paternal educational levels) to T2 child behavioral adjustment (i.e., externalizing and internalizing problems; Table 4).

The standardized coefficients are shown in Fig. 3. Model fit was tested with multiple indices; the model provided a good fit to the data [χ^2 (18) = 31.89, p = .023; CFI = .99; IFI = .99; RMSEA = .02].

In the model, several statistically significant direct and indirect paths were found between the predictors and criterion variables. Family income was found to be a significant predictor of lower levels of destructive marital conflict ($\beta = -.11, p < .001$), lower levels of negative parenting practices ($\beta = -.11, p < .001$), higher levels of constructive marital conflict ($\beta = .09, p < .01$), higher levels of positive parenting practices ($\beta = .09, p < .01$), higher levels of child social skills ($\beta = .09, p < .01$), and lower levels of T2 internalizing problems ($\beta = -.08$,

$p < .001$) and T2 externalizing problems ($\beta = -.06, p < .01$). The indirect paths from family economy to child mental health functioning (i.e., social skills and internalizing and externalizing problems) through marital conflict and parenting practices were also significant.

Maternal education level was found to be a significant predictor of lower levels of negative parenting practices ($\beta = -.07, p < .05$), higher levels of constructive marital conflict ($\beta = .07, p < .05$), higher levels of positive parenting practices ($\beta = .06, p < .05$), and lower levels of T2 internalizing problems ($\beta = -.09, p < .001$) and T2 externalizing problems ($\beta = -.05, p < .05$). The indirect paths from maternal education level to child mental health functioning (i.e., social skills and internalizing and externalizing problems) through marital conflict and parenting practices were also significant.

Paternal education level was found to be a significant predictor of lower levels of destructive marital conflict ($\beta = -.10, p < .001$), lower levels of negative parenting practices ($\beta = -.06, p < .05$), higher levels of constructive marital conflict ($\beta = .10, p < .001$), and higher levels of child social skills ($\beta = .08, p < .01$). The indirect paths from paternal education level to child mental health functioning (i.e., social skills and internalizing and externalizing problems) through marital conflict and parenting practices were also significant.

Notably, in terms of the negative dimension of family processes (marital conflicts and parenting practices), T1 destructive conflict was directly, negatively related to social skills ($\beta = -.11, p < .001$), and indirectly, negatively related to T1 social skills through T1 negative parenting practices. T1 negative parenting practices were directly, negatively related to social skills ($\beta = -.10, p < .001$). Regarding the positive dimension of family processes, T1 constructive conflict was directly, positively related to social skills ($\beta = .09, p < .01$), and indirectly, positively related to T1 social skills through T1 positive parenting practices. T1 positive parenting practices were directly, positively related to social skills ($\beta = .08, p < .01$). In turn, T1 social skills were found to be a direct and significant predictor of lower levels of T2 internalizing problems ($\beta = -.38, p < .001$) and T2 externalizing problems ($\beta = -.45, p < .001$), while controlling for behavior problems at T1.

Therefore, consistent with the hypotheses, each SES indicator was significantly and independently associated with child mental health functioning (i.e., social skills and internalizing/externalizing problems) through positive and negative dimensions of marital conflict and parenting practices. Notably, T1 social skills in preschool, which were affected by T1 family factors, predicted lower levels of T2 behavioral problems in the first grade.

Table 3 Correlations among socioeconomic status, marital conflict, parenting practice, and child social competence and adjustment ($n = 1604$)

Variable	1	2	3	4	5	6	7	8	9	10	11	12
Time 1—Preschool												
Socioeconomic status												
1. Family income	—											
2. Maternal education level	.33***	—										
3. Paternal education level	.30***	.42***	—									
Marital conflict												
4. Destructive marital conflict	−.14***	−.10***	−.14***	—								
5. Constructive marital conflict	.13***	.13***	.14***	−.62***	—							
Parenting practice												
6. Negative parenting practices	−.17***	−.14***	−.14***	.24***	−.16***	—						
7. Positive parenting practices	.14***	.13***	.09***	−.18***	.28***	−.21***	—					
Child social competence												
8. Social skills	.18***	.15***	.16***	−.24***	.23***	−.20***	.17***	—				
Child adjustment												
9. T1 internalizing problems	−.14***	−.12***	−.09***	.23***	−.19***	.19***	−.13***	−.35***	—			
10. T1 externalizing problems	−.16***	−.12***	−.14***	.22***	−.19***	.36***	−.25***	−.44***	.36***	—		
Time 2—First grade												
Child adjustment												
11. T2 internalizing problems	−.18***	−.19***	−.08***	.23***	−.21***	.19***	−.17***	−.44***	.64***	.33***	—	
12. T2 externalizing problems	−.19***	−.18***	−.17***	.24***	−.24***	.31***	−.24***	−.53***	.32***	.74***	.48***	—

[Marital relationship] Destructive marital conflict: QCCS Co-parental Conflict; constructive marital conflict: QCCS Co-parental Support. [Parenting practice] Negative parenting practices: APQ Poor monitoring/supervision, Inconsistent discipline, Corporal punishment; positive parenting practices: APQ Involvement, Positive parenting. [Social competence] Social skills: SSQ Cooperation, Self-control, Assertion

* $p < .05$; ** $p < .01$; *** $p < .001$

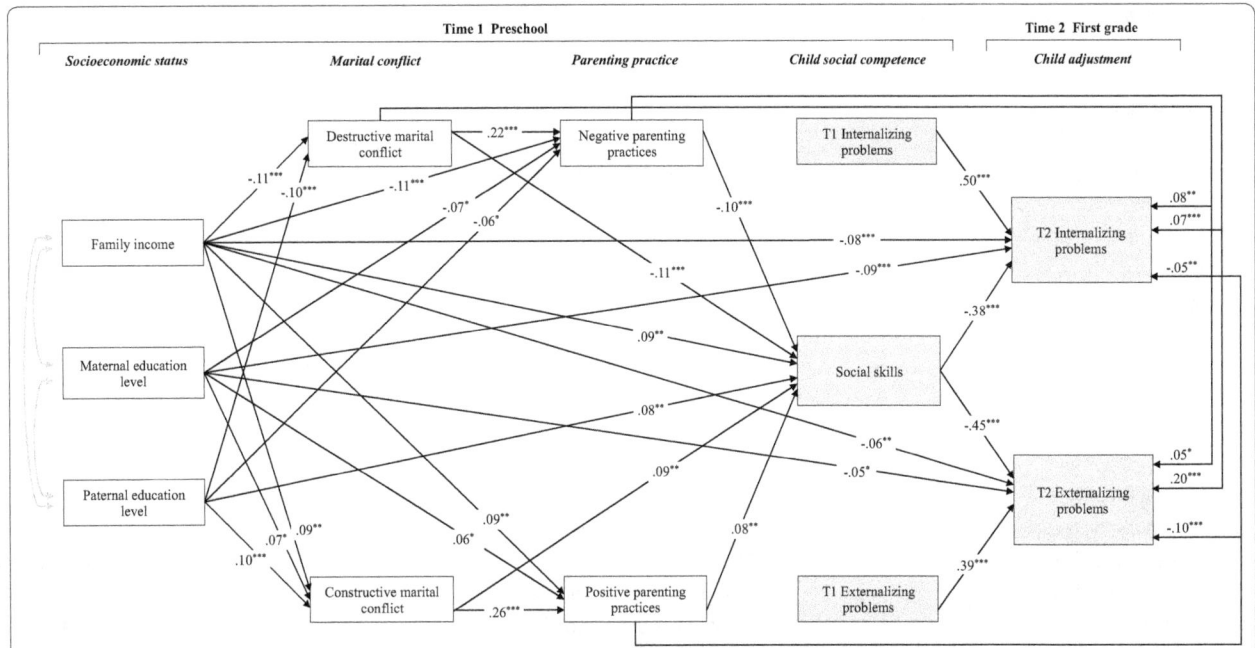

Fig. 3 Statistically significant paths. This model includes the paths that were statistically significant in the hypothesized model. Model fit statistics: $\chi^2 (18) = 31.89$; CFI = .99; IFI = .99; RMSEA = .02. *$p < .05$; **$p < . 01$; ***$p < .001$

Discussion

Our longitudinal study explored, in a comprehensive model, marital conflict (i.e., constructive and destructive marital conflict), parenting practices (i.e., positive and negative parenting practices), and social competence (i.e., social skills) as mediators of the association between SES (i.e., family income, maternal and paternal educational levels) in preschool and child behavioral adjustment (i.e., internalizing and externalizing problems) in the first grade. Our extension of previous research investigating the relationships between SES and child behavioral adjustment comprised the following three points. (1) We included both family income, and maternal and paternal education levels as SES indicators, and as predictors of family processes (i.e., marital conflict and parenting practice) and mental health functioning of children (i.e., social competence and behavioral adjustment), in a unified model. We expected each SES indicator, as predictors, to be differentially associated with family processes and child mental functioning through distinct pathways. (2) We included not only negative mediators (i.e., destructive marital conflict and negative parenting practices), but also positive mediators (i.e., constructive marital conflict and positive parenting), as mediating mechanisms in the link between SES and child mental health functioning. We expected both negative pathways (negative spillover) and positive pathways (positive spillover) in the family process model. (3) We included not only negative child developmental outcomes (i.e., behavioral problems), but

also desirable child developmental outcomes (i.e., social competence) in the relationship between family factors (i.e., SES and family processes) and child mental health functioning. Moreover, we focused on social competence as a mediator of the relationship between family factors and child behavioral problems. We expected social competence in preschool, which was affected by different types of family factors, to be inversely related to the symptoms of behavioral problems in the first grade.

Our main findings were the following. (1) Family income and parental education levels were differentially associated with child mental health functioning through distinct pathways. This result provides evidence that lower SES (i.e., lower family income and lower parental education level) is both directly and indirectly associated with more destructive marital conflict, more use of negative parenting practices, less constructive marital conflict, less use of positive parenting practices, poorer social competence, and more symptoms of behavioral problems. This suggests that, by contrast, higher SES (higher family economy and higher parental education levels) is both directly and indirectly associated with less destructive marital conflict, less use of negative parenting practices, more constructive marital conflict, more use of positive parenting practices, higher social competence, and fewer symptoms of behavioral problems. (2) We identified both negative and positive pathways between SES and child mental health functioning. Positive mediators included constructive marital conflict and positive

Table 4 Path analyses ($n = 1604$)

Construct			B	SE	β
Socioeconomic status					
Family income	→	Destructive marital conflict	− .11	.03	− 3.83***
Family income	→	Constructive marital conflict	.09	.03	3.04**
Family income	→	Negative parenting practices	− .11	.03	− 3.82***
Family income	→	Positive parenting practices	.09	.03	3.05**
Family income	→	Social skills	.09	.03	3.29**
Family income	→	T2 internalizing problems	− .08	.02	− 3.48***
Family income	→	T2 externalizing problems	− .06	.02	− 2.65**
Maternal education level	→	Destructive marital conflict	− .03	.03	− .90
Maternal education level	→	Constructive marital conflict	.07	.03	2.17*
Maternal education level	→	Negative parenting practices	− .07	.03	− 2.28*
Maternal education level	→	Positive parenting practices	.06	.03	2.03*
Maternal education level	→	Social skills	.04	.03	1.18
Maternal education level	→	T2 internalizing problems	− .09	.02	− 3.75***
Maternal education level	→	T2 externalizing problems	− .05	.02	− 2.11*
Paternal education level	→	Destructive marital conflict	− .10	.03	− 3.46***
Paternal education level	→	Constructive marital conflict	.10	.03	3.31***
Paternal education level	→	Negative parenting practices	− .06	.03	− 2.08*
Paternal education level	→	Positive parenting practices	.01	.03	.38
Paternal education level	→	Social skills	.08	.03	2.85**
Paternal education level	→	T2 internalizing problems	−.04	.02	−1.69
Paternal education level	→	T2 externalizing problems	− .02	.02	− .67
Marital conflict					
Destructive marital conflict	→	Negative parenting practices	.22	.03	6.83***
Destructive marital conflict	→	Positive parenting practices	−.01	.03	−.30
Destructive marital conflict	→	Social skills	− .11	.03	− 3.47***
Destructive marital conflict	→	T2 internalizing problems	.08	.03	3.08**
Destructive marital conflict	→	T2 externalizing problems	.05	.02	2.25*
Constructive marital conflict	→	Negative parenting practices	−.01	.03	−.19
Constructive marital conflict	→	Positive parenting practices	.26	.03	8.16***
Constructive marital conflict	→	Social skills	.09	.03	2.68**
Constructive marital conflict	→	T2 internalizing problems	− .03	.03	− 1.09
Constructive marital conflict	→	T2 externalizing problems	− .01	.02	− .54
Parenting practice					
Negative parenting practices	→	Social skills	− .10	.03	− 3.90***
Negative parenting practices	→	T2 internalizing problems	.07	.02	3.30***
Negative parenting practices	→	T2 externalizing problems	.20	.02	10.08***
Positive parenting practices	→	Social skills	.08	.03	3.10**
Positive parenting practices	→	T2 internalizing problems	− .05	.02	− 2.56**
Positive parenting practices	→	T2 externalizing problems	− .10	.02	− 4.90***
Child social competence					
Social skills	→	T2 internalizing problems	− .38	.02	− 18.65***
Social skills	→	T2 externalizing problems	− .45	.02	− 22.75***
Child adjustment					
T1 internalizing problems	→	T2 internalizing problems	.50	.02	27.03***
T1 externalizing problems	→	T2 externalizing problems	.39	.02	21.30***

* $p < .05$; ** $p < .01$; *** $p < .001$

parenting practices. This result suggests that destructive marital conflict is indirectly and negatively related to child mental health functioning through negative parenting practices in the relationship between SES and child mental health functioning. Simultaneously, in that relationship, destructive marital conflict was directly and negatively related to child mental health functioning. By contrast, these results indicate that constructive marital conflict demonstrates an indirect and positive relationship to child mental health functioning through positive parenting practices, as well as a direct positive relationship to child mental health functioning. (3) Social skills, which were associated with different types of family factors (i.e., SES, including family income and parental education levels, and both negative and positive dimensions of family processes), adversely affected later internalizing and externalizing behaviors. This result suggests social skills were lowered by the negative aspects of family processes (i.e., destructive marital conflict and negative parenting practices) and raised by the positive aspects of family processes (constructive marital conflict and positive parenting practices) in preschool, which reduced later symptoms of internalizing and externalizing problem behaviors in the first grade. That is, social skills in preschool played a potentially protective role in preventing later behavioral problems. Therefore, our longitudinal analysis supported the initial hypotheses.

Path of family economic situation, family processes, and child mental health functioning

In this study, family income was directly linked to marital conflict, parenting practices, and in turn, child mental health functioning (i.e., social competence and behavioral problems). This result is consistent with previous research findings identifying a direct path of family income to destructive marital conflict and negative parenting practices, and in turn, child outcomes [7, 28–30, 35, 36, 63]. Furthermore, this result supports the FSM's prediction that family income affects children's socioemotional development through its influence on parents' psychological well-being and, therefore, the inter-parental relationship and parent/child interactions [15]. The result also supports the notion of negative spillover effects and is consistent with family systems theory [17, 18].

Conversely, we found a positive pathway within which a higher family economic status was associated with more constructive marital conflict, and in turn, more use of positive parenting practices, resulting in higher mental health functioning. This result supports the notion of the positive spillover effect, with the positive inter-parental relationship spilling over into the parent/child relationship, resulting in more positive parenting practices.

Similar to negative spillover effects and consistent with family systems theory [18], positive emotions from interparental relationships may transfer to parent/child relationships [82, 83]. This result, that there is a positive spillover effect in the family process model, is an extension of previous studies.

Additionally, we found that family income was directly related to child mental health functioning (i.e., social competence and behavioral problems), while controlling for other variables. There are likely to be other factors that were not accounted for in our model. For example, the Family Investment Model (FIM), which is concerned with the advantages reaped by the developing child because of family wealth [28, 172, 173], may explain this association. The FIM proposes that families with more economic resources can make significant investments in the development of their children, whereas those with lower incomes must invest in more immediate family needs [1, 7, 174]. Income enables families to invest in building their children's human capital. These investments in children involve several dimensions of goods and services, including parents' direct and indirect stimulation of learning (e.g., providing learning materials and activities, and support through advanced training and schools), the family's standard of living (e.g., adequate food, housing, clothing, medical care), and living in a more advantaged neighborhood environment that fosters a child's development [7, 175, 176]. According to this perspective, children in disadvantaged families tend to fare worse because they have limited access to resources that help them develop. Mayer demonstrated that children in disadvantaged families lived under worse conditions, owned fewer stimulating materials, and were less likely to engage in stimulating activities [176]. After controlling for other family background characteristics, these resources were associated with children's developmental outcomes [176]. Therefore, the apparent direct effect of family economic status found in the current study could possibly be mediated by factors that were not accounted for in our model. Future studies should investigate this possibility by including more family factors related to child mental health functioning in their models.

Path of parental educational level, family processes, and child mental health functioning

As mentioned earlier, despite the many studies completed in this area, few studies have simultaneously investigated the influence of family income and maternal and paternal education levels as predictors in the relationships between SES, family processes, and child mental health functioning [6, 7, 28]. Although most of the previous FSM studies have focused primarily on economic conditions, we suspect that they tend to capture a limited scope of the influence of educational achievement. In this study, both maternal and paternal educational levels were independently linked with parental functioning and parent/child interactions, and in turn, with child mental health functioning in a unified model, while controlling for economic conditions. In addition, this result also supports the notion of both positive and negative spillover effects [17, 18], as educational levels were positively related to higher levels of constructive marital conflict, and in turn, higher levels of positive parenting, resulting in better developmental outcomes. Therefore, the results regarding the effects of multiple components of SES, including family income and maternal and paternal education levels on child mental health functioning through distinct pathways, are an extension of those found in previous studies.

In terms of the relationship between educational level and marital conflict, the results of the current study are consistent with those of previous research showing educational attainment to be inversely related to destructive marital conflict [62], and parental educational attainment to be positively related to greater marital satisfaction and marital stability [30, 63–65]. More precisely, paternal education was linked to both destructive and constructive conflict; however, maternal education was linked to only constructive conflict. This might be due to difference of effect of maternal and paternal education on decision-making in the home. As mentioned earlier, previous studies have suggested that higher education helps parents strengthen their communication and problem-solving skills, and promotes effective problem solving between parents [50, 58]. In addition, higher education tends to make fathers positively participate in decision-making in the home, whereas, fathers with lower education negatively participate [177–179]. Therefore, in this study, paternal education might more strongly affect both destructive and constructive than maternal education.

Furthermore, in terms of the relationship between educational level and parental involvement, we found that maternal education was associated with positive parenting practices, but not paternal education; however, both maternal and paternal education were linked to negative parenting practices. This result might indicate that the effects of parental education on involvement is larger for maternal education than for paternal. This might be due to mothers tending to be the main provider of care within the households of Japan. Many studies suggest that mothers assume the primary parenting role, in that mothers were found to be more intrusive toward father/child interactions [180–182]. In addition, this result is consistent with previous research findings. A large number of studies suggest higher maternal educational attainment

to be positively related to positive parenting attitudes, such as talking to children warmly or supportively [72, 73], whereas lower educational levels have been found to be predictors of negative parenting, such as harshness and physical disciplinary tactics [33, 34, 183–185]. However, although many studies suggest maternal educational attainment is related to parenting attitudes, few studies have comparatively investigated the influence of paternal education levels on parental involvement. These results imply the possibility that both maternal and paternal educational levels are independently related to parenting attitudes.

One of the important mechanisms in the effect of parental education levels on family processes and children's development is likely to be parental knowledge about childrearing and child development. Lower levels of parental education are associated with negative parenting attitudes, such as physical and authoritarian disciplinary tactics [33, 34, 183–185]. It has been suggested that this is due to a lack of knowledge concerning the counterproductive outcomes of severe disciplinary responses and appropriate alternatives to harsh discipline [33, 183]. Higher levels of parental education have also been positively associated with sensitivity, positive regard, and cognitive stimulation of children [186]. Further, it has been suggested that higher educational levels are associated with increased knowledge about childrearing and child development, and more supportive parenting [72, 73]. Therefore, both maternal and paternal education levels may influence parenting attitudes, even when controlling for family income, whereas educational attainment affects parenting attitudes through the adverse effects of poor family economic situations on parents' mental well-being. Therefore, we assume that findings related to economic predictions based on the FSM are likely to reflect educational differences in SES as well. Educational levels are likely to play an important role in the relationships among SES, family processes, and child mental health functioning.

In addition, we found a direct association between parental education levels and child mental health functioning (i.e., social competence and behavioral problems), while controlling for other variables. There are likely to be other factors that were unaccounted for in our model. The FIM may also explain this mediating pathway to provide evidence for the plausibility of parental education level as an important aspect of the investment process [1, 7].

The model proposes that, similar to family income, parental education level has an influence on parental investments, and that these investments, in turn, will have a positive relationship with child development. Parents with higher education levels acquire more knowledge about child development, have a greater understanding of strategies to encourage social competence, and may be more effective in teaching children [72, 73, 187]. Families with higher educational levels and more knowledge about childrearing and child development may be more willing to make significant investments in their children's development. Despite the reasonableness of this hypothesized mediating process, there have been limited investigations into the impact of parental education level, in terms of the FIM.

However, some evidence is consistent with the aforementioned ideas. For example, a previous study found education level to be positively correlated with parental investments involving a more enriched and positive child-rearing environment, characterized by the availability of play and learning materials, and the organization and diversity of the physical environment [188].

Investment in this regard is not only material (e.g., reading materials, learning materials, neighborhood, health insurance, and quality of residence), but also emotional (e.g., parenting beliefs and behaviors) [189]. For example, more highly educated parents create a richer and more complex language environment for their children [190]. They also spend more time communicating with their children [173, 191]. A previous study found parental education to be positively related to children's language skills, including vocabulary and reading skills [192]. The richness of the language environment in inter-parental and parent/child interactions may mediate the association between parents' education levels and a child's productive vocabularies, and enhance the children's social competence. Therefore, there are likely to be other factors in family processes that were unaccounted for in our model. This result is likely to support the FIM, including its suggestion of parental educational attainment as an SES indicator.

More precisely, regarding the path between parental education and social competence, we found that paternal education was directly linked to social competence, but maternal education was not. There are likely to be other factors of paternal characteristic roles that were unaccounted for in our model, in addition to factors of the FIM. For instance, paternal involvement tends to be more physical and challenging than maternal [193, 194]. Physical and challenging play is an important component of human socialization [195, 196]. Father/child physical play is likely to help children learn to regulate their own behavior, and practice coping with failure or frustration and interpreting others' emotions. This is because father/child physical play has been linked to children's emotion-regulation and peer competence [196–199]. The positive association between father/child physical play and child social competence is a common empirical finding [195,

200–203]. In addition, several studies have suggested that fathers with higher educational levels tend to be more involved, have more positive engagement, and are more accessible to their children [78–80]. Therefore, fathers with higher educational levels might promote child social competence through not only factors of FIM, but also characteristic parental involvement, such as physical and challenging play.

Moreover, regarding the path between parental education and behavioral problems, we found that maternal education was both directly and indirectly linked to T2 internalizing behavior and externalizing behavior; however, the link for paternal education was only indirect. There are also likely to be other factors of maternal characteristic roles that were unaccounted for in our model. For instance, mothers with higher education tend to have higher quality of mother/child interactions, such as sensitivity and responsiveness [188, 204]. Past researchers have found that maternal sensitivity and responsiveness significantly shape children's cognitive development. Furthermore, cognitive competence deficits have also been reported as a vulnerability factor in causing behavioral problems [205–208]. Therefore, maternal educational achievement might affect behavioral problems through the effect of specific mother/child interactions.

Future studies should investigate the possibilities of the direct effect of parental education levels, as found in this study, being mediated by factors not accounted for in our model. This could be done by including more factors in future models.

The role of social competence in the relationships among SES, family processes, and adjustment

We focused on both negative child developmental outcomes (i.e., behavioral problems) and desirable child developmental outcomes (i.e., social competence) in the relationship between family factors (i.e., SES, marital conflict, and parenting practices) and child mental health functioning. We also highlighted the ways that family processes within the FSM promote positive developmental outcomes.

In the current study, social competence mediated the association between family factors and children's behavioral adjustment in a comprehensive model. SES was positively related to social competence and inversely related to internalizing and externalizing symptomatology, through positive and negative dimensions of parents' marital relationships and parenting styles. This result is an extension of those of previous studies, in which multidimensional family factors (i.e., SES, marital conflict, and parenting style) were related to both negative and positive outcomes in a comprehensive model. This result is consistent with several previous research findings identifying the direct individual path within which marital conflict and parenting practices are associated with child mental health functioning.

In terms of parenting practices and child mental health functioning, in this study, negative parenting practice was directly linked with poorer mental health functioning (i.e., poorer social skills, and more internalizing and externalizing problems). By contrast, positive parenting was directly linked to higher mental health functioning (i.e., better social skills and fewer internalizing and externalizing problems). Previous studies have suggested that negative parenting behaviors, such as harsh discipline, being emotionally neglectful, or demonstrating rejecting behaviors, are often associated with lower sociability-competence and increased problem behaviors in children [16, 25, 143], while positive parenting behaviors, such as emotional expressiveness, responsiveness, and support, have been shown to predict better empathy and social functioning in children [140–143].

Additionally, in terms of marital conflict and child mental health functioning, in this study, marital conflict was not only indirectly related to child outcomes through parenting practices, but also directly related to child outcomes. Parents' destructive marital conflict was directly linked with poorer mental health functioning (i.e., poorer social skills, and more symptoms of internalizing and externalizing problems). By contrast, parents' constructive conflict was directly linked to better mental health functioning (i.e., better social skills), and in turn, fewer symptoms of behavioral problems. These results are consistent with previous studies indicating that exposure to marital conflict is associated with different responses in children, depending on the type of inter-parental relationship [146, 209].

Many previous studies have shown that destructive marital conflict negatively affects social competence [144]. In addition, the relationships between inter-parental destructive conflict and negative psychological adjustment among children (e.g., internalizing symptoms and externalizing problems) are well established [146, 149, 209–211]. That is, destructive marital conflict has been shown to adversely influence children's social competence [212–215], internalizing symptoms [211, 216], and externalizing problems [210, 211]. However, limited research has investigated the impact of constructive marital conflict on child mental health functioning. Therefore, the current result is an extension of those in previous studies, which demonstrated constructive marital conflict's direct association with child social development.

One of the important direct mechanisms of the effect of inter-parental relationship on children's development is likely to be modeling. According to social learning theory, children's social development can be influenced by modeling the behaviors and attitudes of significant persons in their lives, such as parents [217]. Child social development may be both positively and negatively related to parents' social development, due to the effects of modeling [218–220]. Consistent with the modeling mechanism proposed by the spillover hypothesis, children may directly model conflict behavior exhibited by their parents. In the case of destructive marital conflict, children whose parents resolve their problems through aggressive behavior are more likely to learn that aggression is an acceptable way of dealing with disagreements, and thus, may act aggressively when interacting with their peers [149, 221, 222]. Therefore, destructive marital conflict is likely to directly limit children's social development. By contrast, in the case of constructive marital conflict, children whose parents resolve problems through supportive cooperation are more likely to learn from the negotiations between their mothers and fathers during the decision-making process, allowing them a blueprint to communicate more effectively and efficiently when interacting with their peers [150]. Therefore, constructive marital conflict is likely to directly enhance social development.

In addition, in this study, social skills in preschool, which were affected by family factors, inversely predicted later internalizing and externalizing symptomatology in the first grade, after controlling for preschool behavioral symptomatology. This result is consistent with previous research. A number of studies have shown negative correlations between social competence and behavioral problems. Early social competence among children is an important predictor of later social adjustment and psychopathology [223–226]. For example, social competence promotes child development in a number of domains, including social adjustment and interpersonal relationships [223, 227, 228]. Conversely, social competence deficits have been linked to social maladjustment and several problem behaviors, including aggression and delinquency [105, 223, 229–234].

Previous studies have primarily examined individual relationships between different types of SES, marital conflict, parenting practices, social competence, and child outcomes, without considering these associations in a comprehensive model. However, when considering the complex relationships between these variables, social competence was adversely related to later behavioral problems, as a mediating mechanism in the link between SES and child adjustment. Preschool social competence played a potential protective role in preventing later behavioral problems in the first grade. This result is an extension of previous studies, in which social competence was found to influence later adjustment, as shown in the complex relationships among these variables.

The prevailing model of prevention holds that reducing risk factors associated with adverse outcomes, and increasing protective factors that moderate the effects of exposure to risk, will reduce the possibility of later maladjustment [235]. The effectiveness of this approach towards prevention rests on the extent to which identified risk and protective factors are actually causal. Therefore, the current study findings, which focus on multidimensional family factors' simultaneous promotion of social competence among preschoolers, may provide an effective strategy for promoting later social adjustment among children.

Limitations and future directions

Our findings should be interpreted in light of several limitations. First, although this study's design was longitudinal, the design was partially cross-sectional, identifying the relationship between family factors and social competence at T1. The cross-sectional design poses several restrictions that make it difficult to assume causality among the factors. Statistical evidence from studies using a cross-sectional design may not be as informative as longitudinal data [236, 237]. Prior studies have found that children's mental health functioning influences inter-parental relationship and parenting styles, as well as the influence of inter-parental relationship and parenting styles on children's mental health functioning [238–241]. Children's mental health functioning and family factors are likely to influence each other. Furthermore, follow-up period of the current study was only 1 year. Although the transition period from early childhood to elementary school is an important period of mental development for children, 1 year may not be enough follow-up time to estimate the effects that have taken place, leading to the possibility of underestimating the impact of SES. Future studies should primarily focus on longitudinal research to examine the effects of family factors on later social competence. Specifically, it is necessary to have longitudinal research with surveys distributed at least three different time points and more long term to clarify the extent to which family factors flow through social competence to affect later behavioral problems.

Second, the majority of the data in this study (i.e., marital conflict, parenting practices, and child behavioral adjustment) was obtained from only mothers; therefore, there is a risk of reporting bias. This vulnerability to reporting bias can pose a serious potential problem to interpretation of the findings [242–245]. Single respondents views' toward family factors and child mental health functioning may be skewed either more positively or negatively, thus resulting in misleading findings. The arguments for the examination of the complex relationships between components of SES, family processes, and child mental functioning would seem to be not fully realized with data provided only from mothers. Paternal and maternal education levels or other background information may also influence their views of family factors and children's adaptive functioning; several studies have showed there are discrepancies between the views of fathers and mothers [246, 247]. Therefore, this study's data may obscure the extent to which paternal education is associated with the inter-parental relationship, parenting styles, and children's adaptive functioning, since information from the point of view of fathers was absent.

Furthermore, other factors may also influence the views of the informants. For example, regarding the inter-parental relationship, prior studies have shown that views of conflict vary across men and women; women tend to report more conflict episodes than men do, whether for the better or worse [248]. In addition, regarding parenting styles, the data provided by only maternal reports did not reveal information concerning fathers' involvement. Generally, fathers and mothers each have their own parenting styles. Many studies have shown that fathers and mothers play similar or complementary roles in terms of parenting behavior, simultaneously suggesting that their qualities of parenting behavior differ, in particular concerning the amount of physical play; fathering may prove to be more challenging [249–251].

Views of children's adaptive functioning behavior may vary across fathers, mothers, and children's teachers. Many study findings indicate that there are several discrepancies among informants, including fathers, mothers, and children's teachers. These discrepancies are particularly prevalent between children's parents and teachers, in terms of their assessment of the children's psychological well-being [242–245, 252]. The discrepancies may reflect children's symptoms, or the opportunities to observe them. Generally, it is not easy for parents to assess early maladaptive behaviors. In particular, parents have difficulty identifying behavior that is indicative of internalizing problems in young children. For instance, it is difficult for parents to distinguish behavior that is reflective of underlying psychopathology from behavior that is reflective of immaturity in self-regulatory competence. Conversely, teachers have the advantage of having the opportunity to observe the behavior of many other children simultaneously. Furthermore, behavioral problems are likely to be more apparent at school than at home. Therefore, obtaining teacher reports may be particularly important for young children to aid in the assessment and forecasting of their school maladjustment and mental health problems [253]. Furthermore, several studies have suggested that the combination of teacher and parent reports with independent assessments is more sensitive than either assessment alone

[254]. Therefore, in future studies, reports from several dissimilar informants, including those from fathers and teachers, in addition to mothers, will be needed to more precisely evaluate how family factors affect child mental health functioning.

Third, in the current study, we did not consider the interplay between maternal and paternal education, or the interplay between positive and negative aspects of inter-parental functioning. We studied the independent contributions of both maternal and paternal education, and those of the positive and negative aspects of inter-parental functioning; the framework used in this study does not lead to an examination of the actual interplay among any of these factors.

Regarding parental education, we included the independent contributions of both maternal and paternal education level, as we expected each SES indicator, as a predictor, to be differentially associated with family processes and child mental functioning through distinct pathways. However, the argument is incomplete and not generally consistent with theoretical perspectives, including family systems and developmental systems theories [1–5]. Theoretical perspectives suggest there is a more dynamic interplay than the simple additive contribution of maternal and paternal education. Not modeling the interaction between maternal and paternal education achievement may mislead the influence of each maternal and paternal education achievement.

Regarding inter-parental functioning, we also included the independent contributions of both positive and negative aspects of inter-parental functioning, as there are reasons we expected each positive and negative aspect of inter-parental functioning to be differentially associated with other variables through distinct pathways. Most studies empirically investigating the FSM have focused exclusively on the negative aspect of inter-parental functioning [15, 37]. Previous research suggests the interplay between the positive and negative aspects of inter-parental functioning is more complex than simply looking at the independent contributions of each [15, 37]. Previous research also suggests that it is not easy to distinguish the positive and negative aspects of inter-parental functioning, and that children respond to the whole instead of just the parts [29, 37–39]. The model including the independent contributions of both the positive and negative aspects of inter-parental functioning may not precisely assess the influences of each. Therefore, the inclusion of maternal and paternal education, and the positive and negative aspects of inter-parental functioning are both strengths and weaknesses of this study.

Fourth, we could not exactly assess the positive aspects of inter-parental functioning as a constructive marital conflict. As mentioned earlier, we used the Quality of Co-parental Communication (QCCS) measure to assess the positive and negative aspects of inter-parental functioning. The QCCS captures two aspects of the inter-parental relationship: Co-parental Conflict (only the negative side); and Co-parental Support (general helpfulness, resourcefulness, and cooperation) [152]. The Support subscales of this scale measured only "general support"; it has not precisely measured the constructive aspects of conflict. However, in the current study, we treated Co-parental Support, as measured by the Support subscales, as constructive conflict. Thus, the "constructive conflict" we used may not precisely assess the influence of the positive aspects of inter-parental functioning on the other variables. Future studies should investigate this possibility further by using other scales to more precisely assess the constructive aspects of conflict.

Fifth, there are likely to be other factors that were not accounted for in our model. As mentioned earlier, we found a direct association between SES and child mental health functioning, while controlling for other variables. There are likely to be other family environmental factors (e.g., child-rearing environment and more factors of the inter-parental relationship and child/parent interaction). Furthermore, although we found the effects of certain hypothesized family environmental factors on child mental health functioning, we did not consider genetic factors in our model; it is important to realize children's behavioral problems may be influenced by genetic risks, as well as their family's environmental factors. A large body of evidence supports the conclusion that children's behavioral problems are moderately heritable [255–258].

Several studies have suggested the extent to which children's mental health functioning is affected by family environmental factors depends on genetic and early temperamental characteristics; environments help determine how genes express themselves [259–261]. Children with different genetic attributes will respond differentially to the same environmental circumstances. Therefore, it is difficult to distinguish genetic effects from the effects of family environmental factors on child mental health functioning because genetic factors were not examined in this model. Consequently, there are likely to be other family environmental and genetic factors that need to be included in this model. Future studies should investigate this possibility further by including more family environmental factors related to child mental health functioning. Specifically, these studies could include a genetically informative design (e.g., a twin or adoption study design), as these types of studies would be useful in accounting for the interplay between individuals and environmental circumstances.

Furthermore, although we described earlier that the FIM contends that family SES is associated with neighborhood conditions as one aspect of parental investment, our studies did not assess areal characteristics (i.e., neighborhood conditions). Family's socioeconomic resources are likely to largely determine the kind of neighborhood in which they reside [262]. Wealthier parents are expected to reside in areas that have a positive community environment, which provides resources for the developing child, such as parks, good schools, community involvement among residents, and access to conventional friends. Conversely, poor parents are constrained in their choice of neighborhoods. Children reared in neighborhoods without these resources experience a number of negative consequences. Lower income may lead to residing in extremely poor neighborhoods, which are characterized by few resources for child development, such as playgrounds, childcare, health care facilities, and after-school programs. Children who live in areas of disadvantaged neighborhoods tend to have poor physical and mental health [263, 264]. Furthermore, several studies suggest that the affluence of neighborhoods is associated with child outcomes over and above family poverty [265]. Thus, future studies will need to include an assessment of neighborhood quality.

Finally, these findings may not be generalizable to all families, because there is a risk of attrition bias, and the sample was drawn from a limited geographical area in an urban metropolis of Japan. As mentioned earlier, the retention rate from T1 to T2 was 51.6%, and the T2 returning participants tended to be relatively higher in SES than the non-returning participants. This indicates there is a risk of attrition bias. Therefore, there is the possibility that our analyses could not exactly evaluate the mechanism of children with lower SES, and our analyses may underestimate the influence of SES. Furthermore, some characteristics of Japanese society, such as low levels of economic disparity and high education levels among the general population, may have contributed towards the current results. The reproducibility of the current results should be confirmed using data from other regions in a variety of settings. In summary, future research on these topics would benefit from longitudinal designs and samples with higher retention rates (in particular, lower SES participants), and greater demographic and clinical diversity.

Conclusions

Despite the above-mentioned limitations, our findings help advance our understanding of the relationships between different types of SES, marital relationships, parenting styles, and child social competence and behavioral problems. This study highlights the need to simultaneously explore the interrelations between multiple family factors to further our understanding of child mental health functioning.

Emphasis is placed on the importance of examining both family income and educational levels of parents as SES indicators, to elucidate the relationships between family factors and child adjustment. Additionally, consistent with a developmental psychopathology perspective, this study emphasizes the need to explore both positive and negative aspects of family processes (i.e., marital relationships and parenting styles), with a particular focus on the positive dimensions of family functioning. This study also emphasizes social competence as a potential protective factor that prevents later behavioral problems.

The current study advances the understanding of SES, marital conflict, and parenting, utilizing a family systems explanation for child development. (1) This study adds to previous literature concerning the relationship between SES and child mental health outcomes by demonstrating that both family income and parental education levels simultaneously and independently influence child mental health outcomes through marital conflict and parenting practices. In addition, (2) the current study adds to previous literature concerning the relationship between SES and child mental health functioning, by demonstrating the positive pathway where constructive marital conflict was shown to be related to higher levels of affirmative parenting and, in turn, more positive outcomes. The current study supports not only the notion of negative spillover effects, but also of positive spillover effects. In addition, (3) social skills, which were affected by multidimensional family factors (i.e., SES, including family income and parental education levels, and both positive and negative dimensions of family processes), adversely influenced later internalizing and externalizing behaviors. Therefore, our study suggests the possibility that theoretical models, including the FSM, should be included with parental educational levels and positive aspects of family functioning and child outcomes when examining the effects of SES.

These findings offer preliminary evidence for the need to explore SES by including family income and parental educational levels, and both negative and positive aspects of family functioning. They advance our understanding of SES, marital conflict, and parenting practices, using a family systems explanation for child development. Therefore, our results suggest that we should be sensitive to social inequalities in children's mental health problems and developmental outcomes, and strive to reduce social inequalities. In the long-term, it may be necessary to focus not only on economic support, but also on education, as providing equal access to suitable educational opportunities can positively affect the next generation, and is likely to have a more permanent impact on the child-rearing environment than a temporary increase in income. If more parents can become better educated through an improved social system, it might lead to better developmental outcomes for children. In addition, simultaneously focusing on the marital relationship and parenting style in negative and positive domains may be an effective strategy for developing social adjustment among children. The current study suggests that marital relationships and parenting skills in negative and positive domains may be appropriate for interventions promoting social competence among children to prevent later social maladjustment among parents and children who are socioeconomically disadvantaged. Our findings have important clinical and policy implications.

Abbreviations
QCCS: The Quality of Co-parental Communication Scale; APQ: The Alabama Parenting Questionnaire; SSQ: The Social Skills Questionnaire; SDQ: The Strengths and Difficulties Questionnaire.

Authors' contributions
RH designed and managed the study, performed the statistical analyses, and drafted the manuscript. TK administered and supervised the overall conduct of the study. Both authors read and approved the final manuscript.

Author details
[1] School of Nursing, Nagoya City University, Mizuho-cho, Mizuho-ku, Nagoya 467-8601, Japan. [2] Graduate School of Medicine, Kyoto University, Kyoto, Japan.

Acknowledgements
We gratefully acknowledge all the children, parents, and preschool teachers who participated in this study. In addition, we are grateful to the reviewers for their helpful and constructive comments concerning this manuscript.

Competing interests
The authors declare that they have no competing interests.

Funding
This work was supported by JSPS KAKENHI Grant Number 26893224.

References

1. Bradley RH, Corwyn RF. Socioeconomic status and child development. Annu Rev Psychol. 2002;53:371–99. https://doi.org/10.1146/annurev.psych.53.100901.135233.
2. Letourneau NL, Duffett-Leger L, Levac L, Watson B, Young-Morris C. Socioeconomic status and child development: a meta-analysis. J Emot Behav Disord. 2011;21:211–24. https://doi.org/10.1177/1063426611421007.
3. Poulton R, Caspi A, Milne BJ, Thomson WM, Taylor A, Sears MR, et al. Association between children's experience of socioeconomic disadvantage and adult health: a life-course study. Lancet. 2002;360:1640–5. https://doi.org/10.1016/S0140-6736(02)11602-3.
4. Oakes JM, Rossi PH. The measurement of SES in health research: current practice and steps toward a new approach. Soc Sci Med. 2003;56:769–84. https://doi.org/10.1016/S0277-9536(02)00073-4.
5. Haas SA. Health selection and the process of social stratification: the effect of childhood health on socioeconomic attainment. J Health Soc Behav. 2006;47:339–54. https://doi.org/10.1177/002214650604700403.
6. Bøe T, Sivertsen B, Heiervang E, Goodman R, Lundervold AJ, Hysing M. Socioeconomic status and child mental health: the role of parental emotional well-being and parenting practices. J Abnorm Child Psychol. 2014;42:705–15. https://doi.org/10.1007/s10802-013-9818-9.
7. Conger RD, Conger KJ, Martin MJ. Socioeconomic status, family processes, and individual development. J Marriage Fam. 2010;72:685–704. https://doi.org/10.1111/j.1741-3737.2010.00725.x.
8. Castillo J, Welch G, Sarver C. Fathering: the relationship between fathers' residence, fathers' sociodemographic characteristics, and father involvement. Matern Child Health J. 2011;15:1342–9. https://doi.org/10.1007/s10995-010-0684-6.
9. Volling BL, Belsky J. Multiple determinants of father involvement during infancy in dual-earner and single-earner families. J Marriage Fam. 1991;53:461–74. https://doi.org/10.2307/352912.
10. Dearing E, McCartney K, Taylor BA. Change in family income-to-needs matters more for children with less. Child Dev. 2001;72:1779–93. https://doi.org/10.1111/1467-8624.00378.
11. Han W. Maternal nonstandard work schedules and child cognitive outcomes. Child Dev. 2005;76:137–54. https://doi.org/10.1111/j.1467-8624.2005.00835.x.
12. Kohen DE, Brooks-Gunn J, Leventhal T, Hertzman C. Neighborhood income and physical and social disorder in Canada: associations with young children's competencies. Child Dev. 2002;73:1844–60. https://doi.org/10.1111/1467-8624.t01-1-00510.
13. Mills-Koonce WR, Willoughby MT, Garrett-Peters P, Wagner N, Vernon-Feagans L, Family Life Project Key Investigators, The Family Life Project Key Investigators. The interplay among socioeconomic status, household chaos, and parenting in the prediction of child conduct problems and callous-unemotional behaviors. Dev Psychopathol. 2016;28:757–71. https://doi.org/10.1017/S0954579416000298.
14. Schoppe-Sullivan SJ, Schermerhorn AC, Cummings EM. Marital conflict and children's adjustment: evaluation of the parenting process model. J Marriage Fam. 2007;69:1118–34. https://doi.org/10.1111/j.1741-3737.2007.00436.x.
15. Parke RD, Coltrane S, Duffy S, Buriel R, Dennis J, Powers J, et al. Economic stress, parenting, and child adjustment in Mexican American and European American families. Child Dev. 2004;75:1632–56. https://doi.org/10.1111/j.1467-8624.2004.00807.x.
16. Repetti RL, Taylor SE, Seeman TE. Risky families: family social environments and the mental and physical health of offspring. Psychol Bull. 2002;128:330–66. https://doi.org/10.1037/0033-2909.128.2.330.
17. Krishnakumar A, Buehler C. Interparental conflict and parenting behaviors: a meta-analytic review. Fam Relat. 2000;49:25–44. https://doi.org/10.1111/j.1741-3729.2000.00025.x.
18. Sturge-Apple ML, Davies PT, Cummings EM. Impact of hostility and withdrawal in interparental conflict on parental emotional unavailability and children's adjustment difficulties. Child Dev. 2006;77:1623–41. https://doi.org/10.1111/j.1467-8624.2006.00963.x.
19. Gresham FM. Conceptual issues in the assessment of social competence in children. In: Strain P, Guralnick M, Walker H, editors. Children's social behavior: development, assessment, and modification. New York: Academic Press; 1986. p. 143–80.

20. Rubin KH, Rose-Krasnor L. Interpersonal problem solving and social competence in children. In: Van Hasselt VB, Hersen M, editors. Handbook of social development: a lifespan perspective. New York: Plenum; 1992. p. 283–323.

21. Bolger KE, Patterson CJ, Thompson WW, Kupersmidt JB. Psychosocial adjustment among children experiencing persistent and intermittent family economic hardship. Child Dev. 1995;66:1107–29. https://doi.org/10.2307/1131802.

22. Reiss F. Socioeconomic inequalities and mental health problems in children and adolescents: a systematic review. Soc Sci Med. 2013;90:24–31. https://doi.org/10.1016/j.socscimed.2013.04.026.

23. McLoyd VC. Socioeconomic disadvantage and child development. Am Psychol. 1998;53:185–204. https://doi.org/10.1037/0003-066X.53.2.185.

24. Starfield B, Robertson J, Riley AW. Social class gradients and health in childhood. Ambul Pediatr. 2002;2:238–46. https://doi.org/10.1367/1539-4409(2002)002<0238:SCGAHI>2.0.CO;2.

25. Dodge K, Pettit G, Bates J. Socialization mediators of the relation between socioeconomic status and child conduct problems. Child Dev. 1994;65:649–65. https://doi.org/10.2307/1131407.

26. Duncan GJ, Brooks-Gunn J, Klebanov PK. Economic deprivation and early childhood development. Child Dev. 1994;65:296–318. https://doi.org/10.2307/1131385.

27. Raviv T, Kessenich M, Morrison FJ. A mediational model of the association between socioeconomic status and three-year-old language abilities: the role of parenting factors. Early Child Res Q. 2004;19:528–47. https://doi.org/10.1016/j.ecresq.2004.10.007.

28. Conger RD, Donnellan MB. An interactionist perspective on the socioeconomic context of human development. Annu Rev Psychol. 2007;58:175–99. https://doi.org/10.1146/annurev.psych.58.110405.085551.

29. Cutrona CE, Russell DW, Abraham WT, Gardner KA, Melby JN, Bryant C, et al. Neighborhood context and financial strain as predictors of marital interaction and marital quality in African American couples. Pers Relatsh. 2003;10:389–409. https://doi.org/10.1111/1475-6811.00056.

30. Rauer AJ, Karney BR, Garvan CW, Hou W. Relationship risks in context: a cumulative risk approach to understanding relationship satisfaction. J Marriage Fam. 2008;70:1122–35. https://doi.org/10.1111/j.1741-3737.2008.00554.x.

31. Choi H, Marks NF. Marital quality, socioeconomic status, and physical health. J Marriage Fam. 2013;75:903–19. https://doi.org/10.1111/jomf.12044.

32. Gomel JN, Tinsley BJ, Parke RD, Clark KM. The effects of economic hardship on family relationships among African American, Latino, and Euro-American families. J Fam Issues. 1998;19:436–67. https://doi.org/10.1177/019251398019004004.

33. Dietz TL. Disciplining children: characteristics associated with the use of corporal punishment. Child Abuse Negl. 2000;24:1529–42. https://doi.org/10.1016/S0145-2134(00)00213-1.

34. Jansen PW, Raat H, Mackenbach JP, Hofman A, Jaddoe VWV, Bakermans-Kranenburg MJ, et al. Early determinants of maternal and paternal harsh discipline: the generation R study. Fam Relat. 2012;61:253–70. https://doi.org/10.1111/j.1741-3729.2011.00691.x.

35. Hashima PY, Amato PR. Poverty, social support, and parental behavior. Child Dev. 1994;65:394–403. https://doi.org/10.1111/j.1467-8624.1994.tb00758.x.

36. Hart B, Risley TR. American parenting of language-learning children: persisting differences in family-child interactions observed in natural home environments. Dev Psychol. 1992;28:1096–105. https://doi.org/10.1037/0012-1649.28.6.1096.

37. Conger R, Wallace L, Sun Y, Simons R, McLoyd V, Brody G. Economic pressure in African American families: a replication and extension of the family stress model. Dev Psychol. 2002;38:179–93. https://doi.org/10.1037/0012-1649.38.2.179.

38. Conger RD, Conger KJ. Resilience in midwestern families: selected findings from the first decade of a prospective, longitudinal study. J Marriage Fam. 2002;64:361–73. https://doi.org/10.1111/j.1741-3737.2002.00361.x.

39. Cutrona CE, Russell DW, Burzette R, Wesner K, Bryant C. Predicting relationship stability among midlife African American couples. J Consult Clin Psychol. 2011;79:814–25. https://doi.org/10.1037/a0025874.

40. Krieger N, Williams DR, Moss NE. Measuring social class in US public health research: concepts, methodologies, and guidelines. Annu Rev Public Health. 1997;18:341–78. https://doi.org/10.1146/annurev.publhealth.18.1.341.

41. Jefferson AL, Gibbons LE, Rentz DM, Carvalho JO, Manly J, Bennett DA, Jones RN. A life course model of cognitive activities, socioeconomic status, education, reading ability, and cognition. J Am Geriatr Soc. 2011;59:1403–11. https://doi.org/10.1111/j.1532-5415.2011.03499.x.

42. Moretti E. Estimating the social return to higher education: evidence from longitudinal and repeated cross-sectional data. J Econ. 2004;121:175–212. https://doi.org/10.1016/j.jeconom.2003.10.015.

43. Sacerdote B. Peer effects with random assignment: results for Dartmouth roommates. Q J Econ. 2001;116:681–704. https://doi.org/10.1162/00335530151144131.

44. Lewis SK, Ross CE, Mirowsky J. Establishing a sense of personal control in the transition to adulthood. Soc Forces. 1999;77:1573–99. https://doi.org/10.2307/3005887.

45. Gjonça E, Tabassum F, Breeze E. Socioeconomic differences in physical disability at older age. J Epidemiol Commun Health. 2009;63:928–35. https://doi.org/10.1136/jech.2008.082776.

46. Chuang NK, Walker K, Caine-Bish N. Student perceptions of career choices: the impact of academic major. J Fam Consum Sci Educ. 2009;27:18–29.

47. Fujishiro K, Xu J, Gong F. What does "occupation" represent as an indicator of socioeconomic status? Exploring occupational prestige and health. Soc Sci Med. 2010;71:2100–7. https://doi.org/10.1016/j.socscimed.2010.09.026.

48. Becker GS. Human capital: a theoretical and empirical analysis. New York: National Bureau of Economic Research; 1964.

49. Becker GS. A theory of marriage: part II. J Polit Econ. 1974;82:S11–26. https://doi.org/10.1086/260287.

50. Lundberg S, Pollak RA. Efficiency in marriage. Rev Econ Househ. 2003;1:153–67. https://doi.org/10.1023/A:1025041316091.

51. Rossetti S, Tanda P. Human capital, wages and family interactions. Labour. 2000;14:5–34. https://doi.org/10.1111/1467-9914.00122.

52. Huang C, Li H, Liu P, Zhang J. Why does spousal education matter for earnings? Assortative mating and cross-productivity. J Labor Econ. 2009;27:633–52. https://doi.org/10.1086/644746.

53. Tiefenthaler J. The productivity gains of marriage: effects of spousal education on own productivity across market sectors in brazil. Econ Dev Cult Change. 1997;45:633–50. https://doi.org/10.1086/452294.

54. Jepsen LK. The relationship between wife's education and husband's earnings: evidence from 1960–2000. Rev Econ Househ. 2005;3:197–214. https://doi.org/10.1007/s11150-005-0710-4.

55. Lefgren L, McIntyre F. The relationship between women's education and marriage outcomes. J Labor Econ. 2006;24:787–830. https://doi.org/10.1086/506486.

56. Mano Y, Yamamura E. Effects of husband's education and family structure on labor force participation and married Japanese women's earnings. Jpn Econ. 2011;38:71–91. https://doi.org/10.2753/JES1097-203X380303.

57. Benham L. Benefits of women's education within marriage. J Polit Econ. 1974;82:57–71. https://doi.org/10.1086/260291.

58. Mirowsky J, Ross CE. Social causes of psychological distress. 2nd ed. New York: Aldine de Gruyter; 2003.

59. Schudlich T, Norman J, Du Nann B, Wharton A, Block M, Nicol H, Dachenhausen M, Gleason A, Pendergast K. Interparental conflicts in dyadic and triadic contexts: parental depression symptoms and conflict history predict differences. J Child Fam Stud. 2015;2014(24):1047–59. https://doi.org/10.1007/s10826-014-9914-7.

60. Simon RW. Revisiting the relationships among gender, marital status, and mental health. Am J Sociol. 2002;107:1065–96. https://doi.org/10.1086/339205.

61. Dush CMK, Taylor MG, Kroeger RA. Marital happiness and psychological well-being across the life course. Fam Relat. 2008;57:211–26. https://doi.org/10.1111/j.1741-3729.2008.00495.x.

62. Schoen R, Rogers SJ, Amato PR. Wives' employment and spouses' marital happiness: assessing the direction of influence using longitudinal couple data. J Fam Issues. 2006;27:506–28. https://doi.org/10.1177/0192513X05283983.

63. Dakin J, Wampler R. Money doesn't buy happiness, but it helps: marital satisfaction, psychological distress, and demographic differences between low- and middle-income clinic couples. Am J Fam Ther. 2008;36:300–11. https://doi.org/10.1080/01926180701647512.

64. Heaton TB. Factors contributing to increasing marital stability in the United States. J Fam Issues. 2002;23:392–409. https://doi.org/10.1177/0192513X02023003004.

65. Orbuch TL, Veroff J, Hassan H, Horrocks J. Who will divorce: a 14-year longitudinal study of black couples and white couples. J Soc Pers Relatsh. 2002;19:179–202. https://doi.org/10.1177/0265407502192002.

66. Bornstein MH, Hahn C, Suwalsky J, Haynes OM. Socioeconomic status, parenting, and child development: the Hollingshead four-factor index of social status and the socioeconomic index of occupations. In: Bornstein MH, Bradley RH, editors. Socioeconomic status, parenting, and child development. Mahwah: Erlbaum; 2003. p. 29–82.

67. Dix T. The affective organization of parenting: adaptive and maladaptive processes. Psychol Bull. 1991;110:3–25. https://doi.org/10.1037/0033-2909.110.1.3.

68. Cox MJ, Paley B. Families as systems. Annu Rev Psychol. 1997;48:243–67. https://doi.org/10.1146/annurev.psych.48.1.243.

69. Feldman MA, Varghese J, Ramsay J, Rajska D. Relationship between social support, stress and mother–child interactions in mothers with intellectual disabilities. J Appl Res Intellect Disabil. 2002;15:314–23. https://doi.org/10.1046/j.1468-3148.2002.00132.x.

70. Sobolewski JM, Amato PR. Economic hardship in the family of origin and children's psychological well-being in adulthood. J Marriage Fam. 2005;67:141–56. https://doi.org/10.1111/j.0022-2445.2005.00011.x.

71. Brassell AA, Rosenberg E, Parent J, Rough JN, Fondacaro K, Seehuus M. Parent's psychological flexibility: associations with parenting and child psychosocial well-being. J Contextual Behav Sci. 2016;5:111–20. https://doi.org/10.1016/j.jcbs.2016.03.001.

72. Morawska A, Winter L, Sanders MR. Parenting knowledge and its role in the prediction of dysfunctional parenting and disruptive child behaviour. Child Care Health Dev. 2009;35:217–26. https://doi.org/10.1111/j.1365-2214.2008.00929.x.

73. Waylen A, Stewart-Brown S. Factors influencing parenting in early childhood: a prospective longitudinal study focusing on change. Child Care Health Dev. 2010;36:198–207. https://doi.org/10.1111/j.1365-2214.2009.01037.x.

74. Bradley RH, Caldwell BM. Caregiving and the regulation of child growth and development: describing proximal aspects of caregiving systems. Dev Rev. 1995;15:38–85. https://doi.org/10.1006/drev.1995.1002.

75. Barber B, Stolz H, Olsen J, Collins A, Burchinal M. Parental support, psychological control, and behavioral control: assessing relevance across time, culture, and method: abstract. Monogr Soc Res Child Dev. 2005;70:135–7. https://doi.org/10.1111/j.1540-5834.2005.00365.x.

76. Dallaire DH, Weinraub M. The stability of parenting behaviors over the first 6 years of life. Early Child Res Q. 2005;20:201–19. https://doi.org/10.1016/j.ecresq.2005.04.008.

77. Waylen A, Stallard N, Stewart-Brown S. Parenting and health in midchildhood: a longitudinal study. Eur J Public Health. 2008;18:300–5. https://doi.org/10.1093/eurpub/ckm131.

78. Blair SL, Wenk D, Hardesty C. Marital quality and paternal involvement: interconnections of men's spousal and parental roles. J Mens Stud. 1994;2:221–37. https://doi.org/10.3149/jms.0203.221.

79. King V, Harris KM, Heard HE. Racial and ethnic diversity in nonresident father involvement. J Marriage Fam. 2004;66:1–21. https://doi.org/10.1111/j.1741-3737.2004.00001.x.

80. Lerman R, Sorensen E. Father involvement with their nonmarital children: patterns, determinants, and effects on their earnings. Marriage Fam Rev. 2000;29:137–58. https://doi.org/10.1300/J002v29n02_09.

81. Engfer A. The interrelatedness of marriage and the mother–child relationship. In: Hinde RA, Stevenson-Hinde J, editors. Relationships within families: mutual influences. Oxford: Clarendon Press; 1988. p. 104–18.

82. Cox MJ, Paley B. Understanding families as systems. Curr Dir Psychol Sci. 2003;12:193–6. https://doi.org/10.1111/1467-8721.01259.

83. Rinaldi CM, Howe N. Perceptions of constructive and destructive conflict within and across family subsystems. Infant Child Dev. 2003;12:441–59. https://doi.org/10.1002/icd.324.

84. Cummings EM, Goeke-Morey M, Papp L. Children's responses to everyday marital conflict tactics in the home. Child Dev. 2003;74:1918–29. https://doi.org/10.1046/j.1467-8624.2003.00646.x.

85. Goeke-Morey MC, Cummings EM, Harold GT, Shelton KH. Categories and continua of destructive and constructive marital conflict tactics from the perspective of US and Welsh children. J Fam Psychol. 2003;17:327–38. https://doi.org/10.1037/0893-3200.17.3.327.

86. Coln KL, Jordan SS, Mercer SH. A unified model exploring parenting practices as mediators of marital conflict and children's adjustment. Child Psychiatry Hum Dev. 2013;44:419–29. https://doi.org/10.1007/s10578-012-0336-8.

87. McCoy KP, George MRW, Cummings EM, Davies PT. Constructive and destructive marital conflict, parenting, and children's school and social adjustment. Soc Dev. 2013;22:641–62. https://doi.org/10.1111/sode.12015.

88. Du Rocher schudlich TD, Cummings EM. Parental dysphoria and childrens internalizing symptoms: marital conflict styles as mediators of risk. Child Dev. 2003;74:1663–81. https://doi.org/10.1046/j.1467-8624.2003.00630.x.

89. Elliott SN, Busse RT. Social skills assessment and intervention with children and adolescents: guidelines for assessment and training procedures. Sch Psychol Int. 1991;12:63–83. https://doi.org/10.1177/0143034391121006.

90. Gresham FM, Elliott SN. Social skills rating system. Circle Pines: American Guidance Service; 1990.

91. Sheridan SM, Walker D. Social skills in context: considerations for assessment, intervention, and generalization. In: Reynolds CR, Gutkin TB, editors. The handbook of school psychology. 3rd ed. New York: Wiley; 1999. p. 686–708.

92. Birch SH, Ladd GW. The teacher–child relationship and children's early school adjustment. J Sch Psychol. 1997;35:61–79. https://doi.org/10.1016/S0022-4405(96)00029-5.

93. Birch SH, Ladd GW. Children's interpersonal behaviors and the teacher-child relationship. Dev Psychol. 1998;34:934–46. https://doi.org/10.1037/0012-1649.34.5.934.

94. Hamre BK, Pianta RC. Early teacher–child relationships and the trajectory of children's school outcomes through eighth grade. Child Dev. 2001;72:625–38. https://doi.org/10.1111/1467-8624.00301.

95. Ladd GW, Burgess KB. Do relational risks and protective factors moderate the linkages between childhood aggression and early psychological and school adjustment? Child Dev. 2001;72:1579–601. https://doi.org/10.1111/1467-8624.00366.

96. Mischel W, Shoda Y, Peake PK. The nature of adolescent competencies predicted by preschool delay of gratification. J Pers Soc Psychol. 1988;54:687–96. https://doi.org/10.1037/0022-3514.54.4.687.

97. Parker JG, Asher SR. Peer relations and later personal adjustment: are low-accepted children at risk? Psychol Bull. 1987;102:357–89. https://doi.org/10.1037/0033-2909.102.3.357.

98. Coie JD, Dodge KA. Multiple sources of data on social behavior and social status in the school: a cross-age comparison. Child Dev. 1988;59:815–29. https://doi.org/10.1111/j.1467-8624.1988.tb03237.x.

99. Eisenberg N, Fabes R. Prosocial development. In: Damon W, Eisenberg N, editors. Handbook of child psychology. Social, emotional, and personality development, vol. 3. 5th ed. New York: Wiley; 1998. p. 701–78.

100. McClelland MM, Morrison FJ. The emergence of learning-related social skills in preschool children. Early Child Res Q. 2003;18:206–24. https://doi.org/10.1016/S0885-2006(03)00026-7.

101. Campbell S. Hard-to-manage preschool boys: externalizing behavior, social competence, and family context at 2-year follow-up. J Abnorm Child Psychol. 1994;22:147–66. https://doi.org/10.1007/BF02167897.

102. Olson S, Hoza B. Preschool development antecedents of conduct problems in children beginning school. J Clin Child Psychol. 1993;22:60–7. https://doi.org/10.1207/s15374424jccp2201_6.

103. Achenbach TM, Howell CT, Quay HC, Conners CK. National survey of problems and competencies among four- to sixteen-year-olds: parents' reports for normative and clinical samples. Monogr Soc Res Child Dev. 1991;56:1–131. https://doi.org/10.2307/1166156.

104. Allen K, Prior M. Assessment of the validity of easy and difficult temperament through observed mother–child behaviours. Int J Behav Dev. 1995;18:609–30. https://doi.org/10.1177/016502549501800403.

105. Bates J. Conceptual and empirical linkages between temperament and behavior problems: a commentary on the Sanson, Prior, and Kyrios study. Merrill Palmer Q. 1990;36:193–9.

106. Campbell SB. Behavior problems in preschool children: a review of recent research. J Child Psychol Psychiatry. 1995;36:113–49. https://doi.org/10.1111/j.1469-7610.1995.tb01657.x.

107. Campbell SB, Pierce EW, March CL, Ewing LJ, Szumowski EK. Hard-to-manage preschool boys: symptomatic behavior across contexts and time. Child Dev. 1994;65:836–51. https://doi.org/10.1111/j.1467-8624.1994.tb00787.x.

108. Caspi A, Henry B, McGee RO, Moffitt TE, Silva PA. Temperamental origins of child and adolescent behavior problems: from age three to age fifteen. Child Dev. 1995;66:55–68. https://doi.org/10.1111/j.1467-8624.1995.tb00855.x.

109. Caron C, Rutter M. Comorbidity in child psychopathology: concepts, issues and research strategies. J Child Psychol Psychiatry. 1991;32:1063–80. https://doi.org/10.1111/j.1469-7610.1991.tb00350.x.

110. Mathiesen KS, Sanson A. Dimensions of early childhood behavior problems: stability and predictors of change from 18 to 30 months. J Abnorm Child Psychol. 2000;28:15–31. https://doi.org/10.1023/A:1005165916906.

111. Kerr M, Tremblay RE, Pagani L, Vitaro F. Boys' behavioral inhibition and the risk of later delinquency. Arch Gen Psychiatry. 1997;54:809–16. https://doi.org/10.1001/archpsyc.1997.01830210049005.

112. Panak WF, Garber J. Role of aggression, rejection, and attributions in the prediction of depression in children. Dev Psychopathol. 1992;4:145–65. https://doi.org/10.1017/S0954579400005617.

113. Lahey BB, Loeber R, Burke J, Rathouz PJ, McBurnett K. Waxing and waning in concert: dynamic comorbidity of conduct disorder with other disruptive and emotional problems over 7 years among clinic-referred boys. J Abnorm Psychol. 2002;111:556–67. https://doi.org/10.1037/0021-843X.111.4.556.

114. Loeber R, Keenan K. Interaction between conduct disorder and its comorbid conditions: effects of age and gender. Clin Psychol Rev. 1994;14:497–523. https://doi.org/10.1016/0272-7358(94)90015-9.

115. Verhulst FC, Eussen ML, Berden GF, Sanders-Woudstra J, van der Ende J. Pathways of problem behaviors from childhood to adolescence. J Am Acad Child Adolesc Psychiatry. 1993;32:388–96. https://doi.org/10.1097/00004583-199303000-00021.

116. Pine DS, Cohen E, Cohen P, Brook JS. Social phobia and the persistence of conduct problems. J Child Psychol Psychiatry. 2000;41:657–65. https://doi.org/10.1017/S0021963099005764.

117. Lansford JE, Malone PS, Stevens KI, Dodge KA, Bates JE, Pettit GS. Developmental trajectories of externalizing and internalizing behaviors: factors underlying resilience in physically abused children. Dev Psychopathol. 2006;18:35–55. https://doi.org/10.1017/S0954579406000332.

118. Mesman J, Bongers IL, Koot HM. Preschool developmental pathways to preadolescent internalizing and externalizing problems. J Child Psychol Psychiatry. 2001;42:679–89. https://doi.org/10.1111/1469-7610.00763.

119. Olson SL, Brodfeld PL. Assessment of peer rejection and externalizing behavior problems in preschool boys: a short-term longitudinal study. J Abnorm Child Psychol. 1991;19:493–503. https://doi.org/10.1007/BF00919091.

120. Gazelle H, Ladd GW. Anxious solitude and peer exclusion: a diathesis-stress model of internalizing trajectories in childhood. Child Dev. 2003;74:257–78. https://doi.org/10.1111/1467-8624.00534.

121. Larson RW, Raffaelli M, Richards MH, Ham M, Jewell L. Ecology of depression in late childhood and early adolescence: a profile of daily states and activities. J Abnorm Psychol. 1990;99:92–102. https://doi.org/10.1037/0021-843X.99.1.92.

122. Hymel S, Rubin KH, Rowden L, LeMare L. Children's peer relationships: longitudinal prediction of internalizing and externalizing problems from middle to late childhood. Child Dev. 1990;61:2004–21. https://doi.org/10.2307/1130854.

123. Cole DA, Martin JM, Powers B, Truglio R. Modeling causal relations between academic and social competence and depression: a multi-trait-multimethod longitudinal study of children. J Abnorm Psychol. 1996;105:258–70. https://doi.org/10.1037/0021-843X.105.2.258.

124. Dalley MB, Bolocofsky DN, Karlin NJ. Teacher-ratings and self-ratings of social competency in adolescents with low- and high-depressive

125. symptoms. J Abnorm Child Psychol. 1994;22:477–85. https://doi.org/10.1007/BF02168086.

125. Obradovic J, Burt KB, Masten AS. Testing a dual cascade model linking competence and symptoms over 20 years from childhood to adulthood. J Clin Child Adolesc Psychol. 2010;39:90–102. https://doi.org/10.1080/15374410903401120.

126. Coie J, Terry R, Lenox K, Lochman J, Hyman C. Childhood peer rejection and aggression as predictors of stable patterns of adolescent disorder. Dev Psychopathol. 1995;7:697–713. https://doi.org/10.1017/S0954579400006799.

127. Crijnen AA, Achenbach TM, Verhulst FC. Comparisons of problems reported by parents of children in 12 cultures: total problems, externalizing, and internalizing. J Am Acad Child Adolesc Psychiatry. 1997;36:1269–77. https://doi.org/10.1097/00004583-199709000-00020.

128. Fanti KA, Panayiotou G, Fanti S. Associating parental to child psychological symptoms: investigating a transactional model of development. J Emot Behav Disord. 2013;21:193–210. https://doi.org/10.1177/1063426611432171.

129. Rescorla L, Achenbach TM, Ivanova MY, Dumenci L, Almqvist F, Bilenberg N, et al. Epidemiological comparisons of problems and positive qualities reported by adolescents in 24 countries. J Consult Clin Psychol. 2007;75:351–8. https://doi.org/10.1037/0022-006X.75.2.351.

130. Benenson JF, Markovits H, Roy R, Denko P. Behavioural rules underlying learning to share: effects of development and context. Int J Behav Dev. 2003;27:116–21. https://doi.org/10.1080/01650250244000119.

131. Dunn J, Cutting AL. Understanding others, and individual differences in friendship interactions in young children. Soc Dev. 1999;8:201–19. https://doi.org/10.1111/1467-9507.00091.

132. Göncü A. Development of intersubjectivity in the dyadic play of preschoolers. Early Child Res Q. 1993;8:99–116. https://doi.org/10.1016/S0885-2006(05)80100-0.

133. Watson AC, Nixon CL, Wilson A, Capage L. Social interaction skills and theory of mind in young children. Dev Psychol. 1999;35:386–91. https://doi.org/10.1037/0012-1649.35.2.386.

134. Cole PM, Teti LO, Zahn-Waxler C. Mutual emotion regulation and the stability of conduct problems between preschool and early school age. Dev Psychopathol. 2003;15:1–18. https://doi.org/10.1017/S0954579403000014.

135. Stright AD, Gallagher KC, Kelley K. Infant temperament moderates relations between maternal parenting in early childhood and children's adjustment in first grade. Child Dev. 2008;79:186–200. https://doi.org/10.1111/j.1467-8624.2007.01119.x.

136. Eisenberg N, Fabes RA, Spinrad TL. Prosocial development. In: Eisenberg N, Damon W, Lerner RM, editors. Handbook of child psychology, Social, emotional, and personality development, vol. 3. 6th ed. Hoboken: Wiley; 2006. p. 646–718.

137. NICHD Early Child Care Research Network. Early child care and children's development prior to school entry: results from the NICHD study of early child care. Am Educ Res J. 2002;39:133–64. https://doi.org/10.3102/00028312039001133.

138. Vazsonyi AT, Huang L. Where self-control comes from: on the development of self-control and its relationship to deviance over time. Dev Psychol. 2010;46:245–57. https://doi.org/10.1037/a0016538.

139. Tichovolsky MH, Arnold DH, Baker CN. Parent predictors of changes in child behavior problems. J Appl Dev Psychol. 2013;34:336–45. https://doi.org/10.1016/j.appdev.2013.09.001.

140. Parke RD, Buriel R. Socialisation in the family: ethnic and ecological perspective. In: Damon W, Eisenberg N, editors. Handbook of child psychology. Social, emotional and personality development, vol. 3. 5th ed. New York: Wiley; 1998. p. 463–552.

141. Masten A, Coatsworth J. The development of competence in favorable and unfavorable environments: lessons from research on successful children. Am Psychol. 1998;53:205–20. https://doi.org/10.1037/0003-066X.53.2.205.

142. Zhou Q, Eisenberg N, Losoya SH, Fabes RA, Reiser M, Guthrie IK, et al. The relations of parental warmth and positive expressiveness to children's empathy-related responding and social functioning: a longitudinal study. Child Dev. 2002;73:893–915.

143. Barnett MA, Gustafsson H, Deng M, Mills-Koonce WR, Cox M. Bidirectional associations among sensitive parenting, language development,

and social competence. Infant Child Dev. 2012;21:374–93. https://doi.org/10.1002/icd.1750.

144. Finger B, Eiden RD, Edwards EP, Leonard KE, Kachadourian L. Marital aggression and child peer competence: a comparison of three conceptual models. Pers Relatsh. 2010;17:357–76. https://doi.org/10.1111/j.1475-6811.2010.01284.x.

145. El-Sheikh M, Buckhalt J, Mize J, Acebo C. Marital conflict and disruption of children's sleep. Child Dev. 2006;77:31–43. https://doi.org/10.1111/j.1467-8624.2006.00854.x.

146. Cummings EM, Goeke-Morey MC, Papp LM. Everyday marital conflict and child aggression. J Abnorm Child Psychol. 2004;32:191–202. https://doi.org/10.1023/B:JACP.0000019770.13216.be.

147. Grych JH, Fincham FD. Children's appraisals of marital conflict: initial investigations of the cognitive-contextual framework. Child Dev. 1993;64:215–30. https://doi.org/10.2307/1131447.

148. Goodman SH, Barfoot B, Frye AA, Belli AM. Dimensions of marital conflict and children's social problem-solving skills. J Fam Psychol. 1999;13:33–45. https://doi.org/10.1037/0893-3200.13.1.33.

149. Grych JH, Fincham FD. Marital conflict and children's adjustment: a cognitive-contextual framework. Psychol Bull. 1990;108:267–90. https://doi.org/10.1037/0033-2909.108.2.267.

150. McCoy K, Cummings EM, Davies PT. Constructive and destructive marital conflict, emotional security and children's prosocial behavior. J Child Psychol Psychiatry. 2009;50:270–9. https://doi.org/10.1111/j.1469-7610.2008.01945.x.

151. Lengua LJ, Honorado E, Bush NR. Contextual risk and parenting as predictors of effortful control and social competence in preschool children. J Appl Dev Psychol. 2007;28:40–55. https://doi.org/10.1016/j.appdev.2006.10.001.

152. Ahrons CR. The continuing coparental relationship between divorced spouses. Am J Orthopsychiatry. 1981;51:415–28. https://doi.org/10.1111/j.1939-0025.1981.tb01390.x.

153. Ahrons CR, Tanner JL. Adult children and their fathers: relationship changes 20 years after parental divorce. Fam Relat. 2003;52:340–51. https://doi.org/10.1111/j.1741-3729.2003.00340.x.

154. Bonach K, Sales E, Koeske G. Gender differences in perceptions of coparenting quality among expartners. J Divorce Remarriage. 2005;43:1–28. https://doi.org/10.1300/J087v43n01_01.

155. Frick PJ. The Alabama parenting questionnaire. Alabama: University of Alabama; 1991.

156. Shelton KK, Frick PJ, Wootton J. Assessment of parenting practices in families of elementary school-age children. J Clin Child Psychol. 1996;25:317–29. https://doi.org/10.1207/s15374424jccp2503_8.

157. Frick PJ, Dantagnan AL. Predicting the stability of conduct problems in children with and without callous-unemotional traits. J Child Fam Stud. 2005;14:469–85. https://doi.org/10.1007/s10826-005-7183-1.

158. Anme T, Shinohara R, Sugisawa Y, Tanaka E, Watanabe T, Hoshino T. Validity and reliability of the Social Skill Scale (SSS) as an index of social competence for preschool children. J Health Sci. 2013;3:5–11. https://doi.org/10.5923/j.health.20130301.02.

159. Takahashi Y, Okada K, Hoshino T, Anme T. Social skills of preschoolers: stability of factor structures and predictive validity from a nationwide cohort study in Japan. Jpn J Educ Psychol. 2008;56:81–92. https://doi.org/10.5926/jjep1953.56.1_81.

160. Takahashi Y, Okada K, Hoshino T, Anme T. Developmental trajectories of social skills during early childhood and links to parenting practices in a Japanese sample. PLoS ONE. 2015;10:e0135357. https://doi.org/10.1371/journal.pone.0135357.

161. Burt KB, Roisman GI. Competence and psychopathology: cascade effects in the NICHD study of early child care and youth development. Dev Psychopathol. 2010;22:557–67. https://doi.org/10.1017/S0954579410000271.

162. NICHD Early Child Care Research Network. Fathers' and mothers' parenting behavior and beliefs as predictors of children's social adjustment in the transition to school. J Fam Psychol. 2004;18:628–38. https://doi.org/10.1037/0893-3200.18.4.628.

163. Goodman R. The strengths and difficulties questionnaire: a research note. J Child Psychol Psychiatry. 1997;38:581–6. https://doi.org/10.1111/j.1469-7610.1997.tb01545.x.

164. Goodman R. The extended version of the Strengths and Difficulties Questionnaire as a guide to child psychiatric caseness and consequent burden. J Child Psychol Psychiatry. 1999;40:791–9. https://doi.org/10.1111/1469-7610.00494.

165. Goodman R, Ford T, Simmons H, Gatward R, Meltzer H. Using the Strengths and Difficulties Questionnaire (SDQ) to screen for child psychiatric disorders in a community sample. Int Rev Psychiatry. 2003;15:166–72. https://doi.org/10.1080/0954026021000046128.

166. Matsuishi T, Nagano M, Araki Y, Tanaka Y, Iwasaki M, Yamashita Y, et al. Scale properties of the Japanese version of the Strengths and Difficulties Questionnaire (SDQ): a study of infant and school children in community samples. Brain Dev. 2008;30:410–5. https://doi.org/10.1016/j.braindev.2007.12.003.

167. Goodman A, Lamping DL, Ploubidis GB. When to use broader internalising and externalising subscales instead of the hypothesised five subscales on the Strengths and Difficulties Questionnaire (SDQ): data from British parents, teachers and children. J Abnorm Child Psychol. 2010;38:1179–91. https://doi.org/10.1007/s10802-010-9434-x.

168. Bentler PM. Comparative fit indexes in structural models. Psychol Bull. 1990;107:238–46. https://doi.org/10.1037/0033-2909.107.2.238.

169. Bollen KA. Overall fit in covariance structure models: two types of sample size effects. Psychol Bull. 1990;107:256–9. https://doi.org/10.1037/0033-2909.107.2.256.

170. Steiger JH. Structural model evaluation and modification: an interval estimation approach. Multivariate Behav Res. 1990;25:173–80. https://doi.org/10.1207/s15327906mbr2502_4.

171. Byrne BM. Structural equation modeling with LISREL, PRELIS, and SIMPLIS: basic concepts, applications, and programming. Mahwah: Lawrence Erlbaum Associates; 1998.

172. Yeung WJ, Linver MR, Brooks-Gunn JB. How money matters for young children's development: parental investment and family processes. Child Dev. 2002;73:1861–79. https://doi.org/10.1111/1467-8624.t01-1-00511.

173. Conger RD, Dogan SJ. Social class and socialization in families. In: Grusec J, Hastings P, editors. Handbook of socialization: theory and research. New York: Guilford; 2007. p. 433–60.

174. Linver MR, Brooks-Gunn J, Kohen D. Family processes as pathways from income to young children's development. Dev Psychol. 2002;38:719–34.

175. Becker GS, Tomes N. Human capital and the rise and fall of families. J Labor Econ. 1986;4:1–47. https://doi.org/10.1086/298118.

176. Mayer S. What money can't buy: family income and children's life chances. Cambridge: Harvard University Press; 1997.

177. Brown JE, Mann L. The relationship between family structure and process variables and adolescent decision making. J Adolesc. 1990;13:25–37. https://doi.org/10.1016/0140-1971(90)90039-A.

178. Van der Slik FWP, De Graaf ND, Gerris JRM. Conformity to parental rules: asymmetric influences of father's and mother's levels of education. Eur Sociol Rev. 2002;18:489–502. https://doi.org/10.1093/esr/18.4.489.

179. Fulmer KA. Parents' decision-making strategies when selecting child care: effects of parental awareness, experience, and education. Child Youth Care Forum. 1997;26:391–409. https://doi.org/10.1007/BF02589503.

180. Klebanov PK, Brooks-Gunn J, Duncan GJ. Does neighborhood and family poverty affect mothers' parenting, mental health, and social support? J Marriage Fam. 1994;56:441–55. https://doi.org/10.2307/353111.

181. Belsky J, Crnic K, Gable S. The determinants of coparenting in families with toddler boys: spousal differences and daily hassles. Child Dev. 1995;66:629–42. https://doi.org/10.2307/1131939.

182. McHale JP. Coparenting and triadic interactions during infancy: the roles of marital distress and child gender. Dev Psychol. 1995;31:985–96. https://doi.org/10.1037/0012-1649.31.6.985.

183. Barkin S, Scheindlin B, Ip E, Richardson I, Finch S. Determinants of parental discipline practices: a national sample from primary care practices. Clin Pediatr (Phila). 2007;46:64–9. https://doi.org/10.1177/0069922806292644.

184. Frías-Armenta M, McCloskey LA. Determinants of harsh parenting in Mexico. J Abnorm Child Psychol. 1998;26:129–39. https://doi.org/10.1023/A:1022621922331.

185. Jackson S, Thompson RA, Christiansen EH, Colman RA, Wyat J, Buckendahl CW, et al. Predicting abuse-prone parental attitudes and discipline practices in a nationally representative sample. Child Abuse Negl. 1999;23:15–29. https://doi.org/10.1016/S0145-2134(98)00108-2.

186. Tamis-LeMonda CS, Shannon JD, Cabrera NJ, Lamb ME. Fathers and mothers at play with their 2- and 3-year-olds: contributions to language and cognitive development. Child Dev. 2004;75:1806–20. https://doi.org/10.1111/j.1467-8624.2004.00818.x.

187. Bornstein MH, Bradley RH, editors. Socioeconomic status, parenting, and child development. Mahwah: Erlbaum; 2003.

188. Huston AC, Rosenkrantz Aronson S. Mothers' time with infant and time in employment as predictors of mother–child relationships and children's early development. Child Dev. 2005;76:467–82. https://doi.org/10.1111/j.1467-8624.2005.00857.x.

189. Sohr-Preston SL, Scaramella LV, Martin MJ, Neppl TK, Ontai L, Conger R. Parental socioeconomic status, communication, and children's vocabulary development: a third-generation test of the family investment model. Child Dev. 2013;84:1046–62. https://doi.org/10.1111/cdev.12023.

190. Hoff E. The specificity of environmental influence: socioeconomic status affects early vocabulary development via maternal speech. Child Dev. 2003;74:1368–78. https://doi.org/10.1111/1467-8624.00612.

191. Guo G, Harris KM. The mechanisms mediating the effects of poverty on children's intellectual development. Demography. 2000;37:431–47. https://doi.org/10.1353/dem.2000.0005.

192. Bradley RH, Corwyn RF. Age and ethnic variations in family process mediators of SES. In: Bornstein MH, Bradley RH, editors. Socioeconomic status, parenting, and child development. Mahwah: Erlbaum; 2003. p. 161–88.

193. John A, Halliburton A, Humphrey J. Child–mother and child–father play interaction patterns with preschoolers. Early Child Dev Care. 2013;183:483–97. https://doi.org/10.1080/03004430.2012.711595.

194. Carson JL, Burks VM, Parke RD. Parent-child physical play: determinants and consequences. In: MacDonald KB, editor. Parent–child play. Albany: SUNY Press; 1993. p. 197–220.

195. Kerns K, Barth JM. Attachment and play: convergence across components of parent–child relationships and their relations to peer competence. J Soc Pers Relatsh. 1995;12:243–60. https://doi.org/10.1177/0265407595122006.

196. Lindsey EW, Mize J, Pettit GS. Mutuality in parent–child play: consequences for children's peer competence. J Soc Pers Relatsh. 1997;14:523–38. https://doi.org/10.1177/0265407597144007.

197. Barth JM, Parke RD. Parent–child relationship influences on children's transition to school. Merrill-Palmer Q. 1993;39:173–95.

198. Carson JL, Parke RD. Reciprocal negative affect in parent–child interactions and children's peer competency. Child Dev. 1996;67:2217–26. https://doi.org/10.2307/1131619.

199. Sandseter EBH. 'It tickles in my tummy!' Understanding children's risk-taking in play through reversal theory. J Early Child Res. 2010;8:67–88. https://doi.org/10.1177/1476718x09345393.

200. Flanders JL, Leo V, Paquette D, Pihl RO, Séguin JR. Rough-and-tumble play and the regulation of aggression: an observational study of father–child play dyads. Aggress Behav. 2009;35:285–95. https://doi.org/10.1002/ab.20309.

201. Flanders J, Simard M, Paquette D, Parent S, Vitaro F, Pihl R, et al. Rough-and-tumble play and the development of physical aggression and emotion regulation: a five-year follow-up study. J Fam Violence. 2010;25:357–67. https://doi.org/10.1007/s10896-009-9297-5.

202. Fletcher R, StGeorge J, Freeman E. Rough and tumble play quality: theoretical foundations for a new measure of father–child interaction. Early Child Dev Care. 2013;183:746–59. https://doi.org/10.1080/03004430.2012.72343.

203. Martin A, Ryan RM, Brooks-Gunn J. When fathers' supportiveness matters most: maternal and paternal parenting and children's school readiness. J Fam Psychol. 2010;24:145–55. https://doi.org/10.1037/a0018073.

204. Augustine JM, Cavanagh SE, Crosnoe R. Maternal education, early child care and the reproduction of advantage. Soc Forces. 2009;88:1–29. https://doi.org/10.1353/sof.0.0233.

205. Stams GJ, Juffer F, van IJzendoorn MH. Maternal sensitivity, infant attachment, and temperament in early childhood predict adjustment in middle childhood: the case of adopted children and their biologically unrelated parents. Dev Psychol. 2002;38:806–21. https://doi.org/10.1037/0012-1649.38.5.806.

206. Snow C. Enhancing literacy development: programs and research perspectives. Malden: Blackwell Publishing; 1994.

207. Whitehurst GJ, Fischel JE. Practitioner review: early developmental language delay: what, if anything, should the clinician do about it? J Child Psychol Psychiatry. 1994;35:613–48. https://doi.org/10.1111/j.1469-7610.1994.tb01210.x.

208. Guralnick M. Family and child influences on the peer-related social competence of young children with developmental delays. Ment Retard Dev Disabil Res Rev. 1999;5:21–9. https://doi.org/10.1002/(SICI)1098-2779(1999)5:13.3.CO;2-F.

209. Cummings EM, Davies PT. Effects of marital conflict on children: recent advances and emerging themes in process-oriented research. J Child Psychol Psychiatry. 2002;43:31–63. https://doi.org/10.1111/1469-7610.00003.

210. Grych JH, Fincham FD, Jouriles EN, McDonald R. Interparental conflict and child adjustment: testing the mediational role of appraisals in the cognitive-contextual framework. Child Dev. 2000;71:1648–61. https://doi.org/10.1111/1467-8624.00255.

211. El-Sheikh M, Elmore-Staton L. The link between marital conflict and child adjustment: parent-child conflict and perceived attachments as mediators, potentiators, and mitigators of risk. Dev Psychopathol. 2004;16:631–48. https://doi.org/10.1017/S0954579404004705.

212. Camisasca E, Miragoli S, Di Blasio P. Families with distinct levels of marital conflict and child adjustment: which role for maternal and paternal stress? J Child Fam Stud. 2016;2015(25):733–45. https://doi.org/10.1007/s10826-015-0261-0.

213. Marks CR, Glaser BA, Glass JB, Horne AM. Effects of witnessing severe marital discord on children's social competence and behavioral problems. Fam J. 2001;9:94–101. https://doi.org/10.1177/1066480701092002.

214. McCloskey LA, Stuewig J. The quality of peer relationships among children exposed to family violence. Dev Psychopathol. 2001;13:83–96. https://doi.org/10.1017/S0954579401001067.

215. Schudlich TDDR, Shamir H, Cummings EM. Marital conflict, children's representations of family relationships, and childrens dispositions towards peer conflict strategies. Soc Dev. 2004;13:171–92. https://doi.org/10.1111/j.1467-9507.2004.000262.x.

216. Dadds MR, Atkinson E, Turner C, Blums GJ, Lendich B. Family conflict and child adjustment: evidence for a cognitive-contextual model of intergenerational transmission. J Fam Psychol. 1999;13:194–208. https://doi.org/10.1037/0893-3200.13.2.194.

217. Bandura A. Self-efficacy: toward a unifying theory of behavioral change. Psychol Rev. 1977;84:191–215. https://doi.org/10.1037/0033-295X.84.2.191.

218. Frankel LA, Hughes SO, O'Connor TM, Power TG, Fisher JO, Hazen NL. Parental influences on children's self-regulation of energy intake: insights from developmental literature on emotion regulation. J Obes. 2012;2012:327259. https://doi.org/10.1155/2012/327259.

219. Hovell MF, Schumaker JB, Sherman JA. A comparison of parents' models and expansions in promoting children's acquisition of adjectives. J Exp Child Psychol. 1978;25:41–57. https://doi.org/10.1016/0022-0965(78)90037-1.

220. Rubin KH, Hastings P, Chen X, Stewart S, McNichol K. Intrapersonal and maternal correlates of aggression, conflict, and externalizing problems in toddlers. Child Dev. 1998;69:1614–29. https://doi.org/10.2307/1132135.

221. Cassidy J, Parke RD, Butkovsky L, Braungart JM. Family-peer connections: the roles of emotional expressiveness within the family and children's understanding of emotions. Child Dev. 1992;63:603–18. https://doi.org/10.2307/1131349.

222. Brody GH, Henderson RW. Effects of multiple model variations and rationale provision on the moral judgments and explanations of young children. Child Dev. 1977;48:1117–20. https://doi.org/10.2307/1128372.

223. Najaka SS, Gottfredson DC, Wilson DB. A meta-analytic inquiry into the relationship between selected risk factors and problem behavior. Prev Sci. 2001;2:257–71. https://doi.org/10.1023/A:1013610115351.

224. Rose-Krasnor L. The nature of social competence: a theoretical review. Soc Dev. 1997;6:111–35. https://doi.org/10.1111/j.1467-9507.1997.tb00097.x.

225. Han SS, Weisz JR, Weiss B. Specificity of relations between children's control-related beliefs and internalizing and externalizing psychopathology. J Consult Clin Psychol. 2001;69:240–51.

226. Shonk S, Cicchetti D. Maltreatment, competency deficits, and risk for academic and behavioral maladjustment. Dev Psychol. 2001;37:3–17. https://doi.org/10.1037/0012-1649.37.1.3.

227. Ladd GW. Peer relationships and social competence during early and middle childhood. Annu Rev Psychol. 1999;50:333–59. https://doi.org/10.1146/annurev.psych.50.1.333.

228. Ladd GW, Kochenderfer BJ, Coleman CC. Friendship quality as a predictor of young children's early school adjustment. Child Dev. 1996;67:1103–18. https://doi.org/10.2307/1131882.

229. Bornstein MH, Hahn C, Haynes OM. Social competence, externalizing, and internalizing behavioral adjustment from early childhood through early adolescence: developmental cascades. Dev Psychopathol. 2010;22:717–35. https://doi.org/10.1017/S0954579410000416.

230. Walker HM, Stieber S. Teacher ratings of social skills as longitudinal predictors of long-term arrest status in a sample of at-risk males. Behav Disord. 1998;23:222–30.

231. Webster-Stratton C, Hammond M. Conduct problems and level of social competence in head start children: prevalence, pervasiveness, and associated risk factors. Clin Child Fam Psychol Rev. 1998;1:101–24. https://doi.org/10.1023/A:1021835728803.

232. Webster-Stratton C, Lindsay DW. Social competence and conduct problems in young children: issues in assessment. J Clin Child Psychol. 1999;28:25–43. https://doi.org/10.1207/s15374424jccp2801_3.

233. Shaw DS, Keenan K, Vondra JI, Delliquardi E, Giovannelli J. Antecedents of preschool children's internalizing problems: a longitudinal study of low-income families. J Am Acad Child Adolesc Psychiatry. 1997;36:1760–7. https://doi.org/10.1097/00004583-199712000-00025.

234. Eisenberg N, Fabes RA, Murphy B, Maszk P, Smith M, Karbon M. The role of emotionality and regulation in children's social functioning: a longitudinal study. Child Dev. 1995;66:1360–84. https://doi.org/10.1111/j.1467-8624.1995.tb00940.x.

235. Valente E Jr, Dodge KA. Evaluation of prevention programs for children. In: Weissberg RP, Gullotta TP, Hampton RL, Ryan BA, Adams GR, editors. Issues in children's and families' lives. Healthy children 2010: establishing preventive services, vol. 9. Thousand Oaks: Sage; 1997. p. 183–218.

236. Cole DA, Maxwell SE. Testing mediational models with longitudinal data: questions and tips in the use of structural equation modeling. J Abnorm Psychol. 2003;112:558–77. https://doi.org/10.1037/0021-843X.112.4.558.

237. Maxwell SE, Cole DA, Mitchell MA. Bias in cross-sectional analyses of longitudinal mediation: partial and complete mediation under an autoregressive model. Multivariate Behav Res. 2011;46:816–41. https://doi.org/10.1080/00273171.2011.606716.

238. Campbell SB, Pierce EW, March CL, Ewing LJ. Noncompliant behavior, overactivity, and family stress as predictors of negative maternal control with preschool children. Dev Psychopathol. 1991;3:175–90. https://doi.org/10.1017/S0954579400000067.

239. Solantaus T, Leinonen J, Punamaki R. Children's mental health in times of economic recession: replication and extension of the family economic stress model in Finland. Dev Psychol. 2004;40:412–29. https://doi.org/10.1037/0012-1649.40.3.412.

240. Elgar FJ, McGrath PJ, Waschbusch DA, Stewart SH, Curtis LJ. Mutual influences on maternal depression and child adjustment problems. Clin Psychol Rev. 2004;24:441–59. https://doi.org/10.1016/j.cpr.2004.02.002.

241. Feldman R. Mutual influences between child emotion regulation and parent-child reciprocity support development across the first 10 years of life: implications for developmental psychopathology. Dev Psychopathol. 2015;27:1007–23. https://doi.org/10.1017/S0954579415000656.

242. La Greca AM, Silverman WK. Parent reports of child behavior problems: bias in participation. J Abnorm Child Psychol. 1993;21:89–101. https://doi.org/10.1007/BF00910491.

243. Gelfand DM, Teti DM. The effects of maternal depression on children. Clin Psychol Rev. 1990;10:329–53. https://doi.org/10.1016/0272-7358(90)90065-I.

244. Johnston D, Propper C, Pudney S, Shields M. Child mental health and educational attainment: multiple observers and the measurement error problem. J Appl Econom. 2014;29:880–900. https://doi.org/10.1002/jae.2359.

245. Brown JD, Wissow LS, Gadomski A, Zachary C, Bartlett E, Horn I. Parent and teacher mental health ratings of children using primary-care services: interrater agreement and implications for mental health screening. Ambul Pediatr. 2006;6:347–51. https://doi.org/10.1016/j.ambp.2006.09.004.

246. Majdandžić M, de Vente W, Bögels SM. Challenging parenting behavior from infancy to toddlerhood: etiology, measurement, and differences between fathers and mothers. Infancy. 2016;21:423–52. https://doi.org/10.1111/infa.12125.

247. Tavassolie T, Dudding S, Madigan AL, Thorvardarson E, Winsler A. Differences in perceived parenting style between mothers and fathers: implications for child outcomes and marital conflict. J Child Fam Stud. 2016;25:2055–68. https://doi.org/10.1007/s10826-016-0376-y.

248. Schafer J, Caetano R, Clark CL. Rates of intimate partner violence in the United States. Am J Public Health. 1998;88:1702–4. https://doi.org/10.2105/AJPH.88.11.1702.

249. Cabrera NJ, Fitzgerald HE, Bradley RH, Roggman L. The ecology of father–child relationships: an expanded model. J Fam Theory Rev. 2014;6:336–54. https://doi.org/10.1111/jftr.12054.

250. O'Leary SG, Vidair HB. Marital adjustment, child-rearing disagreements, and overreactive parenting: predicting child behavior problems. J Fam Psychol. 2005;19:208–16. https://doi.org/10.1037/0893-3200.19.2.208.

251. Fagan J, Day R, Lamb ME, Cabrera NJ. Should researchers conceptualize differently the dimensions of parenting for fathers and mothers? J Fam Theory Rev. 2014;6:390–405. https://doi.org/10.1111/jftr.12044.

252. Najman JM, Williams GM, Nikles J, Spence S, Bor W, O'Callaghan M, et al. Bias influencing maternal reports of child behaviour and emotional state. Soc Psychiatry Psychiatr Epidemiol. 2001;36:186–94. https://doi.org/10.1007/s001270170062.

253. DeSocio J, Hootman J. Children's mental health and school success. J Sch Nurs. 2004;20:189–96. https://doi.org/10.1177/10598405040200040201.

254. Goodman R, Renfrew D, Mullick M. Predicting type of psychiatric disorder from Strengths and Difficulties Questionnaire (SDQ) scores in child mental health clinics in London and Dhaka. Eur Child Adolesc Psychiatry. 2000;9:129–34. https://doi.org/10.1007/s007870050008.

255. Rhee SH, Waldman ID. Genetic and environmental influences on anti-social behavior: a meta-analysis of twin and adoption studies. Psychol Bull. 2002;128:490–529. https://doi.org/10.1037/0033-2909.128.3.490.

256. Bouchard TJ. Genetic influence on human psychological traits: a survey. Curr Dir Psychol Sci. 2004;13:148–51. https://doi.org/10.1111/j.0963-7214.2004.00295.x.

257. DiLalla LF, Gottesman II. Biological and genetic contributors to violence—Widom's untold tale. Psychol Bull. 1991;109:125–9. https://doi.org/10.1037/0033-2909.109.1.125.

258. Moffitt TE, Caspi A, Rutter M. Strategy for investigating interactions between measured genes and measured environments. Arch Gen Psychiatry. 2005;62:473–81. https://doi.org/10.1001/archpsyc.62.5.473.

259. Boyce WT, Ellis BJ. Biological sensitivity to context: i. an evolutionary-developmental theory of the origins and functions of stress reactivity. Dev Psychopathol. 2005;17:271–301. https://doi.org/10.1017/S0954579405000145.

260. Pluess M, Belsky J. Differential susceptibility to parenting and quality child care. Dev Psychol. 2010;46:379–90. https://doi.org/10.1037/a0015203.

261. Plomin R, Crabbe J. Dna. Psychol Bull. 2000;126:806–28. https://doi.org/10.1037/0033-2909.126.6.806.

262. McBride Murry V, Berkel C, Gaylord-Harden NK, Copeland-Linder N, Nation M. Neighborhood poverty and adolescent development. J Res Adolesc. 2011;21:114–28. https://doi.org/10.1111/j.1532-7795.2010.00718.x.

263. Sonenstein FL. Introducing the well-being of adolescents in vulnerable environments study: methods and findings. J Adolesc Health. 2014;55:S1–3. https://doi.org/10.1016/j.jadohealth.2014.09.008.

264. Wickrama KAS, Noh S. The long arm of community: the influence of childhood community contexts across the early life course. J Youth Adolesc. 2010;39:894–910. https://doi.org/10.1007/s10964-009-9411-2.

265. Brooks-Gunn J, Duncan GJ, Klebanov PK, Sealand N. Do neighborhoods influence child and adolescent development? Am J Sociol. 1993;99(2):353–95. https://doi.org/10.1086/230268.

9

Body image perceptions and symptoms of disturbed eating behavior among children and adolescents in Germany

Kathrin Schuck[1]*⦿, Simone Munsch[2] and Silvia Schneider[1]

Abstract

Theoretical background: Body image distortions such as perception biases are assumed to be precursors of eating disorders (ED). This study aims to investigate body image perceptions and symptoms of disturbed eating behavior among a sample of 11–17 year-old students in Germany.

Methods: A cross-sectional survey study was carried out among 1524 students of twelve secondary schools from all school types in North Rhine-Westphalia (Germany). A naturalistic photograph-rating consisting of photographs of young women's bodies was used to examine children's perceptions of female bodies (i.e., perceived average body size and perceived ideal body size of young women). Also, symptoms of disturbed eating behavior were examined.

Results: Compared to statistical data, children and adolescents underestimated the average body size of young women by more than two BMI-points (estimated average BMI = 20), with no differences between boys and girls. Also, girls and boys generally held a slim female thin-ideal (perceived ideal BMI = 19.5), which is nearly three BMI-points below the average body size in the young female population. Girls showed a slightly stronger female thin-ideal than boys. Among all subgroups, early-adolescent girls (13–14 years) displayed the strongest thin-ideal internalization. Nearly one-third of this group perceived a BMI below 18 as ideal female body size. Symptoms of disturbed eating behavior were common among youth and most frequent among adolescent girls (15–17 years). Girls who displayed a bias towards underestimation of female body size and girls who displayed an underweight female thin-ideal were more likely to report harmful dieting behaviors and psychological distress associated with eating, body, and weight.

Conclusions: This study found that 11–17 year-old girls and boys do not show accurate judgements regarding the average body size of young women. Instead, there is systematic and significant underestimation, indicating considerable perception biases, which may constitute a risk factor for the development and maintenance of ED. Symptoms of disturbed eating behavior were common, especially among girls, and associated with body-related perceptions. Future research will need to clarify the severity and course of these symptoms.

Keywords: Body image, Eating disorders, Cognitive distortion, Children, Adolescents

Background

Body image is a multi-dimensional concept, which describes how we think, feel, perceive, and act with regard to our bodies. Adolescence constitutes a critical period for the development of a healthy or unhealthy body image [1]. A large number of studies have consistently shown that a negative body image, typically measured as body dissatisfaction, is associated with disturbed eating patterns among adolescents [2–6] and one of the strongest risk factors for the development of eating disorders (ED) [7, 8] and other adverse psychological outcomes such as depression [9–11].

Body image disturbances are key characteristics of eating disorders (EDs) such as anorexia nervosa and bulimia nervosa and encompass distortions in cognition, affect, perception, or behavior related to body weight or shape

*Correspondence: kathrin.schuck@rub.de
[1] Mental Health Research and Treatment Center, Ruhr-University Bochum, Massenbergstrasse 9-13, 44787 Bochum, Germany
Full list of author information is available at the end of the article

[12]. They may refer to negative thoughts or negative evaluation regarding one's own body, negative affect in response to one's own body, misperception of body-related stimuli, and specific body-related behaviors (e.g., checking or avoidance). In Western societies, body image disturbances including body dissatisfaction are pervasive problems. Particularly among women, the desire for thinness is so prevalent that it is considered a normative discontent [13]. A growing body of evidence suggests that this body-related discontent may apply to a similar extent to children and adolescents. A large number of studies has shown that body image disturbances (e.g., body dissatisfaction, discrepancy between one's actual and one's ideal body size, weight and shape concerns) frequently occur even before puberty and are reported by up to 50% of children and adolescents [5, 7, 14–23].

Similarly, a growing body of research suggests that symptoms of disturbed eating behavior are common among youth. In a large German study among 7498 students (11–17 years old), nearly one quarter (21.9%) showed symptoms of EDs (e.g., concerns about loss of control over eating, self-induced vomiting, rapid weight loss in the last 3 months). Girls were significantly more often affected than boys (28.9% vs. 15.2%) [24]. Similarly, a study conducted in the United States among 1739 female students (12-18 years) reported that disordered eating attitudes and behaviors (e.g., dieting, binge eating) were present in 27% [25]. Similar numbers have been reported by other studies [17, 20, 21, 26, 27]. The outcomes of eating-disordered attitudes and behaviors in adolescence are severe. Prospective studies show that body dissatisfaction and early ED symptoms (e.g., body image distortions, weight concerns) predict eating-disordered behavior, onset of ED, depressive symptoms, overweight, and obesity in adulthood [3, 26, 28, 29].

While there is consistent evidence that body image disturbances in terms of dysfunctional cognitions (e.g., body dissatisfaction), negative affect (distress in response to weight or shape), and behavioural measures (e.g., symptoms of disturbed eating behavior) already appear in children and adolescents, few data is available regarding body image perceptions. Recent studies have used pictorial figure rating scales to examine body image perceptions, which typically consist of a series of abstract figures ranging from underweight to overweight (for an overview, see [30]). Up to this point, only a handful of studies have employed figure rating scales displaying naturalistic human bodies [31–35] and only one of these studies has been conducted among children [35]. While this study reported discrepancies between children's own body image and ideal body image, normative perceptions of human body sizes (e.g., the ability to correctly perceive human bodies in terms of normality) have not been investigated.

Perceptual distortions may play an important role in the development of EDs [8, 36]. Perceptual distortions are considered a type of cognitive bias, which describe systematic errors in the processing of information (i.e., information processing biases). There is accumulating evidence that cognitive biases may influence the onset and maintenance of eating-related pathology in adolescence and early adulthood [37–42]. Cognitive biases may occur in different domains such as attention, perception, or memory and may foster symptoms of mental disorders, because they determine what people notice, attend to, and remember. In ED, perceptual biases related to body weight or shape (e.g., systematic misperceptions or judgement errors) have been proposed to reinforce disturbed body image experiences [43]. For example, underestimating the average body size may result in a larger perceived discrepancy between oneself and the norm, thereby increasing body dissatisfaction and weight and shape concerns.

The present study aimed to examine normative perceptions (perceived average body size) and thin-ideal perceptions (perceived ideal body size) of female bodies[1] among 11–17 year old children and adolescents using a naturalistic photographic figure rating. Furthermore, symptoms of disturbed eating behavior were studied in relation to these perceptions. We hypothesized that children and adolescents would systematically underestimate the average female body size in comparison to the average statistical body size. We also expected that children and adolescents would display a slim female thin-ideal. In addition, we expected that symptoms of disturbed eating behavior would be associated with a bias towards underestimation of female body size and an underweight thin-ideal.

Methods

Participants and procedure

Study participants were 1524 children and adolescents aged between 11 and 17 years who were recruited from 12 secondary schools from all school types in North Rhine-Westphalia, Germany. Schools were selected from a larger pool of schools and school principals were contacted by telephone by research assistants, who informed them about the study. A total of 119 schools were initially contacted and 12 schools agreed to distribute short questionnaires during school hours to all students in German grades 5–10 (US grades 6–11). Parents received written information about the school's participation in the study

---

[1] The present study solely assessed body image perceptions with regard to female bodies. For male bodies, no photograph material was available for reasons of feasibility. As the stimulus material pertained exclusively to female bodies, only female body image perceptions could be examined.

as well as information about the procedure and aim of the study. All parents were informed that participation in the study was voluntary and received a form to withdraw their child from study participation and a return envelope ('passive consent'). Five children were excluded by their parents from study participation. Data collection took place between April and July 2015. Before the assessment, children were informed about the aim of the study and that participation was voluntary. They received information about the general topic (eating behavior and body image) and the procedure. Questionnaires were filled in anonymously in the presence of an instructed teacher and a research assistant. The study was approved by the ethics committee of the Faculty of Psychology of the Ruhr-University Bochum, Germany.

Measures

Photograph-rating of female bodies

To measure body size perception of female bodies, a photograph figure rating based on the Stunkard Figure Rating Scale [44] was used. The original rating scale consists of silhouette drawings of female bodies ranging from very thin to very large. In the present study, a photographic figure rating was developed using body photographs of women's bodies. As human bodies are quite diverse, the rating consisted of a total of 24 photographs of women varying in body mass index (BMI). The photographs depicted female university students from neck down in different standardized perspectives wearing standardized, beige underwear in front of a white background. The pictures were taken at the Ruhr-University Bochum for the purpose of another study on body image conducted by the first author (material is available upon request). All photographs were released by the former study participants through written consent to be used for research purposes.

A systematic review on pictorial figure rating scale [30] noted that scales often depict unrealistic representations of human body forms (e.g., contour drawings or computerized figures with disproportionately sized or poorly defined body features). Hence, more naturalistic representations of human bodies are needed to increase ecological validity in the assessment of body images. An additional potential limitation of previously used photographic figure rating scales is that few response choices are provided. In previously used scales, one individual body represents one body size, which may be confounded with other variables such as perceived attractiveness, hip-to-waist ratio, or proportions between body features. This methodological artifact ("scale coarseness") limits measurement precision and increases the likelihood of measurement errors [30]. The present study aimed to overcome these methodological limitations by using a photographic figure rating, which consisted of several sets of naturalistic photographs of young women's bodies (four sets each displaying six bodies with varying BMIs), resulting in multiple response choices.

To assess body image perceptions among youth, children and adolescents were presented with four photographic figure rating scales, each consisting of six female bodies differing in BMI from underweight to overweight. Each scale depicted six bodies with the following BMIs: 1) BMI between 16.5 and 18 (underweight), 2) BMI between 18.5 and 20, 3), BMI between 20 and 21 4) BMI between 21.5 and 23, 5) BMI between 23 and 25, and 6) BMI between 25 and 28 (overweight). BMIs were presented in ascending and descending order (the order was counterbalanced within the photograph-rating). The four sets depicted bodies from different perspectives (i.e., the first scale depicted bodies from front view, the second from back view, the third from 90-degree side view, and the fourth from 45-degree side view).

Children and adolescents were asked the following: "Please indicate which of these body sizes is most similar to the ideal body of a young woman", and "Please indicate which of these body sizes is most similar to the average body of a young woman". A mean score and a corresponding BMI for the two variables *average body size* and *ideal body size* was calculated based on the scores endorsed on the four photographic rating scales. To examine perception biases, the perceived average body size of young women reported by children and adolescents was compared to data of the average body size of 18–25 year old women in Germany reported by the Federal Statistical Office. Moreover, we calculated the percentage of children who correctly estimated the average body size of young females, defined as frequently selecting category 4 (BMI: 21.5–23), which displays body sizes closest to the statistical average body size of young females (i.e., selecting category 4 on at least three out of four times on the photographic rating scales). Correspondingly, we also calculated the percentage of children who displayed a bias towards underestimation (i.e., selecting lower BMI categories on average) and a bias towards overestimation (i.e., selecting higher BMI categories on average). To examine pervasive thin-ideal perceptions, we calculated the percentage of children who displayed an underweight thin-ideal, defined as frequently selecting category 1 (BMI: 16.5–18), which displays underweight body sizes according to the World Health Organization (i.e., selecting category 1 at least three out of four time on the photograph rating scales).

To examine construct validity of the photograph-rating, we conducted an "expert-rating" among ten mental health professionals (5 female 5 male). Herefore, a convience sample of ten licensed psychotherapists working at the Mental Health Research and Treatment Center of Ruhr-University Bochum was asked to examine the photographic material used in the present study. Mean age of psychotherapists was 32.1 years (SD = 3.9). All psychotherapists had experience in treating eating disorders, but none of them considered himself to be an expert in this area. The aim was to present a proof-of-concept and an indication of face-validity by examining whether mental health professionals would be able to correctly order the female body photographs by increasing BMI and if they would be able to correctly perceive under- and overweight. Each psychotherapist was presented with the four rating scales consisting of six female bodies each. For the present purpose, the female bodies were presented in quasi-random order. Psychotherapist were asked to re-order the photographs per scale by increasing body weight. Also, they were asked to indicate whether they perceived any of the bodies to be under- or overweight. To examine construct validity, we calculated Cohen's kappa to compare agreement between the correct ranking order and the psychotherapist's ranking order [cf. 31]. In addition, we conducted sensitivity and specificity analyses. Kappa coefficients ranged between .65 and .90 with an average of .79, which indicates good to excellent agreement between actual body size and the psychotherapist's perception of body size. Sensitivity and specificity scores were generally high, indicating that psychotherapists were correctly able to perceive under- and overweight. With the exception of one psychotherapist who never recognized underweight, sensitivity scores for underweight ranged between 75 and 100% (on average 85%), indicating that underweight was correctly perceived in the majority of cases. Specificity scores for underweight were 100% among all psychotherapists, indicating that non-underweight was never falsely perceived as underweight. Sensitivity scores for overweight were 100% for all experts, indicating that overweight was always correctly perceived as overweight. Specificity scores for overweight ranged between 85 and 100% (on average 97%), indicating that non-overweight cases were rarely perceived as overweight. In sum, the present expert-rating indicates good construct validity. In addition, previous research has shown good test–retest validity of photographic figure rating scales as well as good convergent validity with other established measures of eating disorders [31–34].

Eating-related behaviors

To assess eating-related behaviors, participants were asked to respond to the following items previously applied in a large survey study by Micali and colleagues [cf. 20]: "In the past 3 months, did you do any of the following things to influence your weight: "eating less during meals", "skipping meals", "fasting (e.g., not eating for the entire day or almost the entire day)", "exercising to loose weight or to prevent weight gain", "self-induced vomiting", and "taking diet pills or laxatives". To assess symptoms of disturbed eating behavior, participants were asked to respond to the following items [cf. 20]: "Do you feel fat, even though other people tell you that you are not?", "Are you terrified of gaining weight or getting fat?", "Do you avoid certain types of food because you fear weight gain?", "Do you feel upset about your weight or shape?", "Do you feel distressed after eating too much?", "Do you have episodes of binge eating, in which you eat a very large amount of food?", "Do you ever loose control over eating?" Response options for all items were no (0) or yes (1). The items are based on DSM-IV and ICD-10 criteria for ED and they are likely to reflect broader early ED phenotypes, indexing risk for clinical disorders [20]. Previous research has shown that these ED symptoms are associated with psychological outcomes such as social impairment, family burden, and emotional and behavioral disorders. The items have been selected, as they have demonstrated concurrent and predictive validity [20] and can be more easily administered to children than other measures of ED pathology, which may require more complex answers.

Scales indexing risk for ED

In addition to the aforementioned items, we included two scales indexing risk for ED with well-established psychometric properties. The subscale shape concern of the Eating Disorder Examination Questionnaire (EDE-Q; Fairburn & Beglin [45]) consists of eight questions measuring body dissatisfaction and shape concerns. The items refer to the past 28 days and are rated using seven point forced-choice format (1–7). The EDE-Q has a high internal consistency ($\alpha = .97$) and good convergent validity [46]. Responses were added into a mean score with higher score reflecting higher levels of body dissatisfaction and shape concerns. The Sociocultural Attitudes towards Appearance Scale (SATAQ-G, Knauss et al. [47]) assesses the recognition and endorsement of societal appearance standards. The questionnaire consists of 16 items and three subscales: internalization, perceived pressure and awareness of sociocultural appearance standards. Response options range from 1 (strongly disagree) to 5 (strongly agree). Reliability of the subscales is high (Cronbach's alphas = .92–.96; Thompson et al. [48]). The questionnaire has acceptable concurrent validity [47]. Responses were added into a mean score with higher scores reflecting a stronger recognition and endorsement of societal appearance standards.

Strategy for analyses

Analyses were conducted for the total sample and separately for girls and boys. To distinguish between developmental stages, participants were divided into three age groups (pre-adolescents: 11–12 years, early-adolescents: 13–14 years; adolescents: 15–17 years) [cf. 49]. Descriptive statistics (means, standard deviations, frequencies) were used to examine sociodemographic characteristics as well as variables of interest. Statistical comparisons between groups were based on independent sample t-tests for continuous variables and Chi square tests for categorical variables. To examine associations between body image perceptions (average body size and ideal body size) and symptoms of disturbed eating behavior, we compared the frequency distributions of symptoms between samples using Chi square tests. First, we compared girls who displayed a strong bias towards underestimation of average female body size to girls without a strong bias towards underestimation. Therefore, the sample was split in tertiles based on the perceived average female body size on the photograph-rating. Girls scoring within the lowest tertile were compared to girls scoring within the highest tertile.[2] Second, we compared girls who displayed an underweight thin-ideal to girls who did not display an underweight thin-ideal (defined as frequently selecting a BMI below 18 as ideal body size vs. other responses on the photograph-rating).

Results

Descriptive analyses

Table 1 displays descriptive statistics for the total group and for girls and boys separately. On average, participants were 13.6 years ($SD = 1.8$). A total of 828 (55.1%) were girls and 676 (44.9%) were boys. All participants were divided into three developmental groups, respectively pre-adolescents (n = 482, 32%), early-adolescents (n = 495, 32.9%), and adolescents (n = 527, 35.0%). A total of 597 children and adolescents (39.9%) attended the highest (*Gymnasium*) of three German school forms, 151 (10.1%) attended the lowest school form (*Hauptschule*). In comparison to data from the Federal Statistical Office in Germany [50], the characteristics of the present sample resemble population characteristics of students in North-Rhine Westphalia (Germany's most populous state), in terms of school type and age. However, boys were somewhat underrepresented (44.9% vs. 51.0%) in the present study.

Table 1 Descriptive statistics of children and adolescents in the present study

	Total sample	Girls	Boys
Gender (n, %)			
Female	828 (55.1)		
Male	676 (44.9)		
Age group (n, %)			
Pre-adolescent (11–12 years)	482 (32.0)	248 (30.2)	231 (34.5)
Early-adolescent (13–14 years)	495 (32.9)	277 (33.7)	214 (32.0)
Adolescent (15–17 years)	527 (35.0)	297 (36.1)	224 (32.5)
School form (n, %)			
High	597 (39.9)	383 (46.9)	209 (31.2)
Medium	750 (50.2)	377 (46.1)	367 (54.9)
Low	151 (10.1)	57 (7.0)	93 (13.9)
Age (M, SD)			
	13.6 (1.8)	13.7 (1.7)	13.6 (1.8)

M mean, *SD* standard deviation

Body image perceptions

With regard to the average body size, children and adolescents endorsed a mean score of 2.7 on the photographic figure rating scale, which corresponds to a BMI of approximately 20.0. There was no statistically significant difference between girls and boys ($M_{girls} = 2.7$, $M_{boys} = 2.7$, t = − 1.8, p = .07, d = .09). According to the Federal Statistical Office, the average BMI of a young woman (20–25 years) in Germany was 22.4 in the year 2013 [51]. This comparison shows that children and adolescents underestimate the average body size in the population by more than two BMI-points. Only 8.1% of children correctly estimated the average female body size (defined as frequently selecting category 4 on the photograph-rating, which depicts BMIs between 21.5 and 23). In contrast, 88.1% showed a bias towards underestimation of the average female body size, while only 3.8% showed a bias towards overestimation.

With regard to ideal body size, children and adolescents perceived the ideal body size of a young woman to be 2.1 on the photographic figure rating scale, which corresponds to a BMI of approximately 19.5. Comparison between perceived body size ideal and actual body size according to statistical data showed that children and adolescents hold a slim female thin-ideal, which deeds the average body size in the population by nearly three BMI-points. There was a slight, but statistically significant difference between girls and boys ($M_{girls} = 2.0$, $M_{boys} = 2.2$, t = − 5.1, p < .001, d = .27), indicating that the perceived ideal body sizes for young females was slightly lower among girls than among boys.

In addition, we examined the percentage of children and adolescents who display an underweight thin-ideal

---

[2] As a bias towards underestimation of the average female body size was present in nearly the entire sample and a clear cut-off for the definition of a perceptual bias is lacking, we used tertiles to compare groups scoring low compared to high on perception of average female body size.

Table 2 Percentage of children and adolescents who display an underweight thin-ideal by gender and age group

	Total sample	Girls	Boys
Pre-adolescents (11–12 years)	19.2	18.6	20.0
Early-adolescents (13–14 years)	24.7	30.1	17.4
Adolescents (15–17 years)	19.6	24.7	12.6
Total sample (11–17 years)	21.5	24.9	16.8

(i.e., frequently endorsing a BMI below 18 as ideal body size on photograph-rating). Table 2 displays percentages by gender and age group. The proportion of children and adolescents who hold an underweight thin-ideal was generally higher among girls compared to boys (24.9% vs. 16.8%). Among all subgroups, early-adolescent girls held the strongest thin-ideals. Nearly one-third (30.1%) of 13–14 year old girls perceived a BMI below 18 (underweight) as ideal body size. Among 15–17 year old girls, a quarter (24.7%) perceived a BMI below 18 (underweight) as ideal body size.

Symptoms of disturbed eating behavior

Table 3 displays the frequency of symptoms of disturbed eating behavior for the total group as well as by gender and age group. Symptoms of disturbed eating behavior were common and generally higher among girls. Feeling fat, feeling upset about weight or shape, restrictive eating, exercising for weight control, and distress after eating were reported by a quarter to a third of all children

and adolescents. In addition, unhealthy eating behaviors such as skipping meals or fasting were reported by a substantial proportion of youth (21.8 and 15.3%, respectively), especially among adolescent girls (37.4 and 27.7%, respectively). Episodes of binge eating and loss of control over eating were also reported quite frequently by youth (16 and 11%, respectively), again, especially by adolescent girls (24.9 and 14.2%, respectively). Harmful compensatory behaviors (self-induced vomiting or taking dieting pills or laxatives) were generally rare among youth, although a significant percentage of early-adolescent and adolescent girls reported self-induced vomiting within the last 3 months (4.8 and 4.1%, respectively).

Associations between body image perceptions and symptoms of disturbed eating behavior

Associations between perceived average body size and perceived ideal body size and symptoms with disturbed eating behavior among girls are displayed in Table 4. Girls who displayed a strong bias towards underestimation were more likely to report skipping meals (29.7% vs. 23.2%), being terrified of gaining weight (32.8% vs. 22.8%), avoidance of certain food (26.7% vs. 19.3%), feeling upset about weight or shape (48.9% vs 39.3%), distress after eating (38.1% vs. 27.2%, respectively), and perceived loss of control over eating (16.9% vs. 10.7%) compared to girls who did not display a strong bias towards underestimation of female body size. In line with this, they also displayed higher levels of shape concerns (16.4 vs. 13.3, $p < .01$) and a stronger endorsement of societal

Table 3 Symptoms of disturbed eating behavior among children and adolescents by gender and age group

Item	Total sample (%)	Girls			Boys		
		11–12 (years) (%)	13–14 (years) (%)	15–17 (years) (%)	11–12 (years) (%)	13–14 (years) (%)	15–17 (years) (%)
Eating less during meals	34.8	35.1	42.0	46.7	30.0	26.1	22.7
Skipping meals	21.8	13.9	26.8	37.4	14.2	20.5	13.0
Fasting	15.3	11.3	16.6	27.7	9.0	14.2	8.3
Exercising for weight control	58.0	58.7	66.8	65.1	51.6	50.9	62.3
Self-induced vomiting	2.8	1.3	4.8	4.1	2.3	2.4	.9
Taking diet pills or laxatives	1.7	.4	1.5	2.8	1.4	1.4	2.3
Feeling fat	36.0	44.8	48.2	53.6	22.6	21.4	14.5
Terrified of gaining weight	21.9	26.8	25.1	30.7	18.2	13.9	11.9
Avoidance of certain food	20.6	17.9	19.9	28.2	20.7	20.2	15.1
Feeling upset about weight or shape	36.1	38.3	41.9	51.6	24.8	27.3	24.1
Distress after eating	25.7	27.2	32.0	38.2	16.8	18.0	15.3
Episodes of binge eating	16.0	14.3	19.0	24.9	9.1	9.5	14.3
Loss of control over eating	11.0	13.2	14.2	14.2	5.5	6.6	10.1

Results are displayed as absolute percentages

Table 4 Frequency distributions of symptoms among girls in relation to perception biases and an underweight thin-ideal

Symptom	Girls with strong bias towards underestimation (%)	Girls without strong bias towards underestimation (%)	p value	Girls with underweight thin-ideal (%)	Girls without underweight thin-ideal (%)	p value
Eating less during meals	42.7	37.3	.11	44.5	40.5	.19
Skipping meals	29.7	23.2	.05	32.4	25.4	.04
Fasting	21.4	17.6	.14	22.1	18.0	.13
Exercising for weight control	62.5	62.7	.51	65.6	62.0	.21
Self-induced vomiting	4.2	3.2	.36	6.9	2.7	.01
Taking diet pills or laxatives	.7	1.6	.25	1.6	1.6	.61
Feeling fat	47.9	45.5	.31	52.9	47.5	.12
Terrified of gaining weight	32.8	22.8	< .01	31.0	26.3	.13
Avoidance of certain food	26.7	19.3	.02	29.3	20.3	<.01
Feeling upset about weight or shape	48.9	39.3	.01	50.0	42.1	.04
Distress after eating	38.1	27.5	< .01	41.7	30.2	<.01
Episodes of binge eating	17.5	21.1	.15	17.5	20.6	.20
Loss of control over eating	16.9	10.7	.02	14.2	13.2	.40

p values pertain to Chi square tests

appearance standards (44.0 vs. 41.5, $p < .05$) compared to girls did not display a strong bias towards underestimation of female body size.

Girls who displayed an underweight female thin-ideal were more likely to report skipping meals (32.4% vs. 25.4%), self-induced vomiting (6.9% vs. 2.7%), avoidance of certain food (29.3% vs. 20.3%), feeling upset about weight or shape (50.0% vs. 42.1%), and distress after eating (41.7% vs. 30.2%) compared to girls who did not display an underweight female thin-ideal. In line with this, they also displayed higher levels of shape concerns (16.8 vs. 14.1, $p = .02$) and a stronger endorsement of societal appearance standards (47.2 vs. 41.8, $p < .001$) compared to girls who did not display an underweight thin-ideal.

Discussion

The present study aimed to answer the question how accurate children and adolescents judge body sizes of young females in terms of normality and if there is a general bias towards underestimation of female body size among youth. Using a photograph-rating consisting of sets of naturalistic photographs of young women's bodies, body image perceptions (i.e., perceived average female body size and perceived ideal female body size) were examined in a large sample of 11–17 year old German students.

The present study is the first to show that children and adolescents considerably underestimate the average

female body size when judging naturalistic photographs of young female bodies. On average, they underestimated the average body size of a young woman by more than two BMI-points (i.e., they perceived the average BMI of a young woman to be approximately 20, while the average BMI of the reference population is 22.4). Perceptual biases such as normative misperceptions have been found to play an important role in several health-related behaviors such as uptake of smoking or drinking among youth [52, 53]. Similarly, perceptual body-related distortions may influence eating-related attitudes and behaviors by increasing the perceived discrepancy between oneself and the norm, resulting in body dissatisfaction and weight and shape concerns. Research supports these assertions by showing that women who felt discrepant from the norm show more symptoms of ED [54], which may results in more extreme and maladaptive dieting behaviors to achieve an unrealistic and often unattainable body size.

Furthermore, the present study showed that girls and boys generally held a slim female thin-ideal (i.e., they perceived the ideal BMI of a young woman to be approximately 19.5), which represents the lowest quartile of a healthy BMI range (18.5–25). Yet, a substantial proportion of children and adolescents displayed an underweight thin-ideal (24.9% among girls, 16.8% among boys). The results are in line with previous studies. Connolly, Slaughter, and Mealey [55] showed that already 6-year olds have a systematic preference for underweight body shapes. Similarly, Brown and Slaughter [15] showed that children and adolescents across all age groups rate thin female bodies as more attractive than normal bodies. Schneider and colleagues [21] showed that adolescent girls desired a body shape for themselves corresponding to underweight. Similar strong thin-ideals have been observed in adult women [56–59]. In sum, a large body of research indicates that the sociocultural thin-ideal is internalized by a large proportion of the Western population including children and adolescents. The results of the present study strengthen and extend findings of previous studies using pictorial instead of photographic figure rating scales, which may be limited by methodological shortcomings.

Finally, the present study showed that symptoms of disturbed eating behavior among youth were quite common, especially among female adolescents. Feeling fat, feeling upset about weight or shape, restrictive eating, exercising for weight control, and distress after eating were reported by a quarter to a third of all children and adolescents. Also, a substantial proportion of youth reported unhealthy eating behaviors such as skipping meals or fasting (21.8 and 15.3%, respectively), episodes of binge eating (16%), and perceived loss of control over eating (11%). The results are in line with previous research showing that symptoms of disturbed eating behavior are common among youth [17, 20, 21, 24–27]. Importantly, body image perceptions were associated with disordered eating behaviors among youth. Girls who displayed a strong bias towards underestimation of the average female body size and girls who displayed an underweight thin-ideal were more likely to report harmful dieting behavior (e.g., skipping meals, self-induced vomiting) and psychological distress associated with eating and own body weight (e.g., being terrified of gaining weight, feeling upset about weight or shape, distress after eating). Also, they showed significantly elevated scores on well-established measures indexing risk for ED (i.e., higher levels of shape concerns and a stronger recognition and endorsement of societal appearance standards). These associations indicate that both perceptional biases as well as the internalization of a pervasive thin-ideal may constitute risk factors for the onset and maintenance of ED among youth.

In addition, differences between boys and girls were examined. It is reasonable that both boys and girls hold body images, not only for their own but also for the opposite sex (i.e., ideas about how males and females should look like). With regard to the perceived average female body size, boys and girls did not differ (both underestimated the average female body size to a similar extent). However, with regard to the perceived ideal female body size, girls showed a slightly lower thin-ideal than boys.

Previous studies found similar results among adults, showing that men and women differ in attractiveness ratings of female body size, with males being less stringent about female body size than females [60–62]. However, it should be noted that the present study only examined the female body ideal (i.e., thin-ideal), while the male body ideal (i.e., muscular ideal) has not been examined. Therefore, it remains unclear whether females in general are more susceptible than males to adopt and internalize sociocultural body ideals or whether females and males internalize gender-specific sociocultural body ideals to a similar extent. For a comprehensive picture, body ideals of both male and female bodies should be compared between boys and girls.

In addition, differences between developmental groups were examined. Interestingly, the group of early-adolescent girls most often displayed an underweight thin-ideal. Nearly one-third of 13–14 year-old girls perceived a BMI below 18 (underweight) as ideal body size, possibly indicating that early adolescence may constitute a vulnerable developmental period for the onset of disordered eating-related cognitions and attitudes. A potential explanation may be that girls within this developmental phase typically start to experience changes in body composition (i.e., increase in body fat starting with puberty), after a period of typically having a relatively lean body during childhood, which may make this group particularly susceptible for a fear of body fat and the internalization of a pervasive thin-ideal. A general fear of growing or a fear of gaining secondary sex characteristics may also play a role during period and may explain the adoption of a pervasive thin-ideal among early-adolescent girls. With regard to symptoms of disturbed eating behavior, 15–17 year-old girls seemed to be most vulnerable. The results reflect age differences in the onset of different ED. The onset of anorexia (characterized by underweight or severe weight loss) typically lies in early adolescence and the onset of bulimia (characterized by disturbances in eating behavior such as binge eating and inappropriate compensatory behaviors) in late adolescence [63]. The results may reflect a developmental time course, in which cognitive-attitudinal distortions (e.g., adoption of pervasive female thin-ideal) in early-adolescence precede the onset and manifestation of symptoms of disturbed eating behavior during adolescence.

Several limitations should be acknowledged. First, the study has been conducted in a single state of Germany. Although North-Rhine Westphalia is Germany's most populous state, the findings may not be entirely generalizable to the national population level and do not consider culture-related differences in body perceptions and body ideals. Moreover, body image perceptions and symptoms of disturbed eating behavior were self-reported by youth. It is possible that social desirability or response styles may have influenced the results. In addition, the cross-sectional design of the study does not allow to draw conclusions regarding temporal precedence or causality between study variables. While it is intuitive to assume that perceptual distortions precede the development of symptoms of disturbed eating behavior, it is also possible that children and adolescents with disturbed eating behavior develop perceptual distortions as a correlate of eating-related pathology. Moreover, it should be noted that the present study used single items to measure symptoms of ED, which may have limited psychometric properties. Also, the items did not assess the clinical severity of symptoms of disturbed eating behavior, as no clinical rating nor measures of frequency and severity were applied. In addition, it should be noted that the psychometric validity of the photographic figure rating has not been fully established. Yet, an expert-rating among mental health professionals indicated construct validity and previous studies have shown good test–retest validity and convergent validity of similar photographic figure rating scales [31–34]. Finally, it should be acknowledged that the present study did not control for a general underestimation bias. A body of research suggests that individuals tend to display under- instead of overestimation when asked to make judgements regarding size (e.g., when judging package or portion sizes, cf. Ordabayeva & Chandon [64]). Therefore, underestimation biases may constitute normative, hardwired cognitive errors, at least to a certain extent. The present study, however, shows that a strong bias towards underestimation of body size is associated with symptoms of disturbed eating behavior and psychological distress, indicating that strong perception biases are qualitatively different from common, benign errors. The present study also has several strengths including a large, heterogeneous sample of children and adolescents from all school types in Germany's most populous state. In addition, the photographic rating, consisting of a variety of real women's bodies, may have a better ecological validity in the assessment of body image perceptions than figure ratings used in previous studies. As the present rating used a larger number of female body photographs, the risk that a particular confounder was associated with a particular body size is decreased.

The present study suggests several recommendations for future research. First of all, prospective study designs are required to enable conclusions regarding temporal order to improve our understanding of the development and maintenance of ED. Future research may disentangle whether perceptual distortions constitute a risk factor predisposing youth towards the development of ED or merely a symptom of the ED. Furthermore, a better understanding of the frequency and the severity of symptoms of disturbed eating behavior among children and adolescents would be valuable. Future studies may investigate how often these symptoms are experienced by youth and whether they are associated with clinically significant distress or functional impairment. Finally, it would be interesting to investigate if perceptual distortions and symptoms of disturbed eating behavior can be modified by interventions. Possibly, psycho-education and cognitive interventions to modify normative misperceptions and perceptions of the thin-ideal may help to reduce eating-related pathology and prevent the development of ED among youth.

Conclusions

In conclusion, the present study demonstrates that children and adolescents display a considerable perception bias (i.e., bias towards underestimation of female body size). Also, this study suggests the existence of a developmental time course, in which perceptual body-related distortions (e.g., body-related perception biases, internalization of pervasive thin-ideal) in early-adolescence may precede the onset and manifestation of symptoms of disturbed eating behavior during the course of adolescence. However, prospective studies will need to clarify temporal precedence between perceptions, cognitions, and behavior associated with eating-related pathology among youth in the future.

Abbreviation
ED: eating disorders.

Authors' contributions
KS is responsible for the study conception, data collection, data analysis, and report of the study results. SM and SS are supervisors and contributed to the revision of the manuscript. All authors read and approved the final manuscript.

Author details
[1] Mental Health Research and Treatment Center, Ruhr-University Bochum, Massenbergstrasse 9-13, 44787 Bochum, Germany. [2] Department of Psychology, Clinical Psychology and Psychotherapy, University of Fribourg, Rue P.A. de Faucigny 2, 1700 Fribourg, Switzerland.

Compering interests
All authors declare that they have no competing interests.

Funding
KS is supported by a grant from the Deutsche Forschungsgemeinschaft (Deutsche Forschungsgemeinschaft, Grant: SCHN 415/4-1). The German Research Foundation had no role in the study design, collection, analysis, or interpretation of the data, writing the manuscript, or the decision to submit the paper for publication.

References

1. Voelker DK, Reel JJ, Greenleaf C. Weight status and body image perceptions in adolescents: current perspectives. Adolesc Health Med Ther. 2015;6:149–58.
2. Bibiloni Mdel M, Pich J, Pons A, Tur JA. Body image and eating patterns among adolescents. BMC public health. 2013;13:1104.
3. Liechty JM. Body image distortion and three types of weight loss behaviors among nonoverweight girls in the United States. J Adolesc Health. 2010;47(2):176–82.
4. Neumark-Sztainer D, Paxton SJ, Hannan PJ, Haines J, Story M. Does body satisfaction matter? Five-year longitudinal associations between body satisfaction and health behaviors in adolescent females and males. J Adolesc Health. 2006;39(2):244–51.
5. Ricciardelli LA, McCabe MP. Children's body image concerns and eating disturbance: a review of the literature. Clin Psychol Rev. 2001;21(3):325–44.
6. Shroff H, Thompson JK. The tripartite influence model of body image and eating disturbance: a replication with adolescent girls. Body Image. 2006;3(1):17–23.
7. Westerberg-Jacobson J, Edlund B, Ghaderi A. A 5-year longitudinal study of the relationship between the wish to be thinner, lifestyle behaviours and disturbed eating in 9–20-year old girls. Eur Eat Disord Rev. 2010;18(3):207–19.
8. Stice E, Shaw HE. Role of body dissatisfaction in the onset and maintenance of eating pathology: a synthesis of research findings. J Psychosom Res. 2002;53(5):985–93.
9. Holsen I, Kraft P, Roysamb E. The relationship between body image and depressed mood in adolescence: a 5-year longitudinal panel study. J Health Psychol. 2001;6(6):613–27.
10. Stice E, Bearman SK. Body-image and eating disturbances prospectively predict increases in depressive symptoms in adolescent girls: a growth curve analysis. Dev Psychol. 2001;37(5):597–607.
11. Stice E, Hayward C, Cameron RP, Killen JD, Taylor CB. Body-image and eating disturbances predict onset of depression among female adolescents: a longitudinal study. J Abnorm Psychol. 2000;109(3):438–44.
12. Vossbeck-Elsebusch AN, Vocks S, Legenbauer T. Body exposure for eating disorders: technique and relevance for therapy outcome. Psychother Psych Med. 2013;63(5):193–200.
13. Rodin J. Women and weight: a normative discontent. Lincoln: University of Nebraska Press; 1985.
14. Tremblay L. Body image disturbance and psychopathology in children: research evidence and implications for prevention and treatment. Curr Psychiatry Rev. 2009;5:62–72.
15. Brown FL, Slaughter V. Normal body, beautiful body: discrepant perceptions reveal a pervasive 'thin-ideal' from childhood to adulthood. Body Image. 2011;8(2):119–25.
16. Berger U, Schilke C, Strauss B. Weight concerns and dieting among 8 to 12-year-old children. Psychother Psychosom Med Psychol. 2005;55(7):331–8.
17. Cruz-Saez S, Pascual A, Salaberria K, Echeburua E. Normal-weight and overweight female adolescents with and without extreme weight-control behaviours: emotional distress and body image concerns. J Health Psychol. 2015;20(6):730–40.
18. Dohnt H, Tiggemann M. The contribution of peer and media influences to the development of body satisfaction and self-esteem in young girls: a prospective study. Dev Psychol. 2006;42(5):929–36.
19. Jongenelis MI, Byrne SM, Pettigrew S. Self-objectification, body image disturbance, and eating disorder symptoms in young Australian children. Body Image. 2014;11(3):290–302.
20. Micali N, Ploubidis G, De Stavola B, Simonoff E, Treasure J. Frequency and patterns of eating disorder symptoms in early adolescence. J Adolesc Health. 2014;54(5):574–81.
21. Schneider S, Weiss M, Thiel A, Werner A, Mayer J, Hoffmann H, Diehl K, Grp GS. Body dissatisfaction in female adolescents: extent and correlates. Eur J Pediatr. 2013;172(3):373–84.
22. Westerberg-Jacobson J, Edlund B, Ghaderi A. Risk and protective factors for disturbed eating: a 7-year longitudinal study of eating attitudes and psychological factors in adolescent girls and their parents. Eat Weight Disord. 2010;15(4):e208–18.
23. Williamson S, Delin C. Young children's figural selections: accuracy of reporting and body size dissatisfaction. Int J Eat Disord. 2001;29(1):80–4.
24. Holling H, Schlack R. Eating disorders in children and adolescents. First results of the German Health Interview and Examination Survey for Children and Adolescents (KiGGS). Bundesgesundheitsblatt, Gesundheitsforschung, Gesundheitsschutz. 2007;50(5–6):794–9.
25. Jones JM, Bennett S, Olmsted MP, Lawson ML, Rodin G. Disordered eating attitudes and behaviours in teenaged girls: a school-based study. Can Med Assoc J (journal de l'Association medicale canadienne). 2001;165(5):547–52.
26. Loth KA, MacLehose R, Bucchianeri M, Crow S, Neumark-Sztainer D. Predictors of dieting and disordered eating behaviors from adolescence to young adulthood. J Adolesc Health. 2014;55(5):705–12.
27. Tanofsky-Kraff M, Yanovski SZ, Wilfley DE, Marmarosh C, Morgan CM, Yanovski JA. Eating-disordered behaviors, body fat, and psychopathology in overweight and normal-weight children. J Consult Clin Psychol. 2004;72(1):53–61.
28. Rohde P, Stice E, Marti CN. Development and predictive effects of eating disorder risk factors during adolescence: implications for prevention efforts. Int J Eat Disord. 2015;48(2):187–98.
29. Herpertz-Dahlmann B, Dempfle A, Konrad K, Klasen F, Ravens-Sieberer U, BELLA study group. Eating disorder symptoms do not just disappear: the implications of adolescent eating-disordered behaviour for body weight and mental health in young adulthood. Eur Child Adolesc Psychiatry. 2015;24(6):675–84.
30. Gardner RM, Brown DL. Body image assessment: a review of figural drawing scales. Pers Individ Differ. 2010;48(2):107–11.
31. Cohen E, Bernard JY, Ponty A, Ndao A, Amougou N, Said-Mohamed R, Pasquet P. Development and validation of the body size scale for assessing body weight perception in african populations. PLoS ONE. 2015;10(11):e0138983.
32. Swami V, Salem N, Furnham A, Tovee MJ. Initial examination of the validity and reliability of the female photographic figure rating scale for body image assessment. Pers Individ Differ. 2008;44(8):1752–61.
33. Swami V, Stieger S, Harris AS, Nader IW, Pietschnig J, Voracek M, Tovee MJ. Further investigation of the validity and reliability of the photographic figure rating scale for body image assessment. J Pers Assess. 2012;94(4):404–9.
34. Swami V, Taylor R, Carvalho C. Body dissatisfaction assessed by the Photographic Figure Rating Scale is associated with sociocultural, personality, and media influences. Scand J Psychol. 2011;52(1):57–63.
35. Truby H, Paxton SJ. Development of the Children's Body Image Scale. Brit J Clin Psychol. 2002;41:185–203.
36. Williamson DA, White MA, York-Crowe E, Stewart TM. Cognitive-behavioral theories of eating disorders. Behav Modif. 2004;28(6):711–38.
37. Jansen A, Nederkoorn C, Mulkens S. Selective visual attention for ugly and beautiful body parts in eating disorders. Behav Res Ther. 2005;43(2):183–96.
38. Jansen A, Smeets T, Martijn C, Nederkoorn C. I see what you see: the lack of a self-serving body-image bias in eating disorders. Brit J Clin Psychol. 2006;45:123–35.
39. Smeets E, Jansen A, Roefs A. Bias for the (un)attractive self: on the role of attention in causing body (dis)satisfaction. Health Psychol. 2011;30(3):360–7.
40. Smith E, Rieger E. The effect of attentional bias toward shape- and weight-related information on body dissatisfaction. Int J Eat Disord. 2006;39(6):509–15.
41. Smith E, Rieger E. The effect of attentional training on body dissatisfaction and dietary restriction. Eur Eat Disord Rev. 2009;17(3):169–76.
42. Wyssen A, Bryjova J, Meyer AH, Munsch S. A model of disturbed eating behavior in men: the role of body dissatisfaction, emotion dysregulation and cognitive distortions. Psychiatry Res. 2016;246:9–15.
43. Brooks S, Prince A, Stahl D, Campbell IC, Treasure J. A systematic review and meta-analysis of cognitive bias to food stimuli in people with disordered eating behaviour. Clin Psychol Rev. 2011;31(1):37–51.
44. Stunkard A, Sorensen T, Schulsinger F. Use of the Danish Adoption Register for the study of obesity and thinness. Res Publ Assoc Res Nerv Ment Dis. 1983;60:115–20.
45. Fairburn CG, Beglin SJ. Assessment of eating disorder psychopathology. Interview or self-report questionnaire? Int J Eat Disord. 1994;16:363–70.

46. Hilbert A, Tuschen-Caffiert B. Eating disorder examination: Deutschsprachige Übersetzung. Münster: Verlag für Psychotherapy: 2006.

47. Knauss C, Paxton SJ, Alsaker FD. Validation of the German version of the Sociocultural Attitudes Towards Appearance Questionnaire (SATAQ-G). Body Image. 2009;6:113–20.

48. Thompson JK, van den Berg P, Roehrig M, Guarda AS, Heinberg LJ. The sociocultural attitudes towards appearance scale-3 (SATAQ-3): development and validation. Int J Eat Disord. 2004;35:293–304.

49. Israel AC, Ivanova MY. Global and dimensional self-esteem in preadolescent and early adolescent children who are overweight: age and gender differences. Int J Eat Disorder. 2002;31(4):424–9.

50. Bundesamt 2014. Retrieved from: https://www.destatis.de/DE/ZahlenFakten/GesellschaftStaat/BildungForschungKultur/Schulen/Schulen.html. Accessed 19 Jan 2018.

51. Mikrozensus 2013. Retrieved from: https://www.destatis.de/DE/ZahlenFakten/GesellschaftStaat/Gesundheit/GesundheitszustandRelevantesVerhalten/Tabellen/Koerpermasse.html. Accessed 19 Jan 2018.

52. Neighbors C, Dillard AJ, Lewis MA, Bergstrom RL, Neil TA. Normative misperceptions and temporal precedence of perceived norms and drinking. J Stud Alcohol. 2006;67(2):290–9.

53. Otten R, Engels RC, Prinstein MJ. A prospective study of perception in adolescent smoking. J Adolesc Health. 2009;44(5):478–84.

54. Sanderson CA, Darley JM, Messinger CS. "I'm not as thin as you think I am": the development and consequences of feeling discrepant from the thinness norm. Pers Soc Psychol B. 2002;28(2):172–83.

55. Connolly JM, Slaughter V, Mealey L. The development of preferences for specific body shapes. J sex Res. 2004;41(1):5–15.

56. Glauert R, Rhodes G, Byrne S, Fink B, Grammer K. Body dissatisfaction and the effects of perceptual exposure on body norms and ideals. Int J Eat Disord. 2009;42(5):443–52.

57. Winkler C, Rhodes G. Perceptual adaptation affects attractiveness of female bodies. Br J Psychol. 2005;96(Pt 2):141–54.

58. Koscinski K. Assessment of waist-to-hip ratio attractiveness in women: an anthropometric analysis of digital silhouettes. Arch Sex Behav. 2014;43(5):989–97.

59. Crossley KL, Cornelissen PL, Tovee MJ. What is an attractive body? Using an interactive 3D program to create the ideal body for you and your partner. PLoS ONE. 2012;7(11):e50601.

60. Bergstrom RL, Neighbors C, Lewis MA. Do men find "bony" women attractive?: consequences of misperceiving opposite sex perceptions of attractive body image. Body Image. 2004;1(2):183–91.

61. Fallon AE, Rozin P. Sex differences in perceptions of desirable body shape. J Abnorm Psychol. 1985;94(1):102–5.

62. Prantl L, Grundl M. Males prefer a larger bust size in women than females themselves: an experimental study on female bodily attractiveness with varying weight, bust size, waist width, hip width, and leg length independently. Aesthetic Plast Surg. 2011;35(5):693–702.

63. Gowers S, Bryant-Waugh R. Management of child and adolescent eating disorders: the current evidence base and future directions. J Child Psychol Psychiatry. 2004;45(1):63–83.

64. Ordabayeva N, Chandon P. In the eye of the beholder: visual biases in package and portion size perceptions. Appetite. 2016;103:450–57.

10

Dietary behaviour, psychological well-being and mental distress among adolescents in Korea

Seo Ah Hong[1,2] and Karl Peltzer[3,4]* (iD)

Abstract

Background: Dietary intake is important for physical and mental health. The aim of this investigation was to assess associations between dietary behaviours and psychological well-being and distress among school-going adolescents in Korea.

Methods: In a cross-sectional nationally representative survey, 65,212 students (Mean age = 15.1 years, SE = 0.02 and 52.2% male and 47.8% female) responded to a questionnaire that included measures of dietary behaviour, psychological well-being and mental distress.

Results: In logistic regression analyses, adjusted for age, sex, socioeconomic status, school level, school types, Body Mass Index, physical activity, and substance use, positive dietary behaviours (regular breakfast, fruit, vegetable, and milk consumption) were positively and unhealthy dietary behaviours (intake of caffeine, soft drinks, sweet drinks and fast food consumption) were negatively associated with self-reported health, happiness and sleep satisfaction. Positive dietary behaviours (regular breakfast, fruit, vegetable, and milk consumption) were negatively associated with perceived stress and depression symptoms. Unhealthy dietary behaviours (consumption of fast food, caffeine, sweetened drinks and soft drinks) were associated with perceived stress and depression symptoms.

Conclusions: The study found strong cross-sectional evidence that healthy dietary behaviours were associated with lower mental distress and higher psychological well-being. It remains unclear, if a healthier dietary behaviour is the cause or the sequela of a more positive well-being.

Background

Recently, more studies have been trying to link dietary behaviour to psychological well-being and distress [1–6]. Regular fruit, vegetable and breakfast intake (healthy dietary behaviours) have been found positively associated with self-reported health, happiness, and better sleep [1–8], and regular fruit, vegetable and breakfast intake were negatively associated with perceived stress, mental distress and depression [1–3, 9–25]. Further, specific unhealthy dietary behaviours (consumption of soft drinks, fast food, sweets and snacks, skipping breakfast,

and caffeine) were associated with unhappiness, perceived stress, mental or psychological distress, depression or poorer sleep [5, 8, 19, 24–36]. Mixed results were found in relation to the consumption of milk and psychological well-being. One study found that increased milk product consumption was associated with depression [37], Meyer et al. [38] found milk consumption improves sleep quality, and Aizawa et al. [39] found that the frequency of fermented milk consumption was associated with higher Bifidobacterium counts and that patient with major depressive disorder have lower Bifidobacterium and/or Lactobacillus counts.

In a study among Iranian children and adolescents junk food consumption (such as fast foods, sweets, sweetened beverages, and salty snacks) was significantly associated with mental distress, including "worry, depression,

*Correspondence: karl.peltzer@tdt.edu.vn
[3] Department for Management of Science and Technology Development, Ton Duc Thang University, Ho Chi Minh City, Vietnam
[4] Faculty of Pharmacy, Ton Duc Thang University, Ho Chi Minh City, Vietnam
Full list of author information is available at the end of the article

confusion, insomnia, anxiety, aggression, and feelings of being worthless." [26] Fast food consumption was associated with depression among adolescent girls in Korea [32], and among Chinese adolescents, snack consumption was associated with psychological symptoms [34]. The poor nutrient content of junk or fast foods may have an effect on normal brain functioning and, thus, have an effect on negative mood via the synthesis of neurotransmitters such as serotonin [40, 41]. In a study among adolescents in Norway, a J-shaped relationship between soft drink consumption and mental distress was found [42]. The effects of soft drink or sugar consumption on mental health may be mediated through other nutritional or behavioural factors [42]. Among secondary school students in Malaysia, regular breakfast consumption was negatively associated with mild or moderate stress [23]. In a large study of adolescent school-going children (N = 3071) from the United Kingdom, positive relationships between caffeine consumption and anxiety and depression were found [33]. It is possible that students used caffeinated products to cope with stress [33, 43].

We have limited information on the relationship between dietary behaviour, psychological well-being and mental distress among adolescents in Asia, which prompted this study. It was hypothesized that healthy dietary behaviour enhances psychological well-being and reduces mental distress, and unhealthy dietary behaviours reduce psychological well-being and increase mental distress.

Methods

Data sources

The data utilized for this study came from the 2016 12th "Korea Youth Risk Behavior Web-based Survey (KYRBS)" [44]. The KYRBS is an annual anonymous online self-reported cross-sectional survey on various health behaviours that uses a stratified cluster sampling procedure to source middle and high school students that are representative of the adolescent school population in Korea [44], more details under [44]. The online survey was administered during class after survey instructions had been given and written informed consent had been obtained [44]. In 2016, the survey included a total of 798 schools, and a total of 65,528 respondents participated, resulting in a response rate of 96.4% [44].

Measures

Three assessment measures of psychological well-being (self-rated health, happiness, and sleep satisfaction) and two questions on mental distress (perceived stress and depression symptoms) were used in this study.

Self-rated health was assessed with the question: "How healthy do you usually feel?" (Response option ranged from 1 = very healthy to 5 = very unhealthy) [44]. Responses were dichotomized into 1 or 2 = above average health and 3–5 = an average or below average health.

Perceived happiness was measured with the question: "How happy do you usually feel?" (Response options: (1) very happy, (2) happy, (3) average, (4) unhappy, or (5) very unhappy) [44]. Responses were dichotomized into 1–2 = above average happiness and 3–5 = average or below average happiness.

Sleep satisfaction was assessed with the question, "In the past 7 days, did you get adequate sleep to overcome fatigue?" (Response options ranged from 1 = Sufficient to 5 = Not sufficient at all) [44]. Responses were dichotomized into 1–2 = above average sufficient sleep and 3–5 = average or below average sufficient sleep.

Perceived stress was assessed with the question, "To what degree are you usually stressed?" (Response options arranged from 1 = very much to 5 = not at all) [44]. Responses were dichotomized into 1–2 = above average stress and 3–5 = average or below average stress.

Depression symptoms were assessed with the question, "Have you experienced sadness or despair to the degree that you stopped your daily routine for the recent 12 months?" (Response option, "Yes" or "No") [44].

Dietary behaviours

To evaluate dietary behaviours, the regularity of breakfast meal time consumed over the past 7 days was surveyed with eight scales from 0 to 7 days. For food groups consumed over the past 7 days, the participants were asked the frequency of seven food groups, such as (1) soft drinks, (2) highly caffeinated drinks, (3) sweetened drinks, (4) fast food foods (such as pizza, hamburgers, or chicken), (5) fruits (not fruit juices), (6) vegetable dishes (excluding Kimchi), and (7) milk consumption during the past 7 days and the responses were from 1 = none, 2 = 1–2 times/week, 3 = 3–4 times/week, 4 = 5–6 times/week, 5 = once/day, 6 = twice/day, and 7 = 3 times or more/day [44].

Control variables

Sociodemographic variables included gender, age, geolocality (rural area, small or large city), maternal and paternal educational level, perceived socioeconomic status (SES), types of school (Boys only, girls only and mixed), school level (middle school and high school) [44].

The Body Mass Index (BMI) of students was calculated by dividing their self-reported weight in kilogrammes by their height in meters squared (kg/m^2). According to age and gender, the students were categorized into "underweight (< 5th percentile), normal weight (5th ≤ BMI < 85th percentile), overweight (85th ≤ BMI < 95th percentile), and obese (≥ 95th percentile)", following the BMI cut-off criteria set for Korean children by the 2007 Korean Growth Charts [45].

Physical activity was assessed in terms of the frequency of physical activity of ≥ 60 min per day during the past 7 days [44]. Responses were categorised into 1 = no days, 2 = 1–2 days, and 3 = 3–7 days.

Lifetime alcohol and tobacco use was measured with the questions, "Have you ever used alcohol?" and "Have you ever used tobacco?" (Response option, "Yes", "No") [44].

Data analysis
Descriptive statistics were used to present the proportion or mean of general subject characteristics and outcome variables. Logistic regression tests were performed to estimate adjusted odds ratios (ORs) and 95% confidence intervals (CIs) after adjustment for selected covariates. Logistic regression analyses were conducted to calculate the association between the adolescents' well-being and mental distress variables as the main outcome variables and dietary behaviour variables after adjustment for covariates selected from bivariate association analysis with outcome variables. All analyses conducted took the sampling design parameters, weighting, clustering, and stratification of the study survey into account. All values were weighted according to the participant's probability of being chosen by sex-, grade-, and school type-specific distributions for the study region [46]. The "finite population correction (fpc) factor was used to avoid the overestimation, when developing variance estimates for population parameters" [47]. All statistical analyses was done by SAS 9.3 (SAS Institute, Cary, NC).

Results
Sample characteristics
The sample included 65,528 school-going adolescents (Mean age = 15.1 years, SE = 0.02; age range 12–18 years) from Korea. More than half of the sample (52.2%) were male, attended high school (54.6%), and a mixed school (62.0%). More than one-third (37.2%) of the students perceived to have a high or high-middle socio-economic status, 63.4 and 56.0% had a father and had a mother, respectively, with college or higher education. Overall, 17.3% of the students were overweight or obese, 31.3% engaged in 60 min or more physical activity 3–4 times a week, 14.8% ever smoked and 38.8% ever drank alcohol (see Table 1).

Prevalence of well-being and mental distress indicators
Regarding well-being indicators, 26.5% of the students perceived themselves to be "very healthy", 28.1% as "very happy" and 25.8% had sufficient or quite sufficient sleep satisfaction. In terms of mental distress, 37.3% of students reported somewhat or very much "perceived

stress", while 25.5% reported depression symptoms (see Table 2).

Associations between dietary behaviours with well-being and mental distress indicators
Tables 3 and 4 describe the bivariate associations with well-being and mental distress indicators, and Table 5

Table 1 General characteristics of study participants

	Unweighted frequency	Weighted %
Sex		
Boys	33,803	52.2
Girls	31,725	47.8
Age (years), mean (sd)	65,212	15.1 (0.02)
BMI		
Thinness (< 5th percentile)	3586	5.7
Normal weight (5th ≤ BMI < 85th percentile)	48,979	77.0
Overweight (85th ≤ BMI < 95th percentile)	2994	4.5
Obesity (≥ 95th percentile)	8182	12.8
School		
High school	33,309	54.6
Middle school	32,219	45.4
Types of school		
Mixed	41,445	62.0
Boys only	12,032	19.3
Girls only	12,051	18.7
Paternal education level		
High school or less	19,610	36.6
College or higher	31,977	63.4
Maternal education level		
High school or less	23,497	44.0
College or higher	28,860	56.0
Perceived socio-economic status		
High/high-middle	24,244	37.2
Middle	31,056	47.3
Low-middle/Low	10,228	15.6
Place of residence		
Rural area	4856	5.8
Large city	29,046	43.3
Medium-sized city	31,626	50.8
Physical activity (≥ 60 min)		
No	23,817	36.8
1–2/week	20,859	32.0
3+/week	20,852	31.3
Ever smoking in lifetime (yes)	9511	14.8
Ever alcohol drinking in lifetime (yes)	24,804	38.8

All values are presented as weighted Mean (SD) or weighted % as appropriate

Table 2 Prevalence of mental health among adolescents

	Unweighted Frequency	Weighted %
1. Well-being outcomes		
Perceived health		
Very healthy	17,586	26.5
Healthy	29,647	45.3
Fair	14,223	21.9
Poor	3846	6.0
Very poor	226	0.4
Perceived happiness		
Very happy	18,992	28.1
Happy	24,964	38.5
Fair	16,743	25.8
Unhappy	4102	6.4
Very unhappy	727	1.1
Sleep satisfaction (Fatigue recovery from sleep)		
Quite sufficient	5413	7.8
Sufficient	12,081	18.0
So So	20,705	31.7
Not sufficient	18,296	28.4
Not sufficient at all	9033	14.1
2. Mental distress outcomes		
Perceived stress		
Very much	6513	10.0
Somewhat	17,833	27.3
Average	28,021	42.9
Not so much	10,772	16.2
Not at all	2389	3.6
Signs and symptoms of depression during the last year		
No	48,993	74.5
Yes	16,535	25.5

All values are presented as weighted %

the adjusted analysis with well-being and mental distress indicators. In logistic regression analysis, adjusted for potential confounders, positive dietary behaviours (fruit and vegetable consumption, daily breakfast, milk consumption) were positively and unhealthy dietary behaviours (intake of caffeine, soft drinks, sweet drinks and fast food) were negatively associated with happiness or sleep satisfaction or self-reported health. Positive dietary behaviours (fruit and vegetable consumption, having daily breakfast, and milk consumption) were negatively associated with perceived stress and depression symptoms. Unhealthy dietary behaviours (fast food, caffeine, sweetened drinks and soft drinks consumption) were positively associated with perceived stress and depression symptoms (see Tables 3, 4, 5).

Discussion

This study found in agreement with previous studies [1–3] that a dose–response relationship between healthy dietary behaviours (regular fruit, vegetable, breakfast, and milk consumption) and well-being outcomes (perceived health, happiness and sleep satisfaction). In particular, the linear association with positive perceived health and happiness were stronger in fruit and vegetable consumption. A study among ASEAN university students showed a significant association but no dose–response relationship between fruits and vegetable consumption and positive self-rated health status [6]. Hoefelmann et al. [48] also found that higher fruit and vegetables consumption was associated with better sleep quality among Brazilian workers. Reasons for this finding are not clear and need further investigations.

Table 3 Association between covariates and mental health among adolescents

| | Well-being outcomes | | | | | | | | | Mental distress outcomes | | | | | |
| | Perceived health | | | Perceived happiness | | | Sleep satisfaction | | | Perceived stress | | | Depression | | |
	Bad	Good	p-value	Unhappy	Happy	p-value	Insufficient	Sufficient	p-value	Less	Much	p-value	No	Yes	p-value
Sex (boys)	43.2	55.7	<.0001	47.2	54.7	<.0001	47.7	64.8	<.0001	57.9	42.5	<.0001	55.4	42.7	<.0001
Age (years), mean (SD)	15.4 (0.02)	15.0 (0.02)	<.0001	15.4 (0.02)	15.0 (0.02)	<.0001	15.3 (0.02)	15.0 (0.03)	<.0001	15.0 (0.02)	15.3 (0.02)	<.0001	15.0 (0.02)	15.3 (0.02)	<.0001
BMI															
Normal weight	71.4	79.2	<.0001	76.3	77.4	0.008	77.3	76.2	0.0239	77.8	75.6	<.0001	77.0	77.1	0.3670
Thinness	7.3	5.1		5.8	5.6		5.6	6.0		5.8	5.5		5.8	5.5	
Overweight/obesity	21.3	15.7		18.0	17.0		17.1	17.9		16.4	18.8		17.2	17.5	
School level															
High school	62.3	51.6	<.0001	62.4	50.7	<.0001	60.0	39.2	<.0001	51.9	59.2	<.0001	52.9	59.5	<.0001
Middle school	37.7	48.4		37.6	49.3		40.0	60.8		48.1	40.8		47.1	40.5	
Types of school															
Mixed	60.8	62.5	<.0001	61.1	62.5	<.0001	60.6	66.1	<.0001	62.6	61.0	<.0001	61.8	62.6	<.0001
Boys only	16.8	20.3		18.0	19.9		18.5	21.4		21.3	15.9		20.7	15.2	
Girls only	22.4	17.2		21.0	17.6		20.9	12.5		16.0	23.2		17.5	22.1	
Paternal education level															
High school or less	39.8	35.3	<.0001	39.4	35.2	<.0001	37.4	34.1	<.0001	35.7	37.9	<.0001	36.4	37.1	0.1642
College or higher	60.2	64.7		60.6	64.8		62.6	65.9		64.3	62.1		63.6	62.9	
Maternal education level															
High school or less	47.9	42.5	0.0009	47.4	42.4	<.0001	45.3	40.3	<.0001	42.9	45.8	<.0001	44.0	44.2	0.7602
College or higher	52.1	57.5		52.6	57.6		54.7	59.7		57.1	54.2		56.0	55.8	
Socio-economic status															
High/upper middle	27.3	41.0	<.0001	26.4	42.6	<.0001	34.6	44.5	<.0001	39.1	33.8	<.0001	38.0	34.6	<.0001
Middle	50.1	46.1		50.4	45.7		48.5	43.7		48.2	45.7		48.1	44.7	
Lower middle/Low	22.6	12.8		23.2	11.7		16.9	11.8		12.7	20.5		13.8	20.8	
Place of residence															
Rural area	5.4	6.0	0.0016	5.6	6.0	0.006	5.7	6.3	0.2566	5.7	6.1	0.1621	6.0	5.6	<.0001
Large city	42.0	43.8		42.2	43.9		43.3	43.3		43.8	42.6		43.8	44.7	
Medium-sized city	52.6	50.1		52.2	50.1		51.0	50.4		50.5	51.3		50.1	49.7	
Physical activity (≥ 60 min)															
No	42.9	34.3	<.0001	41.0	34.7	<.0001	37.6	34.3	<.0001	35.8	38.4	<.0001	37.2	35.6	0.0011
1-2/week	34.6	30.9		32.7	31.6		32.8	29.6		31.2	33.3		31.6	33.1	
3+/week	22.5	34.7		26.4	33.7		29.6	36.0		33.1	28.3		31.3	31.3	
Ever smoking (yes)	15.7	14.5	0.0013	17.7	13.4	<.0001	15.9	11.9	<.0001	13.9	16.4	<.0001	12.9	20.4	<.0001
Ever alcohol drinking (yes)	42.0	37.5	<.0001	44.4	36.0	<.0001	41.7	30.4	<.0001	36.2	43.1	<.0001	35.5	48.3	<.0001

All values are presented as weighted mean ± SD or weighted % as appropriate

Recent meta-analyses confirmed an inverse association of healthy dietary patterns [49, 50] with poor mental health outcomes, like depression in adults. However, the findings in adolescents remained inconsistent. In agreement with previous studies [1–3, 9–25], this study found that healthy dietary behaviours (regular fruit, vegetable, breakfast, and milk consumption) were negatively associated with perceived stress and depression symptoms, despite no linear associations of consumption of fruit, vegetable, and milk. A population-based study among Swiss people aged 15+ years showed those fulfilling the 5-a-day fruit and vegetable consumption had lower odds of being highly or moderately distressed than individuals consuming less fruit and vegetables (OR = 0.82 for moderate distress, and OR = 0.55, for high distress compared to low distress) [31]. It is possible that due to the consumption of fruits and vegetables, being rich in antioxidants, folic acid and anti-inflammatory components, human optimism or happiness is enhanced [28] and the development of negative mood or depression symptoms decreased [29].

In agreement with previous studies [8, 24–31, 35] unhealthy dietary behaviours (consumption of soft drinks, caffeine, fast food, sweets and snacks, and skipping breakfast) were associated with low self-rated health, unhappiness, and low sleep satisfaction. Although the association became weaker at three or more times consumption of fast foods, increased unhealthy dietary behaviours were inversely associated with positive well-being outcomes, in particular, perceived health and happiness. On the other hand, a dose–response relationship between unhealthy dietary behaviours, such as consumption of soft drinks, highly caffeinated drinks, sweetened drinks, and fast food, and inversely, frequency of breakfast consumption as a health dietary behaviour with depression was observed in this study. These findings are consistent with a prospective Australian adolescents study [51] and a prospective cohort study also showed a positive association of fast food and commercial baked foods with depression in adults [52]. However, in a study among university students in ASEAN countries an inverse dose–response relationship between eating breakfast and sugared coffee/tea and a positive linear association between the consumption of snacks, fast foods, soft drinks and depression symptoms [6]. Although the relationship between sugar consumption and major depression seems to have been confirmed in cross-national observations in Asian countries [53], a study among ASEAN university students has shown an inverse dose–response relationship between sugared coffee/tea consumption and depression symptoms [6]. These findings emphasize the need for further investigations.

Nevertheless, some studies have suggested that an increase in carbohydrate-dense but nutrient-poor foods, such as fast food, sweets and snacks, may be used by individuals to cope with negative mood and elevate mood by increasing brain serotonin levels [42]. Several other studies among adolescents [54] and young adults [55] also found an association between caffeine consumption and low sleep satisfaction or poor sleep quality. A study among adolescents in Germany suggested that later bed and rise times were associated with increased consumption of caffeinated drinks and fast food [56]. The biological mechanism to explain this includes that caffeine increases alertness and increased energy as a function of its interactions with adenosine receptors in the brain [57]. However, caffeine use seems to only reduce sleep quality in individuals that are sensitive to the adenosine effects of caffeine [58]. In addition, the German study reported reduced consumption of dairy products was also associated with later bed and rise times [56]. Our study findings supported this study by showing that frequent milk consumption (once per day or more) was associated with sufficient sleep satisfaction. Further, as the practice of skipping breakfast may increase poor sleep quality [30], our study also showed a positive association between regular breakfast consumption and sleep satisfaction. In terms of fast foods, less frequent consumption of fast foods (less than once per day) showed an inverse association, but among those having once per day or more fast foods the association disappeared. This study may lead to a need for a prospective study to examine the causality, since strong relationships with a dose–response relationship between healthy dietary behaviours and well-being parameters and between unhealthy dietary behaviours and mental distress were found.

Study limitations

The cross-sectional design does not explain if positive well-being promotes a healthier dietary behaviour or healthier dietary patterns lead to more positive well-being. Some of the concepts assessed in this study used single item measures such as depression symptoms, happiness and perceived stress, and future studies should include multiple item measures to assess key concepts. Despite the limitations, the inclusion of data from 65,528 adolescents from a nationally representative sample in South Korea supports the external validity of the study results.

Conclusions

In a large nationally representative sample of adolescent in Korea, strong cross-sectional evidence was found that increased unhealthier dietary behaviour was associated with higher mental distress, while healthier dietary

Table 4 Association between dietary behaviours and mental health among adolescents

Weighted %		Well-being outcomes						Sleep satisfaction			Mental distress outcomes					
		Perceived health			Perceived happiness						Perceived stress			Depression		
		Poor	Good	p-value	Unhappy	Happy	p-value	Insufficient	Sufficient	p-value	Less	Much	p-value	No	Yes	p-value
Breakfast																
0 day	14.9	16.8	14.1	<.0001	17.2	13.7	<.0001	15.5	13.1	<.0001	13.7	16.8	<.0001	14.3	16.7	<.0001
1 day	6.0	7.0	5.6		6.9	5.5		6.3	5.0		5.6	6.6		5.6	6.9	
2 days	7.4	8.4	7.0		8.4	6.9		7.7	6.4		6.9	8.2		6.9	8.6	
3 days	7.5	8.0	7.3		8.5	7.0		7.8	6.8		7.2	8.1		7.3	8.0	
4 days	6.5	7.3	6.2		6.6	6.5		6.8	5.7		6.4	6.7		6.3	7.1	
5 days	10.7	11.7	10.3		11.2	10.4		11.2	9.1		10.5	10.9		10.5	11.2	
6 days	8.6	8.3	8.8		8.3	8.8		8.9	7.9		8.8	8.4		8.7	8.6	
7 days	38.4	32.6	40.8		33.0	41.2		35.8	46.0		40.9	34.3		40.3	32.9	
Soft drinks																
I did not drink	24.2	24.5	24.1	<.0001	24.3	24.1	<.0001	23.8	25.2	<.0001	24.1	24.4	<.0001	24.8	22.4	<.0001
1–2 times/week	48.7	47.0	49.4		46.7	49.8		48.7	49.0		49.7	47.1		49.4	46.7	
3–4 times/week	18.9	19.1	18.7		19.3	18.6		19.1	18.3		18.8	19.0		18.4	20.3	
5–6 times/week	4.3	4.7	4.2		4.9	4.0		4.5	3.9		4.0	4.8		4.0	5.2	
Once/day	2.0	2.3	1.9		2.4	1.9		2.0	2.0		1.8	2.4		1.9	2.5	
Twice/day	0.9	1.1	0.8		1.1	0.8		1.0	0.7		0.8	1.0		0.8	1.2	
3+ times/day	0.9	1.3	0.8		1.3	0.8		1.0	0.8		0.7	1.3		0.7	1.5	
Highly caffeinated drink																
I did not drink	86.2	83.4	87.3	<.0001	83.0	87.8	<.0001	85.2	89.2	<.0001	88.4	82.5	<.0001	88.1	80.7	<.0001
1–2 times/week	9.9	11.2	9.3		11.4	9.1		10.4	8.2		8.7	11.8		8.9	12.7	
3–4 times/week	2.2	2.8	2.0		3.1	1.8		2.5	1.5		1.6	3.2		1.8	3.4	
5–6 times/week	0.8	1.0	0.7		1.1	0.6		0.8	0.6		0.6	1.0		0.6	1.4	
Once/day	0.5	0.8	0.4		0.8	0.4		0.6	0.2		0.3	0.8		0.4	1.0	
Twice/day	0.2	0.4	0.1		0.3	0.1		0.2	0.1		0.1	0.3		0.1	0.4	
3+ times/day	0.2	0.3	0.2		0.3	0.2		0.2	0.2		0.2	0.4		0.1	0.5	
Sweetened drinks																
I did not drink	15.4	15.1	15.5	<.0001	15.5	15.4	<.0001	14.4	18.2	<.0001	16.0	14.5	<.0001	16.3	12.8	<.0001
1–2 times/week	43.2	41.3	43.9		41.5	44.0		42.6	44.7		44.6	40.8		44.2	40.3	
3–4 times/week	26.4	26.4	26.5		26.6	26.4		27.0	24.7		26.1	27.1		25.8	28.5	
5–6 times/week	8.0	8.7	7.7		8.5	7.7		8.4	6.6		7.4	8.9		7.6	9.2	
Once/day	4.3	4.9	4.0		4.5	4.1		4.5	3.5		3.8	5.0		3.9	5.2	
Twice/day	1.5	1.9	1.4		1.8	1.4		1.7	1.1		1.2	2.1		1.3	2.3	
3+ times/day	1.2	1.7	1.0		1.5	1.0		1.2	1.1		0.9	1.7		1.0	1.8	

Table 4 continued

Weighted %	Well-being outcomes									Mental distress outcomes					
	Perceived health			Perceived happiness			Sleep satisfaction			Perceived stress			Depression		
	Poor	Good	p-value	Unhappy	Happy	p-value	Insufficient	Sufficient	p-value	Less	Much	p-value	No	Yes	p-value
Fast foods															
I did not eat	22.8	21.9	23.2	<.0001	22.3	23.1	<.0001	21.8	25.9	<.0001	23.4	22.0	<.0001	23.7	20.3	<.0001
1–2 times/week	60.4	59.1	61.0		58.7	61.3		60.6	60.0		61.2	59.1		61.2	58.4	
3–4 times/week	13.7	15.1	13.1		14.9	13.0		14.4	11.5		12.8	15.1		12.7	16.5	
5–6 times/week	1.9	2.3	1.7		2.4	1.6		2.0	1.5		1.7	2.2		1.6	2.6	
Once/day	0.7	1.0	0.6		1.0	0.6		0.7	0.7		0.6	1.0		0.6	1.2	
Twice/day	0.2	0.3	0.2		0.3	0.2		0.2	0.2		0.2	0.3		0.2	0.4	
3+ times/day	0.2	0.3	0.2		0.4	0.2		0.3	0.2		0.2	0.4		0.1	0.6	
Fruits (excluding fruit juices)															
I did not eat	8.6	11.7	7.4	<.0001	11.8	7.0	<.0001	9.1	7.5	<.0001	7.6	10.5	<.0001	8.3	9.7	<.0001
1–2 times/week	28.7	32.1	27.4		32.3	27.0		30.0	25.1		27.7	30.4		28.3	29.9	
3–4 times/week	27.9	26.5	28.4		26.6	28.5		27.9	27.8		28.8	26.4		28.2	26.9	
5–6 times/week	11.5	10.4	12.0		10.4	12.1		11.3	12.2		11.9	11.0		11.8	10.8	
Once/day	12.6	10.8	13.4		10.6	13.6		12.2	14.0		13.1	11.8		12.8	12.2	
Twice/day	6.1	5.0	6.6		4.5	6.9		5.6	7.7		6.4	5.7		6.3	5.8	
3+ times/day	4.4	3.4	4.8		3.7	4.8		3.9	5.9		4.6	4.2		4.3	4.7	
Vegetable (excluding Kimchi)															
I did not eat	3.8	5.6	3.1	<.0001	5.1	3.1	<.0001	4.0	3.0	<.0001	3.1	5.0	<.0001	3.5	4.5	<.0001
1–2 times/week	15.5	19.4	13.9		18.5	14.0		16.5	12.7		14.7	16.8		15.0	17.0	
3–4 times/week	24.3	26.0	23.6		25.6	23.6		24.8	22.8		24.4	24.0		24.4	23.8	
5–6 times/week	14.2	13.3	14.5		13.6	14.4		14.0	14.5		14.5	13.6		14.4	13.5	
Once/day	13.0	12.0	13.4		12.5	13.3		12.9	13.4		13.4	12.4		13.0	13.0	
Twice/day	14.9	12.4	15.9		12.9	15.9		14.6	15.8		15.3	14.3		15.2	14.3	
3+ times/day	14.3	11.3	15.5		11.7	15.7		13.1	17.9		14.5	14.0		14.5	13.9	
Milk															
I did not drink	16.2	20.7	14.4	<.0001	19.7	14.4	<.0001	17.2	13.2	<.0001	14.4	19.1	<.0001	15.5	18.1	<.0001
1–2 times/week	22.6	25.3	21.5		24.4	21.6		23.8	19.2		21.9	23.7		22.2	23.7	
3–4 times/week	20.2	19.8	20.3		19.8	20.4		20.3	19.8		20.5	19.7		20.2	20.1	
5–6 times/week	14.3	13.1	14.7		13.4	14.7		14.0	15.1		14.8	13.4		14.6	13.2	
Once/day	16.0	12.9	17.2		13.7	17.1		15.3	18.1		16.9	14.4		16.5	14.7	
Twice/day	6.2	4.8	6.7		5.1	6.7		5.6	7.8		6.6	5.5		6.3	5.9	
3+ times/day	4.6	3.3	5.2		3.8	5.0		3.9	6.8		4.9	4.2		4.7	4.4	

All values are presented as weighted %

Table 5 Adjusted odds ratios of well-being and mental distress indicators in relation to dietary behaviours among adolescents

	Well-being outcomes						Mental distress outcomes			
	Perceived health (healthy)		Perceived happiness (happy)		Sleep satisfaction (sufficient)		Perceived stress (much)		Depression (yes)	
	aOR[1]	(95% CI)	aOR[1]	(95% CI)	aOR[2]	(95% CI)	aOR[2]	(95% CI)	aOR[3]	(95% CI)
Dietary behaviors										
Breakfast										
0 day	1.00		1.00		1.00		1.00		1.00	
1 day	0.95	(0.85–1.05)	1.01	(0.92–1.11)	0.96	(0.85–1.09)	0.91	(0.83–1.00)	0.97	(0.89–1.06)
2 days	1.04	(0.95–1.14)	1.06	(0.97–1.15)	0.99	(0.89–1.11)	0.95	(0.87–1.04)	1.02	(0.94–1.10)
3 days	1.06	(0.97–1.17)	1.02	(0.94–1.11)	1.12	(1.01–1.25)	0.91	(0.84–0.99)	0.88	(0.82–0.96)
4 days	0.98	(0.89–1.08)	1.22	(1.11–1.34)	0.99	(0.88–1.11)	0.83	(0.76–0.92)	0.94	(0.87–1.02)
5 days	1.01	(0.94–1.10)	1.16	(1.07–1.25)	0.99	(0.91–1.09)	0.85	(0.79–0.91)	0.89	(0.83–0.96)
6 days	1.22	(1.12–1.34)	1.30	(1.19–1.42)	1.13	(1.03–1.23)	0.76	(0.70–0.82)	0.86	(0.79–0.93)
7 days	1.34	(1.25–1.43)	1.42	(1.34–1.51)	1.45	(1.35–1.56)	0.74	(0.70–0.78)	0.76	(0.72–0.81)
Soft drinks										
I did not drink	1.00		1.00		1.00		1.00		1.00	
1–2 times/week	1.04	(0.99–1.09)	1.08	(1.03–1.13)	0.90	(0.86–0.96)	0.97	(0.93–1.02)	1.05	(1.00–1.09)
3–4 times/week	0.90	(0.84–0.96)	0.95	(0.89–1.01)	0.77	(0.72–0.82)	1.07	(1.01–1.14)	1.24	(1.17–1.31)
5–6 times/week	0.83	(0.74–0.92)	0.82	(0.74–0.91)	0.70	(0.62–0.80)	1.39	(1.25–1.54)	1.44	(1.31–1.58)
Once/day	0.73	(0.63–0.84)	0.76	(0.66–0.88)	0.77	(0.65–0.91)	1.47	(1.28–1.70)	1.57	(1.38–1.79)
Twice/day	0.63	(0.50–0.79)	0.77	(0.62–0.94)	0.58	(0.44–0.77)	1.41	(1.12–1.78)	1.59	(1.34–1.89)
3+ times/day	0.63	(0.50–0.78)	0.67	(0.53–0.84)	0.80	(0.63–1.01)	1.75	(1.41–2.18)	2.07	(1.75–2.44)
Highly caffeinated drink										
I did not drink	1.00		1.00		1.00		1.00		1.00	
1–2 times/week	0.77	(0.72–0.83)	0.73	(0.69–0.78)	0.68	(0.63–0.73)	1.50	(1.42–1.60)	1.50	(1.42–1.59)
3–4 times/week	0.65	(0.57–0.74)	0.55	(0.49–0.62)	0.56	(0.48–0.66)	2.22	(1.96–2.52)	1.91	(1.71–2.13)
5–6 times/week	0.58	(0.46–0.73)	0.55	(0.44–0.68)	0.70	(0.53–0.92)	1.96	(1.58–2.44)	2.66	(2.19–3.23)
Once/day	0.44	(0.33–0.58)	0.43	(0.34–0.55)	0.40	(0.27–0.58)	3.43	(2.67–4.41)	2.62	(2.15–3.20)
Twice/day	0.30	(0.19–0.45)	0.42	(0.26–0.69)	0.49	(0.26–0.96)	3.49	(2.28–5.34)	3.57	(2.38–5.34)
3+ times/day	0.39	(0.25–0.62)	0.43	(0.28–0.68)	0.77	(0.45–1.32)	3.01	(1.85–4.89)	3.25	(2.24–4.71)
Sweetened drinks										
I did not drink	1.00		1.00		1.00		1.00		1.00	
1–2 times/week	1.01	(0.95–1.07)	1.06	(1.00–1.12)	0.87	(0.82–0.93)	0.99	(0.94–1.05)	1.12	(1.06–1.18)
3–4 times/week	0.92	(0.86–0.99)	0.99	(0.93–1.06)	0.77	(0.71–0.83)	1.14	(1.07–1.21)	1.34	(1.26–1.41)
5–6 times/week	0.80	(0.73–0.87)	0.95	(0.87–1.03)	0.63	(0.57–0.71)	1.30	(1.21–1.41)	1.45	(1.35–1.57)
Once/day	0.77	(0.69–0.86)	0.94	(0.84–1.05)	0.66	(0.59–0.75)	1.47	(1.33–1.62)	1.58	(1.44–1.73)
Twice/day	0.65	(0.54–0.78)	0.81	(0.69–0.94)	0.57	(0.47–0.69)	1.82	(1.55–2.14)	2.04	(1.76–2.37)
3+ times/day	0.58	(0.48–0.70)	0.68	(0.57–0.82)	0.82	(0.66–1.01)	2.08	(1.73–2.50)	1.97	(1.67–2.32)
Fast foods										
I did not eat	1.00		1.00		1.00		1.00		1.00	
1–2 times/week	0.97	(0.92–1.02)	1.05	(1.01–1.11)	0.85	(0.81–0.90)	1.01	(0.96–1.05)	1.08	(1.04–1.13)
3–4 times/week	0.80	(0.75–0.86)	0.89	(0.83–0.95)	0.66	(0.62–0.72)	1.24	(1.16–1.32)	1.43	(1.35–1.52)
5–6 times/week	0.69	(0.59–0.81)	0.71	(0.61–0.82)	0.70	(0.59–0.84)	1.49	(1.28–1.72)	1.80	(1.58–2.05)
Once/day	0.50	(0.40–0.63)	0.52	(0.42–0.66)	0.78	(0.58–1.04)	2.03	(1.63–2.54)	2.30	(1.90–2.78)
Twice/day	0.41	(0.25–0.69)	0.50	(0.31–0.82)	0.58	(0.33–1.02)	2.14	(1.35–3.39)	2.36	(1.66–3.37)
3+ times/day	1.32	(0.67–2.59)	0.73	(0.42–1.25)	0.61	(0.32–1.19)	2.09	(1.24–3.52)	3.57	(2.62–4.87)
Fruits (excluding fruit juices)										
I did not eat	1.00		1.00		1.00		1.00		1.00	
1–2 times/week	1.32	(1.21–1.43)	1.45	(1.34–1.57)	1.08	(0.98–1.18)	0.77	(0.72–0.83)	0.88	(0.83–0.94)

Table 5 continued

| | Well-being outcomes | | | | | | Mental distress outcomes | | | |
| | Perceived health (healthy) | | Perceived happiness (happy) | | Sleep satisfaction (sufficient) | | Perceived stress (much) | | Depression (yes) | |
	aOR[1]	(95% CI)	aOR[1]	(95% CI)	aOR[2]	(95% CI)	aOR[2]	(95% CI)	aOR[3]	(95% CI)
3–4 times/week	1.58	(1.46–1.72)	1.76	(1.62–1.90)	1.23	(1.12–1.35)	0.67	(0.62–0.72)	0.83	(0.77–0.88)
5–6 times/week	1.61	(1.46–1.77)	1.77	(1.62–1.94)	1.29	(1.17–1.42)	0.68	(0.63–0.74)	0.83	(0.77–0.90)
Once/day	1.80	(1.64–1.98)	2.04	(1.86–2.23)	1.42	(1.29–1.58)	0.66	(0.61–0.71)	0.86	(0.79–0.92)
Twice/day	1.72	(1.54–1.93)	2.18	(1.95–2.44)	1.56	(1.39–1.75)	0.69	(0.62–0.76)	0.86	(0.78–0.94)
3+ times/day	1.81	(1.58–2.07)	1.89	(1.67–2.14)	1.68	(1.49–1.90)	0.70	(0.63–0.78)	1.05	(0.95–1.17)
Vegetable (excluding Kimchi)										
I did not eat	1.00		1.00		1.00		1.00		1.00	
1–2 times/week	1.35	(1.21–1.51)	1.26	(1.12–1.40)	1.01	(0.88–1.15)	0.69	(0.62–0.77)	0.90	(0.82–1.00)
3–4 times/week	1.68	(1.51–1.87)	1.49	(1.34–1.65)	1.17	(1.03–1.32)	0.63	(0.57–0.70)	0.79	(0.72–0.87)
5–6 times/week	1.90	(1.69–2.14)	1.61	(1.44–1.80)	1.28	(1.12–1.46)	0.62	(0.56–0.70)	0.80	(0.72–0.88)
Once/day	1.93	(1.73–2.16)	1.61	(1.44–1.81)	1.27	(1.11–1.45)	0.62	(0.55–0.69)	0.84	(0.76–0.93)
Twice/day	2.22	(1.97–2.49)	1.87	(1.67–2.10)	1.35	(1.18–1.53)	0.61	(0.55–0.68)	0.78	(0.70–0.86)
3+ times/day	2.21	(1.97–2.48)	1.96	(1.75–2.19)	1.56	(1.37–1.77)	0.66	(0.59–0.74)	0.83	(0.75–0.92)
Milk										
I did not drink	1.00		1.00		1.00		1.00		1.00	
1–2 times/week	1.15	(1.08–1.24)	1.15	(1.08–1.22)	1.00	(0.93–1.08)	0.84	(0.79–0.89)	0.93	(0.88–0.98)
3–4 times/week	1.28	(1.20–1.36)	1.28	(1.20–1.36)	1.09	(1.01–1.18)	0.82	(0.77–0.87)	0.93	(0.88–0.99)
5–6 times/week	1.33	(1.23–1.44)	1.32	(1.23–1.41)	1.07	(0.98–1.16)	0.80	(0.75–0.86)	0.89	(0.84–0.95)
Once/day	1.50	(1.39–1.61)	1.41	(1.32–1.51)	1.18	(1.09–1.28)	0.77	(0.72–0.82)	0.90	(0.85–0.96)
Twice/day	1.48	(1.33–1.64)	1.36	(1.22–1.51)	1.21	(1.10–1.34)	0.83	(0.76–0.91)	1.02	(0.94–1.11)
3+ times/day	1.54	(1.36–1.74)	1.37	(1.22–1.53)	1.46	(1.31–1.63)	0.90	(0.82–1.00)	1.06	(0.96–1.17)

behaviour showed a dose–response relationship with higher psychological well-being. It remains unclear, if a healthier dietary behaviour is the cause or the sequela of a more positive well-being.

Abbreviations

BMI: Body Mass Index; KYRBS: Korea Youth Risk Behavior Web-based Survey.

Authors' contributions

All authors contributed to the conception and design of the study. SAH analysed the data. KP and SAH were involved in writing and revision of the manuscript. Both authors read and approved the final manuscript.

Author details

[1] ASEAN Institute for Health Development, Mahidol University, Salaya, Phuttha-monthon, Nakhon Pathom 73170, Thailand. [2] Institute for Health and Society, Hanyang University, Seoul, Republic of Korea. [3] Department for Management of Science and Technology Development, Ton Duc Thang University, Ho Chi Minh City, Vietnam. [4] Faculty of Pharmacy, Ton Duc Thang University, Ho Chi Minh City, Vietnam.

Competing interests

The authors declare that they have no competing interests.

References

1. Blanchflower DG, Oswald AJ, Stewart-Brown S. Is psychological well-being linked to the consumption of fruit and vegetables? Soc Indic Res. 2013;114(3):785–801. https://doi.org/10.1007/s11205-012-0173-y.
2. Mujcic R, Oswald JA. Evolution of well-being and happiness after increases in consumption of fruit and vegetables. Am J Public Health. 2016;106(8):1504–10. https://doi.org/10.2105/AJPH.2016.303260.
3. Lesani A, Mohammadpoorasl A, Javadi M, Esfeh JM, Fakhari A. Eating breakfast, fruit and vegetable intake and their relation with happiness in college students. Eat Weight Disord. 2016;21(4):645–51. https://doi.org/10.1007/s40519-016-0261-0.
4. Liu X, Yan Y, Li F, Zhang D. Fruit and vegetable consumption and the risk of depression: a meta-analysis. Nutrition. 2016;32(3):296–302. https://doi.org/10.1016/j.nut.2015.09.009.

5.   Khalid S, Williams CM, Reynolds SA. Is there an association between diet and depression in children and adolescents? A systematic review. Br J Nutr. 2016;116(12):2097–108. https://doi.org/10.1017/S0007114516004359.

6.   Peltzer K, Pengpid S. dietary behaviors, psychological well-being, and mental distress among University students in ASEAN. Iran J Psychiat Behav Sci. 2017;11(2):e10118. https://doi.org/10.5812/ijpbs.10118.

7.   Franckle RL, Falbe J, Gortmaker S, Ganter C, Taveras EM, Land T, Davison KK. Insufficient sleep among elementary and middle school students is linked with elevated soda consumption and other unhealthy dietary behaviors. Prev Med. 2015;74:36–41. https://doi.org/10.1016/j.ypmed.2015.02.007.

8.   Katagiri R, Asakura K, Kobayashi S, Suga H, Sasaki S. Low intake of vegetables, high intake of confectionary, and unhealthy eating habits are associated with poor sleep quality among middle-aged female Japanese workers. J Occup Health. 2014;56(5):359–68.

9.   Conner TS, Brookie KL, Richardson AC, Polak MA. On carrots and curiosity: eating fruit and vegetables is associated with greater flourishing in daily life. Br J Health Psychol. 2015;20(2):413–27. https://doi.org/10.1111/bjhp.12113.

10. Lengyel CO, Tate RB, Obirek Blatz AK. The relationships between food group consumption, self-rated health, and life satisfaction of community-dwelling Canadian older men: the Manitoba follow-up study. J Nutr Elder. 2009;28(2):158–73. https://doi.org/10.1080/01639360902950182.

11. Fararouei M, Brown IJ, Akbartabar Toori M, Estakhrian Haghighi R, Jafari J. Happiness and health behaviour in Iranian adolescent girls. J Adolesc. 2013;36(6):1187–92. https://doi.org/10.1016/j.adolescence.2013.09.006.

12. Peltzer K, Pengpid S, Sodi T, Mantilla Toloza SC. Happiness and health behaviours among university students from 24 low, middle and high income countries. J Psychol Afr. 2017;27(1):61–8. https://doi.org/10.1080/14330237.2016.1219556.

13. Piqueras JA, Kuhne W, Vera-Villarroel P, van Straten A, Cuijpers P. Happiness and health behaviours in Chilean college students: a cross-sectional survey. BMC Public Health. 2011;11:443. https://doi.org/10.1186/1471-2458-11-443.

14. Peltzer K, Pengpid S. Subjective happiness and health behavior among a sample of university students in India. Soc Behav Personal. 2013;41(6):869–80.

15. Grant N, Wardle J, Steptoe A. The relationship between life satisfaction and health behavior: a cross-cultural analysis of young adults. Int J Behav Med. 2009;16(3):259–68. https://doi.org/10.1007/s12529-009-9032-x.

16. White BA, Horwath CC, Conner TS. Many apples a day keep the blues away—daily experiences of negative and positive affect and food consumption in young adults. Br J Health Psychol. 2013;18(4):782–98. https://doi.org/10.1111/bjhp.12021.

17. El Ansari W, Berg-Beckhoff G. Nutritional correlates of perceived stress among University Students in Egypt. Int J Environ Res Public Health. 2015;12(11):14164–76. https://doi.org/10.3390/ijerph121114164.

18. Kingsbury M, Dupuis G, Jacka F, Roy-Gagnon MH, McMartin SE, Colman I. Associations between fruit and vegetable consumption and depressive symptoms: evidence from a national Canadian longitudinal survey. J Epidemiol Commun Health. 2016;70(2):155–61. https://doi.org/10.1136/jech-2015-205858.

19. Kim TH, Choi JY, Lee HH, Park Y. Associations between dietary pattern and depression in Korean adolescent girls. J Pediatr Adolesc Gynecol. 2015;28(6):533–7. https://doi.org/10.1016/j.jpag.2015.04.005.

20. Mikolajczyk RT, El Ansari W, Maxwell AE. Food consumption frequency and perceived stress and depressive symptoms among students in three European countries. Nutr J. 2009;8:31. https://doi.org/10.1186/1475-2891-8-31.

21. Richard A, Rohrmann S, Vandeleur CL, Mohler-Kuo M, Eichholzer M. Associations between fruit and vegetable consumption and psychological distress: results from a population-based study. BMC Psychiatry. 2015;15:213. https://doi.org/10.1186/s12888-015-0597-4.

22. Roohafza H, Sarrafzadegan N, Sadeghi M, Rafieian-Kopaei M, Sajjadi F, Khosravi-Boroujeni H. The association between stress levels and food consumption among Iranian population. Arch Iran Med. 2013;16(3):145–8.

23. Tajik E, Latiffah AL, Awang H, Siti Nur'Asyura A, Chin YS, Azrin Shah AB, Patricia Koh CH, Mohd Izudin Hariz CG. Unhealthy diet practice and symptoms of stress and depression among adolescents in Pasir

Gudang, Malaysia. Obes Res Clin Pract. 2016;10(2):114–23. https://doi.org/10.1016/j.orcp.2015.06.001.

24. Papier K, Ahmed F, Lee P, Wiseman J. Stress and dietary behaviour among first-year university students in Australia: sex differences. Nutrition. 2015;31(2):324–30. https://doi.org/10.1016/j.nut.2014.08.004.

25. Chang HH, Nayga RM. Childhood obesity and unhappiness: the influence of soft drinks and fast food consumption. J Happiness Stud. 2009;11(3):261–75. https://doi.org/10.1007/s10902-009-9139-4.

26. Zahedi H, Kelishadi R, Heshmat R, Motlagh ME, Ranjbar SH, Ardalan G, et al. Association between junk food consumption and mental health in a national sample of Iranian children and adolescents: the CASPIAN-IV study. Nutrition. 2014;30(11–12):1391–7. https://doi.org/10.1016/j.nut.2014.04.014.

27. El Ansari W, Adetunji H, Oskrochi R. Food and mental health: relationship between food and perceived stress and depressive symptoms among university students in the United Kingdom. Cent Eur J Public Health. 2014;22(2):90–7. https://doi.org/10.21101/cejph.a3941.

28. Liu C, Xie B, Chou CP, Koprowski C, Zhou D, Palmer P, et al. Perceived stress, depression and food consumption frequency in the college students of China Seven Cities. Physiol Behav. 2007;92(4):748–54. https://doi.org/10.1016/j.physbeh.2007.05.068.

29. Moor I, Lampert T, Rathmann K, Kuntz B, Kolip P, Spallek J, et al. Explaining educational inequalities in adolescent life satisfaction: do health behaviour and gender matter? Int J Public Health. 2014;59(2):309–17. https://doi.org/10.1007/s00038-013-0531-9.

30. Wang L, Qin P, Zhao Y, Duan S, Zhang Q, Liu Y, Hu Y, Sun J. Prevalence and risk factors of poor sleep quality among Inner Mongolia Medical University students: a cross-sectional survey. Psychiatry Res. 2016;244:243–8. https://doi.org/10.1016/j.psychres.2016.04.011.

31. Richard A, Rohrmann S, Vandeleur CL, Mohler-Kuo M, Eichholzer M. Associations between fruit and vegetable consumption and psychological distress: results from a population-based study. BMC Psychiatry. 2015;15:213. https://doi.org/10.1186/s12888-015-0597-4.

32. Kim TH, Choi JY, Lee HH, Park Y. Associations between dietary pattern and depression in Korean adolescent girls. J Pediatr Adolesc Gynecol. 2015;28(6):533–7. https://doi.org/10.1016/j.jpag.2015.04.005.

33. Richards G, Smith A. Caffeine consumption and self-assessed stress, anxiety, and depression in secondary school children. J Psychopharmacol. 2015;29(12):1236–47. https://doi.org/10.1177/0269881115612404.

34. Weng TT, Hao JH, Qian QW, Cao H, Fu JL, Sun Y, Huang L, Tao FB. Is there any relationship between dietary patterns and depression and anxiety in Chinese adolescents? Public Health Nutr. 2012;15(4):673–82. https://doi.org/10.1017/S1368980011003077.

35. Liu C, Xie B, Chou CP, Koprowski C, Zhou D, Palmer P, Sun P, Guo Q, Duan L, Sun X, Anderson Johnson C. Perceived stress, depression and food consumption frequency in the college students of China Seven Cities. Physiol Behav. 2007;92(4):748–54.

36. Hayward J, Jacka FN, Skouteris H, Millar L, Strugnell C, Swinburn BA, Allender S. Lifestyle factors and adolescent depressive symptomatology: associations and effect sizes of diet, physical activity and sedentary behaviour. Aust NZ J Psychiatry. 2016;50(11):1064–73.

37. Takada M, Nishida K, Gondo Y, Kikuchi-Hayakawa H, Ishikawa H, Suda K, Kawai M, Hoshi R, Kuwano Y, Miyazaki K, Rokutan K. Beneficial effects of Lactobacillus casei strain Shirota on academic stress-induced sleep disturbance in healthy adults: a double-blind, randomised, placebo-controlled trial. Benef Microbes. 2017;8(2):153–62. https://doi.org/10.3920/BM2016.0150.

38. Meyer BJ, Kolanu N, Griffiths DA, Grounds B, Howe PR, Kreis IA. Food groups and fatty acids associated with self-reported depression: an analysis from the Australian National Nutrition and Health Surveys. Nutrition. 2013;29(7–8):1042–7. https://doi.org/10.1016/j.nut.2013.02.006.

39. Aizawa E, Tsuji H, Asahara T, Takahashi T, Teraishi T, Yoshida S, Ota M, Koga N, Hattori K, Kunugi H. Possible association of Bifidobacterium and Lactobacillus in the gut microbiota of patients with major depressive disorder. J Affect Disord. 2016;202:254–7. https://doi.org/10.1016/j.jad.2016.05.038.

40. Bellisle F. Effects of diet on behaviour and cognition in children. Br J Nutr. 2004;92(Suppl 2):S227–32.

41. Bamber D, Stokes C, Stephen A. The role of diet in the prevention and management of adolescent depression. Nutr Bull. 2007;32:90–9.

42. Lien L, Lien N, Heyerdahl S, Thoresen M, Bjertness E. Consumption of soft drinks and hyperactivity, mental distress, and conduct problems among

adolescents in Oslo, Norway. Am J Public Health. 2006;96(10):1815–20. https://doi.org/10.2105/AJPH.2004.059477.

43. Ríos JL, Betancourt J, Pagán I, Fabián C, Cruz SY, González AM, González MJ, Rivera-Soto WT, Palacios C. Caffeinated-beverage consumption and its association with socio-demographic characteristics and self-perceived academic stress in first and second year students at the University of Puerto Rico Medical Sciences Campus (UPRMSC). Puerto Rico Health Sci J. 2013;32:95–100.

44. Korea Centers for Disease Control and Prevention. Korea Youth Risk Behavior Web-based Survey (KYRBS). http://yhs.cdc.go.kr. Accessed 1 June 2017.

45. Lee SY, Nam CM, Kim JH, Oh KW, Kim YN, Kang YJ, et al. Development of growth curves and the criteria of obesity in Korean children and adolescents. Final report. Gwacheon: Ministry of Health and Welfare (Korea); 2007.

46. Ministry of Education, Ministry of Health and Welfare, Korea Centers for Disease Control and Prevention. The Twelfth Korea Youth Risk Behavior Web-based Survey 2016. Cheongwon: Korea Centers for Disease Control and Prevention; 2016.

47. Ministry of Education, Ministry of Health and Welfare, Korea Centers for Disease Control and Prevention. The Twelfth Korea Youth Risk Behavior Web-based Survey 2016. Cheongwon: Korea Centers for Disease Control and Prevention; 2016.

48. Hoefelmann LP, Lopes Ada S, Silva KS, Silva SG, Cabral LG, Nahas MV. Lifestyle, self-reported morbidities, and poor sleep quality among Brazilian workers. Sleep Med. 2012;13(9):1198–201. https://doi.org/10.1016/j.sleep.2012.05.009.

49. Lai JS, Hiles S, Bisquera A, Hure AJ, McEvoy M, Attia J. A systematic review and meta-analysis of dietary patterns and depression in community-dwelling adults. Am J Clin Nutr. 2014;99(1):181–97.

50. Psaltopoulou T, Sergentanis TN, Panagiotakos DB, Sergentanis IN, Kosti R, Scarmeas N. Mediterranean diet, stroke, cognitive impairment, and depression: a meta-analysis. Ann Neurol. 2013;74(4):580–91.

51. Jacka FN, Kremer PJ, Berk M, et al. A prospective study of diet quality and mental health in adolescents. PLoS ONE. 2011;6(9):e24805.

52. Sánchez-Villegas A, Toledo E, De Irala J, et al. Fast-food and commercial baked goods consumption and the risk of depression. Public Health Nutr. 2012;15(3):424–32.

53. Westover AN, Marangell LB. A cross-national relationship between sugar consumption and major depression? Depress Anxiety. 2002;16(3):118–20. https://doi.org/10.1002/da.10054.

54. Galland BC, Gray AR, Penno J, Smith C, Lobb C, Taylor RW. Gender differences in sleep hygiene practices and sleep quality in New Zealand adolescents aged 15–17 years. Sleep Health. 2017;3(2):77–83. https://doi.org/10.1016/j.sleh.2017.02.001.

55. Lohsoonthorn V, Khidir H, Casillas G, Lertmaharit S, Tadesse MG, Pensuksan WC, Rattananupong T, Gelaye B, Williams MA. Sleep quality and sleep patterns in relation to consumption of energy drinks, caffeinated beverages, and other stimulants among Thai college students. Sleep Breath. 2013;17(3):1017–28. https://doi.org/10.1007/s11325-012-0792-1.

56. Fleig D, Randler C. Association between chronotype and diet in adolescents based on food logs. Eat Behav. 2009;10(2):115–8. https://doi.org/10.1016/j.eatbeh.2009.03.002.

57. Bjorness TE, Greene RW. Adenosine and sleep. Curr Neuropharmacol. 2009;7(3):238–45.

58. Landolt HP. "No Thanks, Coffee Keeps Me Awake": individual caffeine sensitivity depends on ADORA2A Genotype. Sleep. 2012;35(7):899–900.

11

Comorbidities and correlates of conduct disorder among male juvenile detainees in South Korea

Bum-Sung Choi[1], Johanna Inhyang Kim[2], Bung-Nyun Kim[2] and Bongseog Kim[3*]

Abstract

Background: The purpose of this study was to examine the rate and distribution of comorbidities, severity of childhood maltreatment, and clinical characteristics of adolescents with conduct disorder detained in a juvenile detention center in South Korea.

Methods: In total, 173 juvenile detainees were recruited. We analyzed the distribution of psychiatric disorders among the sample and compared the rate of comorbidities between groups with and without conduct disorder. We compared the two groups in terms of demographic and clinical characteristics, as well as severity of childhood maltreatment and psychiatric problems, using the Young Self Report (YSR) scale.

Results: A total of 95 (55%) of the detainees were diagnosed with conduct disorder, and 93 (96.9%) of them had at least one comorbid axis I psychiatric disorder. Detainees with conduct disorder had a higher number of comorbid psychiatric disorders; a higher rate of violent crime perpetration; had suffered more physical, emotional, and sexual abuse; and showed higher total YSR scores and externalizing behavior, somatic complaints, rule-breaking behavior, and aggressive behavior YSR subscale scores.

Conclusions: Conduct disorder is a common psychiatric disorder among juvenile detainees in South Korea, who tend to commit more violent crimes and show more psychopathology than detainees who do not have conduct disorder. These findings highlight the importance of diagnosing and intervening in conduct disorder within the juvenile detention system.

Background

Juvenile offenders constitute 5.1% of all criminal offenders in South Korea. Approximately 8272 juvenile offenders are newly detained in juvenile detention centers every year [1]. Previous studies reported that 40–90% of juvenile offenders had at least one psychiatric disorder [2–6], which represents an approximately three- to fourfold higher prevalence of psychiatric illness compared with the general population [7–9]. The prevalence of different psychiatric disorders varies by study; in a metaregression analysis of 13,778 boys and 2972 girls, 3.9–7.3% of the boys had major depression, 4.1–19.2% had attention deficit hyperactivity disorder (ADHD), and 40.9–64.7% had conduct disorder. Among the girls, 21.9–36.5% had major depression, 9.3–27.7% had ADHD, and 32.4–73.2% had conduct disorder [10].

Despite the high rate of psychiatric illnesses among juvenile offenders, research on the psychiatric health of this population in Asian countries, including South Korea, is limited. Park et al. [1] reported that, among 1700 inmates of three prisons, 28.1% were classified as being at high risk for depression, 33.6% had suicidal ideation, and 39.1% were diagnosed with alcohol abuse. Another study reported higher rates of depression, paranoia, antisociality, and Minnesota Multiphasic Personality Inventory (MMPI) scale hypomania among 1155 juvenile offenders compared to the general population [11]. Both studies used self-rated questionnaires,

*Correspondence: kimbs328@paik.ac.kr
[3] Department of Psychiatry, Sanggye Paik Hospital, Inje University College of Medicine, 1342 Dong-il Street, Seoul 01757, Republic of Korea
Full list of author information is available at the end of the article

and only the latter targeted a juvenile population. To our knowledge, no South Korean study has estimated the prevalence of psychiatric disorders among juvenile offenders using Diagnostic and Statistical Manual for Mental Disorders (DSM) or International Classification of Diseases (ICD)-based criteria.

Conduct disorder is one of the most common psychiatric disorders among juvenile offenders, with the prevalence ranging from 31 to 77% [12, 13]. In previous studies, conduct disorder showed high comorbidity with substance use disorders and ADHD; all of these disorders are risk factors for higher psychiatric disorders.

The purpose of this study was to investigate the prevalence of psychiatric disorders among juvenile detainees in South Korea, and to assess patterns of comorbidity and psychopathology among those with conduct disorder.

Methods
Participants and procedure
In total, 200 detainees who were sentenced to 6 or 12-month detainment in a single male juvenile detention center in Seoul, South Korea, were recruited from December 2015 to January 2016. A total of 27 detainees over the age of 19 were excluded from the study, giving 173 participants. Subjects were eligible for inclusion in the study regardless of psychiatric diagnosis, degree of drug or alcohol intoxication, or fitness to stand trial. Exclusion criteria included refusal or inability to cooperate or understand the study procedures. Written informed consent was obtained from the participants after the study procedures were explained. This study protocol was approved by the Institutional Review Board of Sanggye Paik Hospital (IRB No. SGPAIK 2015-06-022-002).

Psychiatric diagnoses were confirmed using the Mini-International Neuropsychiatric Interview (MINI), which is a short, structured psychiatric interview that can detect a wide range of DSM-IV and ICD-10 psychiatric disorders [14]. The MINI has been applied for the assessment of psychiatric disorders in various criminal justice settings [15, 16]. The Korean version has well-established validity and reliability [17]. In cases of disorders not covered by the MINI, the Kiddie-Schedule for affective disorders and Schizophrenia-Present and Lifetime Version-Korean Version (K-SADS-PL-K) were used; the reliability and validity of the K-SADS-PL-K have been confirmed [18]. Diagnoses of ADHD, ODD, CD, and tic disorders were based on the behavioral disorder supplement of the K-SADS-PL-K.

The presence and degree of childhood maltreatment were evaluated using the Korean version of the Childhood Trauma Questionnaire (CTQ) [19], which has good validity and reliability [20]. The CTQ consists of 28 items;

each item is rated on a five-point Likert scale and higher scores indicate more severe childhood maltreatment. The results are presented as total scores, and as scores on each of five subscales (emotional neglect, emotional abuse, physical neglect, physical abuse, and sexual abuse). We applied a moderate-to-severe cut-off score for each subscale [21, 22], and individuals who exceeded the cut-off score were categorized as juvenile detainees with a history of childhood maltreatment.

Various psychiatric symptoms were screened for using the Youth Self Report (YSR) scale, which is used widely for the assessment of emotional and behavioral problems and comprises 112 items [23]. The Korean version was standardized by Oh et al. [24]. All subscale scores were converted into T-scores, with higher scores indicating more severe symptoms. In the present study, we included the subscales of total problem behavior, internalizing, externalizing, anxiety/depression, withdrawal/depression, somatic complaints, thought problems, attention problems, rule-breaking behaviors, and aggressive behaviors.

Statistical analysis
The demographic and clinical characteristics were compared between detainees with and without conduct disorder using independent t-tests for continuous variables and Chi square or Fisher's exact test for categorical variables (such as psychiatric comorbidity status). The association between type of childhood maltreatment and conduct disorder was analyzed using logistic regression. We used multiple linear regression to evaluate the association between conduct disorder and YSR subscale scores.

All statistical analyses were performed using SPSS software (ver. 22.0; SPSS Inc., Chicago, IL, USA), and a two-tailed p-value <0.05 was considered significant.

Results
The demographic and judicial characteristics of the whole sample, and of the detainees with and without conduct disorder, are presented in Table 1. The mean age was 17.5 ± 1.1 years, and all participants were male. In total, 42 (24.3%) of the participants had dropped out of school, and 104 (60.1%) were from a family with a yearly income exceeding $2500. A majority of the detainees had been living in a single parent home (n = 97, 56.1%), and 57 (32.9%) had been living with both parents; 19 (11.0%) had not been living with their parents. Property crime was the most common type of crime (n = 86, 49.7%), followed by violent crime (n = 68, 39.3%), traffic offenses (n = 42, 24.3%), and sex crimes (n = 34, 19.7%).

There were no significant differences between the groups with versus without conduct disorder in demographic or judicial characteristics, except for a higher

Table 1 Demographic and clinical characteristics of the detainees with and without conduct disorder

Characteristic	Whole sample (n = 173)	With conduct disorder (n = 96)	Without conduct disorder (n = 77)	p value
Age (years), mean (SD)	17.5 (1.1)	17.4 (1.2)	17.6 (1.1)	0.171
School drop out, N (%)	42 (24.3)	23 (24)	19 (24.7)	0.913
Yearly family income > $2500, N (%)	104 (60.1)	59 (61.5)	45 (58.4)	0.687
Paternal education ≥ college education, N (%)	25 (14.5)	13 (19.1)	12 (21.4)	0.750
Maternal education ≥ college education, N (%)	20 (11.6)	10 (16.7)	10 (18.2)	0.830
Living arrangements, N (%)				0.928
With both parents	57 (32.9)	31 (32.3)	26 (33.8)	
With a single parent	97 (56.1)	55 (57.3)	42 (54.5)	
No parents	19 (11.0)	10 (1.4)	9 (11.7)	
Recidivism, N (%)	154 (89)	88 (91.7)	66 (85.7)	0.213
Number of crime, mean (SD)	3.2 (1.8)	3.4 (1.9)	3.1 (1.6)	0.243
Type of crime, N (%)				
Property crime	86 (49.7)	48 (49)	40 (51.9)	0.696
Violent crime	68 (39.3)	48 (50)	20 (26)	0.001
Sex crime	34 (19.7)	14 (14.6)	20 (26.3)	0.055
Drug crime	1 (0.6)	0 (0)	1 (1.3)	0.445
Domestic violence	1 (0.6)	1 (1.0)	0 (0)	1.00
Traffic offenses	42 (24.3)	23 (24.0)	19 (24.7)	0.913
Obstruction of justice	7 (4.0)	4 (4.2)	3 (3.9)	1.00
Drunk driving	2 (1.2)	2 (2.1)	0 (0)	0.503
Others	20 (11.6)	13 (13.5)	7 (9.1)	0.363

SD standard deviation

rate of violent crimes in the conduct disorder group (p = 0.001; Table 1).

Data on psychiatric disorder prevalence and comorbidity with conduct disorder are shown in Table 2. In total, 157 (90.8%) participants had at least one psychiatric diagnosis, and the most common axis I psychiatric disorder was alcohol use disorder (n = 100, 57.8%), followed by conduct disorder (n = 96, 55.5%), bipolar disorder (n = 82, 47.4%), and ADHD (n = 61, 35.3%). Antisocial personality traits were present in 83 (48%) detainees.

Table 2 Prevalence of psychiatric disorders among detainees and comorbidity with conduct disorder

Diagnosis	Whole sample (n = 173)	With conduct disorder (n = 96)	Without conduct disorder (n = 77)	p value
Any psychiatric disorder, except conduct disorder	154 (89.0)	93 (96.9)	61 (79.2)	<0.001
Number with diagnosis, N (%)				
Major depressive disorder	50 (28.9)	41 (21.9)	9 (11.7)	0.079
Bipolar disorder	82 (47.4)	59 (61.5)	23 (29.9)	<0.001
Alcohol use disorder	100 (57.8)	66 (68.8)	34 (44.2)	0.001
Substance use disorder	8 (4.6)	4 (4.2)	4 (5.2)	1.00
Schizophrenia	19 (11.0)	11 (11.5)	8 (10.4)	0.823
Eating disorder	6 (3.5)	6 (6.3)	0 (0)	0.026
ADHD	61 (35.3)	40 (41.7)	21 (27.3)	0.049
Tic disorder	47 (27.2)	24 (25.0)	23 (29.9)	0.474
ODD	14 (8.1)	0 (0)	14 (18.2)	<0.001
Antisocial personality trait	83 (48.0)	62 (64.6)	21 (27.3)	<0.001
Anxiety disorder	44 (25.4)	30 (31.3)	14 (18.2)	0.050

AHDH attention deficit hyperactivity disorder, *ODD* oppositional defiant disorder

In total, 96 (55.5%) detainees had a diagnosis of conduct disorder, of whom 93 (96.9%) had at least one comorbid axis I psychiatric disorder. Detainees with conduct disorder had a higher rate of comorbidity compared to those without ($p < 0.001$), and the most common axis I comorbid disorder was alcohol use disorder ($n = 66$, 68.8%), followed by bipolar disorder ($n = 59$, 61.5%) and ADHD ($n = 40$, 41.7%). All of the psychiatric disorders—except for major depressive disorder, substance use disorder, tic disorders, and anxiety disorders—were more frequently diagnosed in the conduct disorder than in the non-conduct disorder group (all $p < 0.05$).

The detainees with conduct disorder showed significant associations with emotional abuse [odds ratio (OR) = 1.26, 95% confidence interval (CI) 1.06–1.43; $p = 0.009$], sexual abuse (OR = 1.23, 95% CI 1.03–1.46; $p = 0.022$), and physical abuse (OR = 1.23, 95% CI 1.06–1.43; $p = 0.008$), and all associations remained significant after adjusting for age, living arrangements,

socioeconomic status, and the presence of psychiatric comorbidities (Table 3).

Scores on YSR subscales were higher in the conduct disorder versus non-conduct disorder group, including total problem behavior ($\beta = 1.57$, 95% CI 0.47–2.67; $p = 0.005$), externalizing behavior ($\beta = 2.33$, 95% CI 1.27–3.40; $p < 0.001$), somatic complaints ($\beta = 0.58$, 95% CI 0.01–1.16; $p = 0.047$), rule-breaking behavior ($\beta = 1.41$, 95% CI 0.78–2.03; $p < 0.001$), and aggressive behavior ($\beta = 1.15$, 95% CI 0.45–1.85; $p = 0.001$) after adjusting for age and the presence of psychiatric comorbidities (Table 4).

Discussion

Research on the prevalence of psychiatric disorders among detained adolescents is still limited in comparison to analogous research in adults. Nevertheless, reports of psychiatric prevalence studies of adolescents have been published with increasing frequency over the past few years.

Table 3 Association of childhood maltreatment and conduct disorder

Variables	Whole sample (n = 173	With conduct disorder (n = 96)	Without CD (n = 77)	Unadjusted OR	95% CI	p value	Adjusted OR[a]	95% CI	p value
Child maltreatment	136 (78.6)	76 (79.2)	60 (77.9)	1.019	0.849–1.223	0.843	1.01	0.82–1.24	0.942
Type of childhood maltreatment									
Emotional abuse	54 (31.2)	38 (39.6)	16 (20.8)	1.257	1.059–1.492	0.009	1.252	1.04–1.51	0.018
Sexual abuse	49 (28.3)	34 (35.4)	15 (19.5)	1227	1.029–1.462	0.022	1.209	1.00–1.46	0.048
Physical abuse	87 (50.3)	57 (59.4)	30 (39.0)	1.230	1.055–1.434	0.008	1.271	1.07–1.51	0.006
Emotional neglect	92 (53.2)	49 (51.0)	42 (55.8)	0.953	0.820–1.108	0.529	1.370	0.70–2.70	0.364
Physical neglect	93 (53.8	49 (51.0)	44 (57.1)	0.940	0.809–1.093	0.424	0.934	0.79–1.10	0.418

[a] Adjusted for age, living arrangements, SES, and presence of psychiatric disorders

Table 4 Association of YSR scores with conduct disorder

Variables	With conduct disorder (n = 96)	Without conduct disorder (n = 77)	β	95% CI	p value
Total problem behavior	57.2 (14.2)	49.9 (13.3)	1.57	0.47 to 2.67	0.005
Internalizing	51.6 (13.4)	46.6 (12.9)	1.034	−0.10 to 2.08	0.052
Externalizing	65.6 (13.5)	55.3 (13.5)	2.332	1.27 to 3.40	<0.001
Anxious/depressed	55.3 (7.5)	53.6 (6.3)	0.39	−0.16 to 0.95	0.166
Withdrawn/depressed	55.4 (7.3)	54.0 (6.4)	0.26	−0.29 to 0.81	0.353
Somatic complaints	56.1 (8.2)	53.7 (5.7)	0.581	0.01 to 1.16	0.047
Thought problems	56.2 (7.9)	53.8 (6.0)	0.553	−0.1 to 1.12	0.055
Attention problems	55.6 (7.5)	53.9 (8.0)	0.35	−0.27 to 0.97	0.261
Rule-breaking behavior	69.7 (7.4)	63.5 (8.6)	1.41	0.78 to 2.03	<0.001
Aggressive behavior	59.6 (10.0)	54.5 (7.1)	1.15	0.45 to 1.85	0.001

Adjusted for age and presence of psychiatric comorbidity

YSR the Youth Self Report scale

The main objectives of this study were to document the rate and distribution of comorbidities, severity of childhood maltreatment, and clinical characteristics of adolescents with conduct disorder detained in a juvenile detention center in South Korea.

Many of the juvenile offenders in our study had psychiatric disorders, including alcohol use disorder, conduct disorder, bipolar disorder, and ADHD. The percentage of detainees with at least one psychiatric axis I disorder was 90.8%, which is very high compared to the rates reported among the general adolescent population, and is in the range reported in previous studies. Alcohol abuse (57.8%) was the most common disorder, followed by conduct disorder (55.5%), bipolar disorder (47.4%), and ADHD (35.3%). Additionally, antisocial personality traits were identified in 48% of the participants. Previous studies have shown that personality disorder is highly prevalent in incarcerated juvenile populations [25]. However, a diagnosis of antisocial personality disorder is still possible above 18 years of age if there is evidence of conduct disorder with an onset prior to 15 years of age; thus the term 'trait' was used rather than 'disorder'. These findings are similar to the results of Collins et al., in that the mean prevalence of any disorder was 69.9% (95% CI 69.5–70.3), with conduct disorder occurring most frequently (46.4%; 95% CI 45.6–47.3), followed by substance use disorder (45.1%; 95% CI 44.6–45.5), oppositional defiant disorder (19.8%; 95% CI 9.2–20.3), and ADHD (13.5%; 95% CI 13.2–13.9) [26]. In a meta-analysis by Fazel et al., high rates of psychotic illness (male adolescents, 3.3%), major depression (10.6%), ADHD (11.7%), and CD (male adolescents, 52.8%) were described [10]. Despite methodological differences between the two studies, overall prevalence rates for ADHD (Fazel et al., 11.7%, compared with 13.6% in our study), CD (52.8% vs. 38.8%), and major depression (10.6% vs. 10.0%) were similar [10]. As expected, conduct disorder was the most prevalent of the disorders studied, with a similar prevalence in both sexes of slightly more than 50% [10]. A report by the American Academy of Pediatrics estimated the prevalence ranges as follows: 1–6% for psychosis, up to 50% for ADHD, and 20–60% for conduct disorder [27]. Thus, the risk of conduct disorder is five to tenfold higher than that of the general population [10].

Another finding of the current study was that the rate of violent crimes among the conduct disorder group was higher than that of the non-conduct disorder group. Out of a total of 96 (55.5%) detainees who had a diagnosis of conduct disorder, 93 (96.9%) had at least one comorbid axis I psychiatric disorder. Those with conduct disorder had a higher rate of comorbidities than those without, and the most common axis I comorbid disorder was alcohol use disorder, followed by bipolar and ADHD. With

the exceptions of major depressive disorder, substance use disorder, tic disorders, and anxiety disorders, all psychiatric conditions were more frequently diagnosed in the conduct disorder than in the non-conduct disorder group. One main implication arises from these findings: mental disorders are markedly more common among adolescents in detention than among age-equivalent individuals in the general population. The largest increase in risk among detainees is for conduct disorder; for male adolescent detainees, the risk of conduct disorder is five- to tenfold higher than that of the general population [10].

Regarding the YSR subscales, including total problem behavior, externalizing behavior, somatic complaints, rule-breaking behavior, and aggressive behavior, after adjusting for age and the presence of psychiatric comorbidities, scores for the conduct disorder group were consistently higher. No significant differences were found on the other subscales, including internalizing behavior, anxious/depressed behavior, withdrawn/depressed behavior, thought problems, and attention problems, after adjusting for age and the presence of psychiatric comorbidities. Additionally, Rosenblatt et al. [28] reported that juvenile offenders displayed increased functional impairment due to conduct and externalizing behavioral problems compared to the general adolescent population.

Although conduct disorder is a psychiatric condition commonly observed among juvenile detainees in South Korea, available psychiatric interventions of for this population remain limited. The present results confirm that detainees with conduct disorder had higher rates of comorbid axis I psychiatric disorders and violent crime perpetration, and had suffered more physical, emotional, and sexual abuse than those without conduct disorder. These findings suggest that the diagnosis of, and interventions for, conduct disorder within the juvenile detention system are important for the prevention of further damage to juvenile detainees.

The present study also demonstrated that detainees with conduct disorder had more severe psychopathologies than those without conduct disorder; thus, designing intervention programs will be necessary. Furthermore, additional research on the treatment of youth detainees with conduct disorder will be necessary. Subsequent studies aimed at identifying the traits of youth detainees with conduct disorder, such as callous unemotional traits, may lead to the development of more effective treatments for juvenile detainees with these characteristics.

There were some noteworthy limitations to this study. First, we included only male subjects, as the juvenile detention center from which the participants were drawn was for males only; this may limit the generalizability of the findings. Second, the detainees without conduct disorder also had high rates of psychiatric comorbidity, and there were insufficient detainees without a psychiatric disorder to act as a control group for the conduct disorder detainees. Therefore, further studies including control groups (which could be detainees without any psychiatric disorder or adolescents drawn from the general population) could help to clarify the results. Third, because we conducted the study inside the detention center, the detainees were the only informants and we were unable to obtain information from any other source. Fourth, rather than the MINI KID, the MINI was used to diagnose psychiatric disorders. The use of an adult assessment tool may be a limitation in that it does not fully cover child and adolescent psychiatric diagnoses. Finally, the detainees were drawn from a single detention center; further large-scale studies including detainees from other areas and detention centers are thus warranted.

Conclusions

Almost all of the juvenile detainees that we recruited from a detention center in South Korea had at least one psychiatric disorder. The most common disorder was alcohol use disorder, followed by conduct disorder and antisocial personality disorder. The detainees with conduct disorder had higher rates of comorbid axis I psychiatric disorders and violent crime perpetration; had suffered more physical, emotional, and sexual abuse; and exhibited more severe psychopathology than those without conduct disorder. These findings highlight the importance of diagnosing and intervening in conduct disorder within the juvenile detention system.

Authors' contributions
BSC, JIK, BNK and BK were responsible for study concept and design. BK contributed to the acquisition of data. BSC and JIK were involved in the interpretation of the data. BSC was responsible for drafting the manuscript, and all authors were involved in critical revisions of the manuscript. All authors read and approved the final manuscript.

Author details
[1] Department of Psychiatry, Medical Research Institute, Pusan National University Yangsan Hospital, 20 Geumo-ro, Yangsan, Mulgeum-eup 50612, Republic of Korea. [2] Division of Child and Adolescent Psychiatry, Department of Psychiatry, Seoul National University College of Medicine, 101 Daehak-no, Chongno-gu, Seoul 03080, Republic of Korea. [3] Department of Psychiatry, Sanggye Paik Hospital, Inje University College of Medicine, 1342 Dong-il Street, Seoul 01757, Republic of Korea.

Acknowledgements
None.

Competing interests
The authors declare that they have no competing interests.

Funding
This study was supported by a grant of the Korean Mental Health Technology R&D Project, Ministry of Health & Welfare, Republic of Korea (HM15C1040).

References
1. Park JI, Kim YJ, Lee SJ. Mental health status of prisoners in correctional institutions. J Korean Neuropsychiatr Assoc. 2013;52:454–62.
2. Ulzen TPM, Hamilton H. The nature and characteristics of psychiatric comorbidity in incarcerated adolescents. Can J Psychiatry. 1998;43:57–63.
3. Teplin LA, Abram KM, McClelland GM, Dulcan MK, Mericle AA. Psychiatric disorders in youth in juvenile detention. Arch Gen Psychiatry. 2002;59:1133–43.
4. Abram KM, Teplin LA, McClelland GM, Dulcan MK. Comorbid psychiatric disorders in youth in juvenile detention. Arch Gen Psychiatry. 2003;60:1097–108.
5. Vreugdenhil C, Doreleijers TAH, Vermeiren R, Wouters LFJM, Van den Brink W. Psychiatric disorders in a representative sample of incarcerated boys in the Netherlands. J Am Acad Child Adolesc Psychiatry. 2004;43:97–104.
6. Harzke AJ, Baillargeon J, Baillargeon G, Henry J, Olvera RL, Torrealday O, et al. Prevalence of psychiatric disorders in the texas juvenile correctional system. J Correct Health Care. 2012;18:143–57.
7. Cocozza K. Youth with mental disorders: issues and emerging responses. Off Juv Justice Delinq Prev J. 2000;7:3–13.
8. McReynolds LS, Wasserman GA, DeComo RE, John R, Keating JM, Nolen S. Psychiatric disorder in a juvenile assessment center. Crime Delinq. 2008;54:313–34.
9. Steiner H, Silverman M, Karnik NS, Huemer J, Plattner B, Clark CE, et al. Psychopathology, trauma and delinquency: subtypes of aggression and their relevance for understanding young offenders. Child Adolesc Psychiatry Mental Health. 2011;5:21.
10. Fazel S, Doll H, Langstrom N. Mental disorders among adolescents in juvenile detention and correctional facilities: a systematic review and metaregression analysis of 25 surveys. J Am Acad Child Adolesc Psychiatry. 2008;47:1010–9.
11. Park S. A study on relation between vioent crimes juveniles and mental disorder disposition. Korean Police Stud Rev. 2009;8:3–42.
12. Ruchkin V, Koposov R, Vermeiren R, Schwab-Stone M. Psychopathology and age at onset of conduct problems in juvenile delinquents. J Clin Psychiatry. 2003;64:913–20.
13. Copur M, Turkcan A, Erdogmus M. Substance abuse, conduct disorder and crime: assessment in a juvenile detention house in Istanbul, Turkey. Psychiatry Clin Neurosci. 2005;59:151–4.
14. Sheehan DV, Lecrubier Y, Sheehan KH, Amorim P, Janavs J, Weiller E, et al. The mini-international neuropsychiatric interview (M.I.N.I.): the development and validation of a structured diagnostic psychiatric interview for dsm-iv and icd-10. J Clin Psychiatry. 1998;59(Suppl 20):22–33.
15. Black DW, Arndt S, Hale N, Rogerson R. Use of the mini international neuropsychiatric interview (mini) as a screening tool in prisons: results of a preliminary study. J Am Acad Psychiatry. 2004;32:158–62.
16. Marzano L, Faze S, Rivlin A, Hawton K. Psychiatric disorders in women prisoners who have engaged in near-lethal self-harm: case control study. Br J Psychiatry. 2010;197:219–26.
17. Yoo S, Kim Y, Noh J, Oh K, Kim C, Namkoong K, et al. Validity of korean version of the mini international neuropsychiatric interview. Anxiety Mood. 2006;2:50–5.
18. Kim YS, Cheon K, Kim BN, Chang S, Yoo HJ, Kim J, et al. The reliability and validity of kiddie-Schedule for affective disorders and schizophrenia-present and lifetime version-Korean version (K-SADS-PL-K). Yonsei Med J. 2004;45(1):81–9.
19. Bernstein DP, Fink L, Handelsman L, Foote J, Lovejoy M, Wenzel K, et al. Initial reliability and validity of a new retrospective measure of child abuse and neglect. Am J Psychiatry. 1994;151:1132–6.
20. Yu J, Park J, Park D, Ryu S, Ha J. Validation of the Korean childhood trauma questionnaire: the practical use in counselling and therapeutic intervention. Korean J Health Psychol. 2009;14:563–78.

21. Choi JY, Choi YM, Kim B, Lee DW, Gim MS, Park SH. The effects of child-hood abuse on self-reported psychotic symptoms in severe mental illness: mediating effects of posttraumatic stress symptoms. Psychiatry Res. 2015;229:389–93.
22. De Sanctis VA, Nomura Y, Newcorn JH, Halperin JM. Childhood mal-treatment and conduct disorder: independent predictors of criminal outcomes in adhd youth. Child Abuse Negl. 2012;36:782–9.
23. Achenback T, Rescorla, L. The manual for the aseba school-age forms and profiles. Burling: University of Vermont (Research center for children, youth and families); 2001.
24. Oh KJ, Ha EH, Lee HR, Hong KE. K-YSR, Korean Youth Self Report. Seoul: Chung Ang Aptitude pressing; 2001.
25. Robison BD. Comorbidity of conduct disorder and personality disorders in an incarcerated juvenile population. Am J Psychiatry. 1993;1(50):1233.
26. Colins O, Vermeiren R, Vreugdenhil C, van den Brink W, Doreleijers T, Broe-kaert E. Psychiatric disorders in detained male adolescents: a systematic literature review. Can J Psychiatry. 2010;55:255–63.
27. American Academy of Pediatrics Committee on Adolescence. Health care for children and adolescents in the juvenile correctional care system. Pediatrics. 2001;107:799Y803.
28. Rosenblatt JA, Rosenblatt A, Biggs EE. Criminal behavior and emotional disorder: comparing youth served by the mental health and juvenile justice systems. J Behav Health Serv Res. 2000;27:227–37.

12

Mental health status, and suicidal thoughts and behaviors of migrant children in eastern coastal China in comparison to urban children: a cross-sectional survey

Jingjing Lu[1†], Feng Wang[1†], Pengfei Chai[2], Dongshuo Wang[3], Lu Li[1*] and Xudong Zhou[1*]

Abstract

Purpose: Although adolescents' mental health problems and self-injurious thoughts and behaviors (SITBs) have been a serious public health concern worldwide, descriptions of risk factors for SITBs often fail to take migration into account. There are roughly 35.8 million migrant children in China who, with their parents, moved from original rural residence to urban areas. Little is known about migrant children's mental health status and levels of SITBs. This study aims to explore the mental health status and SITBs of migrant children living in eastern coastal China in comparison to their urban counterparts.

Methods: This study was a cross-sectional survey conducted in 13 schools. Mental health status and SITBs were measured via self-administered questionnaires. Associations between strengths and difficulties questionnaire outcomes and SITBs were investigated.

Results: Data from 4217 students (1858 migrant children and 2359 urban children) were collected. After controlling for gender, age, family economic status, parent's education level and parents' marital status, migrant children scored higher for total difficulties (p < 0.001) and externalizing problems (p < 0.001) than did urban children and reported higher rates of suicidal ideation (p < 0.05) and self-injurious behaviors (p < 0.05).

Conclusions: Migrant children, compared with urban children, have a higher risk of externalizing problems and SITBs. It is urgent to address these problems by providing both mental health services at migrant-exclusive schools and equitable education and social welfare to migrant children.

Keywords: Migrant children, SDQ, Suicide ideation, Self-injurious behavior

Background

Since the mid-1980s when China started to implement the reform and opening-up policy, a growing number of people have migrated from rural to urban areas in search of better jobs and living conditions. In recent years, an increasing number of migrant workers have made the choice to raise their children in cities, creating a new generation of migrant children.

In China, migrant children are defined as "children under 18 who have left their original residence and migrated to a big city for at least 6 months" [1]. According to the most recent statistics, the number of migrant children in China aged between 0 and 17 years is about 35.80 million [2], and this number continues to grow [3]. Because of the *Hukou*, China's system of household registration, most migrant children are unable to enroll in public schools or utilize the same social welfare provided to urban children. Unregistered schools specifically set up for migrant children, usually called migrant-exclusive

*Correspondence: lilu@zju.edu.cn; zhouxudong@zju.edu.cn
†Jingjing Lu and Feng Wang are co-first authors
[1] The Institute of Social and Family Medicine, School of Public Health, Zhejiang University, 866 Yuhangtang Rd., Hangzhou 310058, Zhejiang, People's Republic of China
Full list of author information is available at the end of the article

schools, are typically small and often lack qualified teachers, standard teaching materials and adequate sanitation facilities [4]. A minority of migrant children can attend public schools due to regional policies, for example, if their parents migrated to a city because of a regional labor-importing policy. However, these migrant children may be socially excluded in their classrooms, treated unjustly by their teachers and discriminated against by the parents of their urban classmates [5]. As such, migrant children experience inequitable health conditions, both physically and mentally, in the process of adapting to a new environment, making them extremely vulnerable.

Because of these precarious circumstances, there is great concern regarding the health condition of migrant children, but only limited data at the population-level have been collected regarding the mental health status of migrant children using standardized tools in China. Although the strengths and difficulties questionnaire (SDQ) is a standardized measure of mental health in children and adolescents, with established reliability and validity [6, 7], studies of the mental health status of migrant children using SDQ in China are rarely conducted. Existing studies on the subject reported mixed results. One study conducted in Guangdong found that migrant children scored significantly higher in every SDQ outcome compared to normative scores in China [8]. Another study conducted in Hubei found that migrant children only reported significantly higher scores in emotional symptoms, conduct problems, hyperactivity and peer problems [9] when compared to urban children. Meanwhile, when compared to rural left-behind children who were still living in rural areas, migrant children reported significantly lower scores in emotional symptoms and total difficulties [10].

Despite these studies demonstrating the detrimental effect of migrant status on children's mental health, gaps remain in the existing literature; these studies had small sample sizes, and did not include an appropriate comparison group to verify the impact of migrant status on mental health.

Another concern regarding migrant children and adolescents' health conditions is self-injurious thoughts and behaviors (SITBs), which is a serious public health concern worldwide [11]. In children and adolescents, two particular types of SITBs are notable: suicidal ideation, referring to thoughts of ending one's own life, and non-suicidal self-injury (NSSI), defined as the direct and deliberate destruction of one's body tissue without the intent to die [12]. Previous international studies have already confirmed migrant status as a risk factor for suicidal ideation [13] and self-injurious behaviors [14]. In China, it is estimated that between 14.01 and 26.03% of

children and adolescents report suicidal ideation [15, 16]; however, studies investigating this phenomenon seldom investigate the impact of migrant status on these behaviors in children and adolescents [17]. Only one study [18], conducted in Shanghai, examined the prevalence of suicidal ideation in migrant adolescents, and found the rate to be 36.80%, without a comparison to their urban counterparts.

The present study aims to investigate the mental health status of migrant children living in eastern coastal China in comparison to their urban counterparts, and SITBs among this sample. Based on the aforementioned review of the literature, two major hypotheses were developed: firstly, compared to urban children, migrant children would score significantly higher in all SDQ outcomes and secondly, migrant children would report significantly more SITBs.

Methods
Sample
A cross-sectional survey was conducted in a migrant receiving urban city, the Yinzhou district of Ningbo, Zhejiang Province, between May and June 2013. The region has an estimated population of 136 million, of whom 46.60% are migrants. There are two kinds of schools available for migrant children: migrant-exclusive schools, utilized by the majority of migrant children; and public schools, utilized by migrant children whose parents are relatively socio-economically advantaged. As roughly 30% of migrant children in this area attend public schools, 5 migrants' schools and 8 public schools were randomly selected from the school roster of the District Education Bureau to ensure the comparability of sample size between the two groups.

In each school, all selected students were between grades 5 and 9. Across the 13 schools, 4217 students (1858 migrant children and 2359 urban children) out of 4409 eligible enrolled students completed the questionnaire, representing a response rate of 95.65%.

Procedure
Study information was sent to the head of each school and the District Education Bureau by mail, and approvals from both parties were obtained. Information packs (an information letter and a consent form) were distributed to parents by school staff to gain verifiable parental consent. The study was performed during lunch breaks and course recesses, during which students with parental consent were assessed collectively by two well-trained investigators. Before filling out the questionnaire, students' verbal agreement to participate was obtained after a simplified study introduction given by the investigators. The questionnaire was strictly self-administered by

students under investigators' uniform instruction, and teachers were off-site to ensure anonymity.

The study was approved by the Ethics Committee of Zhejiang University (Ref no. ZGL201412-2).

Measures
Socio-demographics
Socio-demographic characteristics included: age, gender, migrant status, family economic status, parents' education level and parents' marital status. Family economic status was measured by possession of a number of household items, such as an air conditioner, refrigerator, washing machine, computer and private car [19, 20]. This variable was then coded as low- (zero to two item), moderate- (three to four items), and high-income (five items). Parents' education level referred to the highest education level of one parent.

The strengths and difficulties questionnaire
Child psycho-social wellbeing was measured with the self-reported version of the strengths and difficulties questionnaire (SDQ), which has been validated in China [21]. The SDQ consists of five subscales: emotional symptoms, conduct problems, hyperactivity, peer problems and prosocial behavior; each subscale contains five items in the form of statements requiring a response via a three-point Likert response scale: 1 (not true); 2 (somewhat true); or 3 (certainly true) [6]. The Cronbach's alpha for the emotional symptoms in this study was 0.76; 0.72 for the conduct problems; 0.77 for the hyperactivity; 0.67 for the peer problems; and 0.79 for the prosocial behavior. Emotional symptoms and peer problems were combined to form a single "internalizing" subscale, conduct problems and hyperactivity were combined to form a single "externalizing" subscale, and the third subscale, "prosocial behavior," remained unchanged. The total difficulties score was calculated by adding the scores of the internalizing and externalizing subscales. Higher scores on the total difficulties, internalizing and externalizing subscales represent higher levels of psychological problems; while higher scores on the prosocial behavior subscale represent lower levels of psychological problems.

Self-injurious thoughts and behaviors (SITBs)
SITBs, including non-suicidal self-injury, suicidal thoughts, suicide attempts and death by suicide, are widely used to obtain information regarding adolescent suicidality [22]. In this study, the SITBs we assessed were suicidal ideation and non-suicidal self-injury. These two items were assessed with the following questions: "Did you have suicidal thoughts during the past 2 weeks?" and "Did you hurt yourself deliberately during the past year?" The following statements were identified as a "yes"

answer for suicidal ideation: "During the last 2 weeks, I had thoughts of killing myself" and "During the last 2 weeks, I had thoughts of killing myself but I wouldn't carry them out". The following statements were identified as a "yes" answer for self-injurious behaviors: "During the past year, I hurt myself deliberately once" and "During the past year, I hurt myself deliberately more than once".

Data analysis
Chi square tests and t-tests were conducted to compare sample characteristics between migrant and urban children. Multiple linear regression and binary logistic regressions models were applied to examine the associations between the psycho-social outcomes and migrant-urban status. Suicidal ideation and self-injurious behavior and SDQ outcomes were included as dependent variables and migrant-urban status was examined as an independent variable. Analyses were adjusted for age, gender, family economic status, parents' education level and parents' marital status. All analyses were performed using SPSS 20.0 version and assumed a statistical significance level of $p < 0.05$.

Results
Table 1 presents the differences in socio-demographic characteristics and the psychological outcomes between migrant children and urban children. There were significantly more males among migrant children (55.90%) than urban children (49.04%). The mean age of migrant children was 13.67 (SD = 1.52) and the mean age of urban children was 13.92 (SD = 1.30). Migrant children had a generally lower family economic status ($\chi^2 = 1031.00$; $p < 0.001$), with parents who were less educated compared to urban children ($\chi^2 = 576.80$; $p < 0.001$). Compared to urban children's parents (6.45%), fewer migrant children's parents (4.29%) were divorced ($\chi^2 = 9.24$; $p < 0.01$).

Migrant children had significantly higher mean scores for total difficulties ($t = 47.84$, $p < 0.001$), internalizing problems ($t = 65.81$; $p < 0.001$) and externalizing problems ($t = 81.15$; $p < 0.001$), and lower mean scores on the prosocial behavior scale ($t = 53.35$; $p < 0.001$) compared to urban children. Migrant children reported significantly higher rates of self-injurious behaviors ($\chi^2 = 4.86$; $p < 0.05$).

Table 2 shows the linear regression analyses of SDQ outcomes and the binary logistic regression analyses of SITBs outcomes. After controlling for gender, age, family economic status, parent's education level and parents' marital status, migrant children scored higher for total difficulties ($\beta = 0.46$; 95% CI = 0.06, 0.85; $p < 0.05$) and externalizing problems ($\beta = 0.50$; 95% CI = 0.26, 0.74; $p < 0.001$) than did urban children. Migrant children

Table 1 The social-demographic characteristics, SDQ and SITBs of migrant compared to urban children

	Migrant children n = 1858 N (%)	Urban children n = 2359 N (%)	χ^2 or t	p value
Gender			18.41	< 0.001
Male	966 (55.90)	1100 (49.04)		
Female	762 (44.10)	1143 (50.96)		
Age, mean (SD)	13.67 (1.52)	13.92 (1.30)	34.23	< 0.001
Family economic status			1031.00	< 0.001
Poor	566 (31.03)	53 (2.26)		
Fair	821 (45.01)	711 (30.35)		
Wealthy	437 (23.96)	1579 (67.39)		
Parents' education level			576.80	< 0.001
Illiteracy or primary school	319 (17.68)	89 (3.90)		
Middle school	1100 (60.98)	975 (42.71)		
High school	329 (18.24)	754 (33.03)		
College or above	56 (3.10)	465 (20.37)		
Are your parents divorced?			9.24	0.003
Yes	79 (4.29)	151 (6.45)		
No	1761 (95.71)	2189 (93.55)		
Total difficulties, mean (SD)	12.28 (5.19)	11.12 (5.56)	47.84	< 0.001
Emotional symptoms, mean (SD)	3.09 (2.00)	3.03 (2.12)	7.40	0.007
Conduct problems, mean (SD)	2.43 (1.63)	2.18 (1.60)	4.43	0.035
Hyperactivity, mean (SD)	3.92 (2.16)	3.36 (2.20)	6.17	0.013
Peer problems, mean (SD)	2.84 (1.60)	2.55 (1.65)	2.73	0.098
Prosocial behavior, mean (SD)	6.93 (2.02)	7.39 (2.10)	53.35	< 0.001
Internalizing problems, mean (SD)	5.93 (2.88)	5.58 (3.06)	65.81	< 0.001
Internalizing problems (> 8)	326 (17.55)	418 (17.72)	0.02	0.903
Externalizing problems, mean (SD)	6.35 (3.30)	5.54 (3.30)	81.15	< 0.001
Externalizing problems (> 10)	1796 (96.66)	2231 (94.57)	10.54	0.001
Suicidal ideation			1.70	0.200
Yes	492 (26.67)	584 (24.89)		
No	1353 (73.33)	1762 (75.11)		
Self-injuries behavior			4.86	0.030
Yes	189 (10.47)	193 (8.45)		
No	1616 (89.53)	2091 (91.55)		

reported significantly higher rates of suicidal ideation (OR = 1.23; 95% CI = 1.03, 1.46; p < 0.05) and self-injurious behaviors (OR = 1.32; 95% CI = 1.01, 1.72; p < 0.05).

Discussion

As China's economy grows, migrant populations will continue to expand. Migration is a carefully weighed family decision [23]. While migrant children may benefit from staying with their parents, their well-being may be harmed from limited access to social welfare and other social services [24]. This study sought to explore the mental health status and SITBs in migrant children living in eastern coastal China in comparison to their urban counterparts. We found that migrant children, compared

to urban children, are more likely to experience externalizing problems (conduct problems and hyperactivity) and SITBs (suicidal thoughts and behaviors).

Partly in line with our first hypothesis, after controlling for socio-demographic variables, migrant children reported higher mean scores in total difficulties and externalizing problems (conduct problems and hyperactivity) compared to urban children but not in internalizing problems (emotional symptoms and peer problems). Low familial socioeconomic status (SES) is one of the several environmental adversities that has been found to increase the risk of mental health problems in this age group [25, 26]. Coleman [27] has proposed that three types of capital influence youth's well-being: parents who

Table 2 Regression coefficients for SDQ outcomes and SITBs on children group with adjustment for socio-demographic characteristics

	Emotional symptoms β (95% CI)	Conduct problems β (95% CI)	Hyperactivity β (95% CI)	Peer problems β (95% CI)	Internalizing problems β (95% CI)	Externalizing problems β (95% CI)	Prosocial behavior β (95% CI)	Total difficulties β (95% CI)	Suicidal ideation OR (95% CI)	Self-injurious behavior OR (95% CI)
Group										
Urban children	1.00	1.00	1.00	1.00	1.00	1.00	1.00	1.00	1.00	1.00
Migrant children	−0.09 (− 0.24, 0.07)	0.15 (0.03, 0.27)*	0.35 (0.19, 0.51)***	0.04 (− 0.08, 0.16)	−0.05 (− 0.27, 17)	0.50 (0.26, 0.74)***	−0.10 (− 0.25, 0.05)	0.46 (0.06, 0.85)*	1.23 (1.03, 1.46)*	1.32 (1.01, 1.72)*
Gender										
Male	1.00	1.00	1.00	1.00	1.00	1.00	1.00	1.00	1.00	1.00
Female	0.36 (0.23, 0.49)***	−0.40 (− 0.49, − 0.29)***	−0.45 (− 0.59, − 0.32)***	−0.36 (− 0.46, − 0.25)***	0.01 (− 0.18, 0.19)	−0.85 (− 1.00, − 0.64)***	0.61 (0.48, 0.74)***	−0.84 (− 1.17, − 0.51)***	1.11 (0.97, 1.30)	1.09 (0.87, 1.36)
Age	0.08 (0.03, 0.12)**	0.02 (− 0.02, 0.06)	0.17 (0.12, 0.22)***	0.01 (− 0.03, 0.04)	0.08 (0.01, 0.15)*	0.19 (0.12, 0.27)***	−0.01 (− 0.05, 0.04)	0.27 (0.15, 0.39)***	1.22 (1.16, 1.29)***	1.11 (1.02, 1.20)*
Family economic status										
Poor	1.00	1.00	1.00	1.00	1.00	1.00	1.00	1.00	1.00	1.00
Fair	−0.19 (− 0.40, 0.02)	0.05 (− 0.11, 0.21)	−0.04 (− 0.25, 0.18)	−0.19 (− 0.35, − 0.03)*	−0.38 (− 0.68, − 0.09)*	0.02 (− 0.31, 0.34)	0.17 (− 0.03, 0.38)	−0.36 (− 0.89, 0.17)	1.09 (0.87, 1.38)	0.83 (0.59, 1.17)
Wealthy	−0.24 (− 0.46, − 0.02)*	−0.30 (− 0.20, 0.14)	−0.20 (− 0.43, 0.03)	−0.38 (− 0.55, − 0.21)***	−0.62 (− 0.93, − 0.30)**	−0.23 (− 0.58, 0.12)	0.50 (0.29, 0.72)***	−0.85 (− 1.42, − 0.28)**	1.29 (1.01, 1.65)*	1.07 (0.74, 1.54)
Parents' education level										
Illiteracy/primary school	1.00	1.00	1.00	1.00	1.00	1.00	1.00	1.00	1.00	1.00
Middle school	−0.43 (− 0.64, − 0.22)***	−0.26 (− 0.42, − 0.09)**	−0.33 (− 0.55, − 0.11)**	−0.27 (− 0.43, − 0.10)**	−0.69 (− 0.99, − 0.39)***	−0.59 (− 0.91, − 0.26)**	0.32 (0.11, 0.52)**	−1.28 (− 1.82, − 0.74)***	0.68 (0.54, 0.85)**	0.73 (0.53, 1.01)
High school	−0.45 (− 0.69, − 0.22)***	−0.24 (− 0.42, − 0.06)**	−0.44 (− 0.68, − 0.19)***	−0.34 (− 0.52, − 0.15)***	−0.79 (− 1.13, − 0.45)***	−0.68 (− 1.05, − 0.31)***	0.49 (0.26, 0.72)***	−1.47 (− 2.07, − 0.86)***	0.68 (0.53, 0.88)**	0.69 (0.47, 1.02)
College or above	−0.78 (− 1.06, − 0.50)***	−0.40 (− 0.61, − 0.18)***	−0.82 (− 1.11, − 0.53)***	−0.61 (− 0.83, − 0.39)***	−1.39 (− 1.79, − 0.99)***	−1.22 (− 1.65, − 0.77)***	0.77 (0.50, 1.04)***	−2.60 (− 3.32, − 1.88)***	0.74 (0.54, 1.02)	0.90 (0.58, 1.40)
Parental martial status										
Married	1.00	1.00	1.00	1.00	1.00	1.00	1.00	1.00	1.00	1.00
Divorced	0.26 (− 0.02, 0.54)	0.36 (0.14, 0.57)**	0.58 (0.29, 0.88)***	0.15 (− 0.07, 0.37)	0.41 (0.01, 0.82)*	0.94 (0.50, 1.38)***	−0.12 (− 0.39, 0.16)	1.35 (0.63, 2.08)***	1.70 (1.27, 2.28)***	1.32 (0.86, 2.04)

* p < 0.05, ** p < 0.01, *** p < 0.001

are educated (human capital) are assumed to have a better economic status (financial capital) and are more likely to be communicative with their children (social capital). Under this framework, our findings suggest that better family economic status and parental education levels can mitigate against the adverse psychological experiences caused by migration with parents, indicating that material and family support can work as important factors supporting children's psychological well-being. Essentially, migrant children from lower-income families with less-educated parents are susceptible to additional risks for psychosocial disadvantages.

Previous studies also have suggested that SES is more closely related to the externalizing than to the internalizing domain [28, 29]. As a possible explanation for this, some scholars suggest that, as children age, they become more exposed to influences outside of the family, which may reduce their internalizing problems [30]. Migrant and urban children in our study were close in age and lived in similar neighborhoods, which may explain why migrant children in our study didn't report higher mean scores of internalizing problems (emotional symptoms and peer problems) than did their urban counterparts.

Previous studies have suggested that externalizing problems (conduct problems [31, 32] and hyperactivity [33]) in youth are associated with low family cohesion and the low intellectual/cultural orientation of the family. Families with low levels of intellectual/cultural orientation can only offer limited opportunities for socialization and access to community resources to their children, which may increase children's externalizing problems [34]. Likewise, the strong negative influence of parental divorce highlights the importance of family cohesion on children's mental health [35]. Parental divorce will impair the bonds between family members, which may exert negative influences on a child's development of children.

After adjusting for relevant variables, migrant children reported significantly higher rates of suicidal ideation and self-injurious behaviors than did urban children in the present study, supporting our second hypothesis. As noted, externalizing problems are associated with SITBs in adolescents [36, 37]. The risk of suicide is 30–50 times higher in populations with SITBs than in the general population [38]. Thus, migrant children with suicidal ideation or non-suicidal self-injurious behaviors are at high risk for suicide. In recent years, a growing number of scholars have argued that the existing measures being implemented for youth suicide prevention do not have the same efficiency in migrant children as they do in urban children [39], as migrant workers are too busy to take care of their children [40] and migrant-exclusive schools are usually under-provisioned. Therefore, to prevent suicide among migrant children more effectively,

greater importance should be attached to their SITBs and appropriate follow up management should be implemented.

Several limitations in the present study were identified when interpreting the study findings, in light of its design and methodological characteristics. Firstly, the sample size was large, yet the study was conducted in a single district within one eastern coastal city of China. Therefore, it is inappropriate to extrapolate the results to the whole country. Secondly, to understand the condition of mental health and SITBs of migrant children, more factors should be taken into consideration, including domestic violence and parents' history of mental illness. Adolescents who have experienced family violence were at higher risk of developing externalising problems [41]. Since young children may be reluctant to answer some of these questions, we didn't include them in the questionnaire. Thirdly, our exclusive reliance on adolescents' self-reporting may result in the under-reporting of mental health problems [6]. Consequently, mental health problems and SITBs may be underestimated in the present study.

Conclusion
A comparison of the migrant children and urban children reveals that migrant children are highly likely to face externalizing problems (conduct problems and hyperactivity) and SITBs (suicidal thoughts and behaviors). Actions should be taken to identify migrant children's externalizing problems and SITBs, improve the communication between teachers and parents, and provide mental health services at migrant-exclusive schools. The migration policy should be changed to improve access to equitable education and social welfare for migrant children.

Abbreviations
SDQ: strengths and difficulties questionnaire; SITBs: self-injurious thoughts and behaviors; NSSI: non-suicidal self-injurious; SES: socioeconomic status.

Authors' contributions
JL analyzed and interpreted the data; and drafted the manuscript. FW and DW drafted the manuscript. PC participated in the coordination of the study. LL participated in critical review of the manuscript; and participated in the conception and design of the study. XZ participated in critical review of the manuscript; and participated in the conception, design and coordination of the study. All authors read and approved the final manuscript.

Author details
[1] The Institute of Social and Family Medicine, School of Public Health, Zhejiang University, 866 Yuhangtang Rd., Hangzhou 310058, Zhejiang, People's Republic of China. [2] Yinzhou District CDC, 1221 Xueshi Rd., Ningbo 315199, Zhejiang, People's Republic of China. [3] Oxford Road, SG16 Samuel Alexander Building, Manchester M13 9PL, UK.

Acknowledgements
Not applicable.

Competing interests
The authors declare that they have no competing interests.

Funding
The survey was conducted with funding from Zhejiang University Zijin Talent Project and infrastructure support from Yinzhou District CDC. Funders had no role in study design; collection, analysis and interpretation of data; and in writing the manuscript.

References

1. Liang Z, Guo L, Duan C. Migration and the well-being of children in China. Yale-China Health J. 2008;5:25–46.
2. All China Women's Federation. China's rural left-behind children, rural and urban migrant children research report. 2013. http://acwf.people.com.cn/n/2013/0510/c99013-21437965.html.
3. Xu LL. A study on the social integration dilemma of migrant children. Contemp Econ. 2016;20:12–3.
4. Wong DFK, Li CY, Song HX. Rural migrant workers in urban China: living a marginalised life. Int J Soc Welf. 2007;16(1):32–40.
5. Guo Z. Exceeding the discrimination: the use of anti-discriminatory practice of social work in mental health on movable children. J South Yangtze Univ. 2007;1:006.
6. Goodman R, Meltzer H, Bailey V. The strengths and difficulties questionnaire: a pilot study on the validity of the self-report version. Eur Child Adolesc Psychiatry. 1998;7(3):125–30.
7. Goodman R. Psychometric properties of the strengths and difficulties questionnaire. J Am Acad Child Adolesc Psychiatry. 2001;40(11):1337–45.
8. Lu T, Guo L, Zhu QZ, et al. The difficult experience of the early adolescence migrant children and analyzed of its relevant factors. Chin J Women Child Health. 2014;2:008.
9. Luan W, Lu H, Tong Y, et al. Family ties and the mental health of migrant children. Stud Early Childhood Educ. 2013;2:27–35.
10. Wang F, Zhou X, Hesketh T. Psychological adjustment and behaviours in children of migrant workers in China. Child Care Health Dev. 2017;43(6):884–90.
11. Kim YK. Suicide & suicidal behavior. Epidemiol Rev. 2008;30(1):133–54.
12. Nock MK. Self-injury. Ann Rev Clin Psychol. 2010;6:339–63.
13. Blum R, Sudhinaraset M, Emerson MR. Youth at risk: suicidal thoughts and attempts in Vietnam, China, and Taiwan. J Adolesc Health. 2012;50(3):S37–44.
14. Plener PL, Munz LM, Allroggen M, et al. Immigration as risk factor for non-suicidal self-injury and suicide attempts in adolescents in Germany. Child Adolesc Psychiatry Ment Health. 2015;9(1):34.
15. Chen LI, Hong WA, Jin LI. Suicidal ideation among adolescents in chongqing and its influencing factors. Chin Gen Pract. 2012;34:030.
16. Guo WH, Cao YJ. Analysis of suicidal intention and its influencing factors among teenagers in Qinghai province. Chin J School Health. 2012;33:937–41.
17. Qiu WT, Feng W. Review and forecast on research of adolescents suicide in the past decades in China. Mod Prev Med. 2009;11:042.
18. Shuang C. Suicidal ideation of migrant children in Shanghai. Youth Rep. 2015;2:92–6.
19. Laska-Mierzejewska T, Olszewska E. Anthropological assessment of changes in living conditions of the rural population in Poland in the period 1967–2001. Ann Hum Biol. 2007;34(3):362.
20. Kumar R, Bhave A, Bhargava R, et al. Prevalence and risk factors for neurological disorders in children aged 6 months to 2 years in northern India. Dev Med Child Neurol. 2013;55(4):348–56.
21. Lai KYC, Luk ESL, Leung PWL, et al. Validation of the Chinese version of the strengths and difficulties questionnaire in Hong Kong. Soc Psychiatry Psychiatr Epidemiol. 2010;45(12):1179–86.
22. Castellví P, Lucas-Romero E, Miranda-Mendizábal A, et al. Longitudinal association between self-injurious thoughts and behaviors and suicidal behavior in adolescents and young adults: a systematic review with meta-analysis. J Affect Disord. 2017;215:37.
23. Bloom DE, Stark O. In the new economics of labour migration. Am Econ Rev. 1985;75(2):173–8.
24. Wu Q, Lu D, Kang M. Social capital and the mental health of children in rural China with different experiences of parental migration. Soc Sci Med. 1982;2015(132):270–7.
25. Velez CN, Johnson J, Cohen P. A longitudinal analysis of selected risk factors for childhood psychopathology. J Am Acad Child Adolesc Psychiatry. 1989;28(6):861–4.
26. Oort FVAV, Ende JVD, Wadsworth ME, et al. Cross-national comparison of the link between socioeconomic status and emotional and behavioral problems in youths. Soc Psychiatry Psychiatr Epidemiol. 2011;46(2):167–72.
27. Coleman JS. Social capital in the creation of human capital. Am J Sociol. 1988;94:95–120.
28. Kapi A, Veltsista A, Kavadias G, Lekea V, et al. Social determinants of self-reported emotional and behavioral problems in Greek adolescents. Soc Psychiatry Psychiatr Epidemiol. 2007;42(7):594–8.
29. Lahelma E, Laaksonen M, Martikainen P, et al. Multiple measures of socioeconomic circumstances and common mental disorders. Soc Sci Med. 2006;63(5):1383.
30. Bengi-Arslan L, Verhulst FC, Ende JVD, et al. Understanding childhood (problem) behaviors from a cultural perspective: comparison of problem behaviors and competencies in Turkish immigrant, Turkish and Dutch children. Soc Psychiatry Psychiatr Epidemiol. 1997;32(8):477–84.
31. Haddad JD, Barocas R, Hollenbeck AR. Family organization and parent attitudes of children with conduct disorder. J Clin Child Adolesc Psychol. 1991;20(2):152–61.
32. Slee PT. Family climate and behavior in families with conduct disordered children. Child Psychiatry Hum Dev. 1996;26(4):255.
33. Crea TM, Chan K, Barth RP. Family environment and attention-deficit/hyperactivity disorder in adopted children: associations with family cohesion and adaptability. Child Care Health Dev. 2014;40(6):853–62.
34. George C, Herman KC, Ostrander R. The family environment and developmental psychopathology: the unique and interactive effects of depression, attention, and conduct problems. Child Psychiatry Hum Dev. 2006;37(2):163–77.
35. Strohschein L. Parental divorce and child mental health trajectories. J Marriage Fam. 2005;67(5):1286–300.
36. Kovess-Masfety V, Pilowsky DJ, Goelitz D, et al. Suicidal ideation and mental health disorders in young school children across Europe. J Affect Disord. 2015;177:28–35.
37. Hurtig T, Taanila A, Moilanen I, et al. Suicidal and self-harm behaviour associated with adolescent attention deficit hyperactivity disorder—a study in the Northern Finland Birth Cohort 1986. Nord J Psychiatry. 2012;66(5):320–8.
38. Cooper J, Kapur N, Webb R, et al. Suicide after deliberate self-harm: a 4-year cohort study. Am J Psychiatry. 2005;162(2):297–303.
39. Donath C, Graessel E, Baier D, et al. Is parenting style a predictor of suicide attempts in a representative sample of adolescents? BMC Pediatr. 2014;14(1):1–13.
40. Yang H, He F, Wang TH, et al. Health-related lifestyle behaviors among male and female rural-to-urban migrant workers in Shanghai, China. PLoS ONE. 2015;10(2):e0117946.
41. Ajduković M, Rajhvajn Bulat L, Sušac N. The internalising and externalising problems of adolescents in Croatia: socio-demographic and family victimisation factors. Int J Soc Welf. 2017;3:88–100.

13

Examining changes in personality disorder and symptomology in an adolescent sample receiving intensive mentalization based treatment: a pilot study

Kirsten Hauber[1,3]* ⓘ, Albert Eduard Boon[1,2,3] and Robert Vermeiren[3,4]

Abstract

Objective: To examine changes in personality disorders and symptomology and the relation between personality disorder variables and treatment outcomes in an adolescent sample during partial residential mentalization based treatment.

Methods: In a sample of 62 (out of 115) adolescents treated for personality disorders, assessment was done pre- and post-treatment using the Structured Clinical Interview for DSM personality disorders and the Symptom Check List 90.

Results: Significant reductions in personality disorder traits ($t = 8.36, p = .000$) and symptoms ($t = 5.95, p = .000$) were found. During pre-treatment, 91.8% ($n = 56$) of the patients had one or more personality disorders, compared to 35.4% ($n = 22$) at post-treatment. Symptom reduction was not related to pre-treatment personality disorder variables.

Conclusion: During intensive psychotherapy, personality disorders and symptoms may diminish. Future studies should evaluate whether the outcomes obtained are the result of the treatment given or other factors.

Background

Relatively little research has been conducted on personality disorders in adolescents; specifically, research regarding effective treatments is limited [1–5]. This is an omission, as the psychosocial and the economic burdens of adolescents with (traits of) personality disorders are high [3, 6]. Interestingly, the direct mental health and medical costs for adolescents in the year prior to treatment for personality disorders were demonstrated to be substantially higher than for adults [6, 7]. Timely detection and treatment of (traits of) personality disorders during adolescence are for that reason important. Therefore, the aim of this cohort pilot study is to examine the changes in a group of adolescents with clinically diagnosed personality disorders who received an intensive mentalization based treatment (MBT) with partial

hospitalisation [8–10]. Mentalizing refers to the ability to understand and differentiate between the mental states of oneself and others and to acknowledge the relation between underlying mental states and behaviour [8, 11].

Doubts regarding the permanence of personality disorders in adolescents are considered to be the main problem underlying the lag in research on this topic [2, 3, 12, 13]. Despite guidelines [14] advising professionals to diagnose personality disorders (with the exception of antisocial personality disorder during adolescence), most psychologists and psychiatrists are hesitant to diagnose personality disorders in minors. As a result, minors are not offered specific treatments. This is partly understandable as, during adolescence, normal emotional maturation is characterised by an interplay between progression and regression [15], which complicates the diagnostic process of personality disorders. In addition, diagnosing personality disorders might stigmatise adolescents. However, the reluctance of professionals to diagnose (traits of) personality disorders in adolescents is likely to delay

*Correspondence: k.hauber@dejutters.com
[1] De Jutters B.V, Centre for Youth Mental Healthcare Haaglanden, The Hague, The Netherlands
Full list of author information is available at the end of the article

research and thus the development of effective treatments for this group of patients.

According to current research, the primary information used to treat personality disorders in adolescents is based on randomised controlled trials of treatments developed for adults, mostly treatments for borderline personality disorder (BPD). The few studies that have been conducted on adolescents with (traits of) BPD have yielded mixed results. Two studies showed no advantages over treatment as usual [16, 17]; one study showed only a short term effect [18]; while another found a better outcome compared to treatment as usual [19]. All treatments were associated with improvements over time, which may partially reflect the natural course of BPD in adolescents. Whether existing adult treatment programmes are useful for adolescents with personality disorders other than BPD is mostly unknown, as research is scarce. One study investigated the treatment outcome of a 12 month inpatient psychotherapy intervention for adolescents with personality disorders. Only 51 patients of a total sample of 109 completed the research protocol, of whom 29% recovered fully in terms of the level of symptom severity, 12% improved, while 49% showed no significant change and 10% showed deterioration [20]. Furthermore, none of the specific personality disorders or clusters of personality disorders (A, B, C and NOS) predicted treatment outcome. In conclusion, the results of the few studied treatments for adolescents with (traits of) personality disorders have shown mixed results; however, the most severe sample studied, the inpatient group, showed moderate results.

Difficulties in establishing randomised clinical trials (RCTs) in clinical practice—especially in a high risk adolescent sample with comorbidity—is another reason that potentially explains the scarcity of research in adolescents with personality disorders. Although RCTs are essential for studying the comparative effectiveness of treatments and have a high internal validity, trials dictate strict protocol adherence and often have a low external validity [21]. Furthermore, randomising carries ethical and practical ramifications in a high risk adolescent group in need of an inpatient programme due to family dynamics, suicidal actions, self-injury and prolonged school absenteeism. Randomisation on the individual level within an inpatient treatment programme is even more intricate, as it implies training half of the treatment staff to follow a study protocol and compare the effect of their interventions with the effect of the interventions of the non-trained half. Moreover, as populations and circumstances differ significantly, the results of RCTs may have limited relevance to clinical practice. Therefore, nonrandomised evaluations of inpatient programmes focusing on external validity, in order to obtain generalisable knowledge of the patient group and treatment evaluation, are needed. The transparent reporting of evaluations with nonrandomised designs (TREND) group [22] has developed a 22 items checklist to improve the reporting standards of nonrandomised evaluations of behavioural and public health interventions.

In this study, we provide treatment evaluation data following the TREND guidelines [22] from a prospective pilot study of 115 adolescents with clinically diagnosed personality disorders, of whom 62 (54%) completed the treatment protocol and filled out questionnaires during pre- and post-treatment. This group received intensive MBT with partial hospitalisation [8–10]. The external validity is tested. Furthermore, the predictive power of personality disorder variables on treatment outcomes concerning symptomology is explored.

Methods
Setting
The present study was conducted from January 2008 until December 2014 at a residential psychotherapeutic institution for adolescents in the urban area of The Hague in the Netherlands. This facility offers a 5 days a week intensive MBT with partial hospitalisation for adolescents between the ages of 16 and 23 years with personality disorders. This structured and integrative psychodynamic group psychotherapy programme is manualised, adapted to adolescents [8–10] and facilitated by a multidisciplinary team trained in MBT. The major difference with the MBT programme for adolescents in England [19] is the psychodynamic group psychotherapy approach. The mentalizing focus of the different therapies in the programme is on the adolescent's subjective experience of himself or herself and others and on the relationships with the group members and therapists. The programme offers weekly verbal and non-verbal group psychotherapies, such as group psychotherapy, art therapy and psychodrama therapy, in combination with individual and family psychotherapy. The average duration of treatment is 1 year with a maximum of 18 months. Commonly, the treatment starts with hospitalisation and continues as day treatment later on during the programme. Medication is prescribed if necessary by a psychiatrist working in the therapy programme, according to protocol. Referrals come non-systematically from other mental health professionals from within and outside our mental health care institution.

Subjects
In total, 115 adolescents with clinically diagnosed personality disorders were studied with a mean age at the start of treatment of 18.2 ($SD = 1.6$, range $= 15–22$; females 80.9%). Most of the participants had other comorbid

axis-I disorders (mood disorder 58%; anxiety disorder, including PTSD 31%; eating disorder 13%; ADHD 8%; substance dependence 7%; dissociative disorder 3%; and obsessive compulsive disorder 2%). The average duration of treatment was 277.8 days ($SD = 166.1$, range $= 3–549$), with an average of 186.1 days ($SD = 146.1$) of hospitalisation. Intelligence was estimated based on the level of education and was average to above average. All patients followed the treatment on a voluntary basis and were fluent in the Dutch language.

Of the 115 adolescents who were included in this study, 13 were considered treatment dropouts because they withdrew or were sent away before their treatment duration exceed the diagnostic phase of 2 months (61 days) [23, 24]. These 13 dropouts did not differ significantly from the rest in age, gender or severity of symptoms or personality disorders. The remaining sample consisted of 102 respondents, with 83 females (81.4%) and 19 males (18.6%). While all were assessed by the SCID-II interview initially, only 62 (60.8%) post-treatment SCID-II interviews were administered. One adolescent did not complete the SCID-II interview at pre-treatment but did at post-treatment. The average duration of treatment of adolescents who only participated in a pre-treatment SCID-II interview was shorter (202.1 days; $SD = 115.2$, 61–526), with an average of 146.4 ($SD = 124.9$, 0–20) days of hospitalisation, compared to those who also participated in a post-treatment SCID-II interview (378.6 days; $SD = 126.0$, 120–549), with an average of 246.0 ($SD = 139.4$, 0–547) days of hospitalisation ($p = 0.000$; $t = 7.406$). Of the respondents who only participated in a pre-treatment SCID-II interview, 43% completed the treatment according to protocol, as compared to 92% of the adolescents who also participated in a post-treatment SCID-II interview. The number and type of personality disorders did not differ between these groups. Missing post-treatment research data was caused by respondents who failed to complete the set of web-based questionnaires during post-treatment or repeatedly failed to show up at the final SCID-II interview appointment.

Measures

The participating adolescents completed a set of web-based questionnaires at the beginning and end of treatment, including the Dutch Questionnaire for Personality Characteristics (Vragenlijst voor Kenmerken van de Persoonlijkheid) (VKP) [25] and the Symptom Check List 90 (SCL-90) [26, 27]. Subjects were interviewed using the Structured Clinical Interview for DSM personality disorders (SCID-II) [28].

VKP

The VKP is a questionnaire consisting of 197 questions with the answer categories 'true' or 'false'; its purpose is to screen for personality disorders according to the DSM-IV. The VKP is known for its high sensitivity and low specificity [25] and is recommended [29, 30] as a pre-assessment instrument before administering the Dutch version of the SCID-II. Presumed and certain indications of a personality disorder on the VKP indicate which SCID-II personality disorder sections should be applied. The test–retest reliability (Cohen's Kappa) of the VKP on categorical diagnoses was moderate ($k = .40$) [25].

SCL-90

An authorised Dutch version of the SCL-90 [26] is a questionnaire consisting of 90 questions with a 5-point rating scale (ranging from 1 'not at all' to 5 'extreme'). This questionnaire assesses general psychological distress and specific primary psychological symptoms of distress. Outcome scores are divided into nine symptom subscales: anxiety; agoraphobia; depression; somatisation; insufficient thinking and handling; distrust and interpersonal sensitivity; hostility; sleeping disorders; and a rest subscale. The total score (range 90–450) is calculated by adding the scores of the subscales. The test–retest reliability was reasonable to good ($k = .62$ to .91) [26].

SCID-II

The SCID-II [28] is a semi-structured interview consisting of 134 questions. The purpose of this interview is to establish the ten DSM-IV personality disorders, and depressive and passive-aggressive personality disorders. In line with the DSM-IV criteria, the depressive and passive-aggressive personality disorders are covered by the 'personality disorder not otherwise specified' (NOS). The language and diagnostic coverage make the SCID-II most appropriate for adults (age 18 or over), while with slight modification it can be used for younger adolescents [28]. Only the sections that were indicated by the outcome of the VKP were applied in the clinical interview. The SCID-II was administered by trained psychologists. The inter-rater reliability (Cohen's Kappa) of the SCID-II for categorical diagnoses was reasonable to good ($k = .61$–1.00) [31], and the test–retest reliability was also reasonable to good ($k = .63$) [32].

Procedures

From 2008, 115 newly admitted patients were asked to participate in the study. The data of patients ending treatment before the end of 2014 were used. Following a verbal description of the treatment protocol to the subjects, written informed consent was obtained according to legislation, the institution's policy and the Dutch law

[33]. All patients ($N = 115$) agreed to participate and, in accordance with the institutional policy, they participated without receiving incentives or rewards. All procedures in this study were in accordance with the 1964 Declaration of Helsinki and its later amendments or comparable ethical standards. According to the treatment protocol, the patients completed a set of web-based questionnaires, including the VKP and the SCL-90 during the first and last weeks of treatment. The participants filled out the questionnaires by themselves and were not aware of the study's objective.

Statistical analysis

All analyses were performed using the Statistical Package for the Social Sciences, version 20.0 [34]. A Wilcoxon Signed-Rank Test was performed between the number of pre-treatment SCID-II personality disorders and the number of post-treatment SCID-II personality disorders. To compare the total score on the SCL-90 across the number of SCID-II personality disorders at pre- and post-treatment an ANOVA was used. A Pearson correlation test was performed to compare the length of treatment with changes in the SCL-90 and paired t test were performed to compare the SCL-90 and number of SCID- II personality disorders between two groups based on length of treatment. A linear regression analysis was used to explore the relationship between the predictor variables (VKP, SCID-II scales) at $t − 1$ and the SCL-90 outcome at post-treatment.

Results

Pre- and post-treatment personality disorders SCID-II

In Table 1, the number of patients who met the criteria for a personality disorder according to the VKP and the SCID-II at pre- and post-treatment are shown.

When comparing the number of pre-treatment versus post-treatment SCID-II personality disorders, a significant decrease was found ($t − 1$: $M = 1.42$, $SD = 1.21$, range 0–4; $t − 2$: $M = 0.48$, $SD = 0.78$, range 0–4; $z = 5.76$, $p = .000$). The effect size for this analysis ($d = 0.92$, 95% CI [0.77–1.26]) was found to exceed Cohen's (1988) convention for a large effect ($d = .80$). At pre-treatment, 91.8% ($n = 56$) of the patients had one or more personality disorders, compared to 35.4% at post-treatment ($n = 22$). The majority, 74.1% ($n = 46$) of patients, showed a decrease in the number of SCID-II personality disorders at the end of treatment; 19.4% ($n = 12$) retained the same number; and 6.5% ($n = 4$) had more personality disorders at the end of the treatment. Although clinical judgment indicated a personality disorder, at the start of treatment, six (9.6%) patients were free of any personality disorder on the SCID-II. One adolescent out of the six deteriorated to having one SCID-II personality disorder at the end.

Pre- and post-treatment personality disorders and SCL-90

Of the 62 adolescents who participated in pre- and post-treatment SCID-II interviews, 56 (90.3%) completed the SCL-90 at both points in time. A significant symptom reduction was observed ($t = 5.95$, $p = .000$). The

Table 1 Number of patients with personality disorders according to the VKP and the SCID-II at $t − 1$ and $t − 2$ (N = 62)

| | $t − 1$ | | | | $t − 2$ | | | |
| | VKP* | | SCID-II | | VKP* | | SCID-II | |
	N	%	N	%	N	%	N	%
No PD	3	4.8	6	9.7	15	24.2	40	64.5
Paranoid PD	31	50.0	13	20.9	11	17.7	5	8.1
Schizoid PD	11	17.7	2	3.2	3	4.8	0	0.0
Schizotypal PD	12	19.4	0	0.0	1	1.6	0	0.0
Antisocial PD	6	9.7	1	1.6	1	1.6	0	0.0
Borderline PD	18	29.0	23	37.1	5	8.1	7	11.3
Histrionic PD	4	6.4	0	0.0	2	3.2	0	0.0
Narcissistic PD	1	1.6	0	0.0	0	0.0	0	0.0
Avoidant PD	41	66.1	34	54.8	19	30.6	11	17.7
Dependant PD	19	30.7	3	4.8	6	9.7	1	1.6
Obsessive compulsive PD	15	24.2	8	12.9	5	8.1	3	4.8
Depressive PD	32	51.6	29	46.8	8	12.9	9	14.5
Passive aggressive PD	5	8.1	2	3.2	2	3.2	0	0.0
PD NOS			2	3.2			1	1.6

PD personality disorder

* Certain indications of a personality disorder according to the VKP. The presumed indications of a personality disorder according to the VKP were left out of this table

mean t − 1 total score of 241.0 (SD = 51.8) on the SCL-90 declined to 189.8 (SD = 64.8) at t − 2 (d = .87, 95% CI [33.9–68.4]). A significant correlation was found at pre- and post-treatment between the number of SCID-II personality disorders and the total score on the SCL-90 ($t − 1$: N = 61, F = 4.71, p = .005; $t − 2$: N = 57, F = 10.64, p = .000) (Fig. 1).

The group with one or more SCID-II personality disorders (n = 51) differed significantly on the total SCL-90 score between pre- (247.73, SD = 47.38) and post-treatment (191.92, SD = 63.77; t = 6.29, p = .000, d = .87, 95% CI [35.9–68.7]). Moreover, the separate groups of SCID-II personality disorders reported significantly fewer symptoms at post-treatment in comparison to their initial levels (Table 2). The group without SCID-II personality disorders at the start of treatment reported fewer symptoms both pre- and post-treatment in comparison to the SCID-II groups, and it showed no symptom decrease (n = 5, $t − 1$: 172.20, SD = 48.90; $t − 2$: 168.20, SD = 78.84, t = 0.15, p = .891, d = .06, 95% CI [− 72.2 to 80.2]).

Length of treatment and changes in the SCL-90 and the SCID-II

No significant correlation was found between the length of treatment and symptom reduction on the total SCL-90

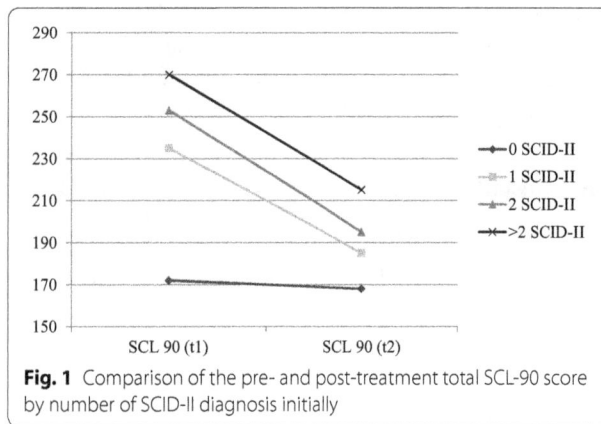

Fig. 1 Comparison of the pre- and post-treatment total SCL-90 score by number of SCID-II diagnosis initially

(r = 0.168; n = 64; p = .184). The total group was divided in three groups based on length of treatment, resulting in a less than 234 days group (N = 8), a 235–364 days group (N = 22) and a more than 365 days group (N = 32). The less than 234 days group (N = 8) was to small for analyses and had to be excluded. The two remaining groups based on length of treatment, the 235–364 days group and the more than 365 days group, were compared by using the total SCL-90 scores and the number of SCID-II personality disorders at the beginning and the end of treatment. The 235–364 days group (symptoms: n = 23, $t − 1$: 233.00, SD = 47.76; $t − 2$: 190.87, SD = 61.44, t = 3.68, p = .001, d = .77; personality disorders: n = 22, $t − 1$: 1.73, SD = 1.03; $t − 2$: .59, SD = .73, t = 4.74, p = .000, d = 1.28) and the more than 365 days (symptoms: n = 31, $t − 1$: 247.45, SD = 55.16; $t − 2$: 183.84, SD = 64.21, t = 5.15, p = .000, d = 1.06; personality disorders: n = 32, $t − 1$: 1.97, SD = 1.23; $t − 2$: .63, SD = 1.16, t = 6.29, p = .000, d = 1.12) showed approximately equal symptom and number of personality disorders reduction. No significant differences were found between the two length of treatment groups on the different SCID-II personality disorders.

Predictive value of personality disorder variables on treatment outcome

The scales of the pre-treatment VKP and pre-treatment SCID-II were entered in a logistic regression with age, gender and duration of treatment as control variables and SCL-90 outcome as a dependent variable. None of the independent variables contributed significantly to the outcome.

Discussion

Our pilot study indicates that, during intensive psychotherapeutic treatment including partial hospitalisation, the number of personality disorders and symptoms may decrease substantially. At the end of the treatment, approximately three quarters of the participants showed a lower number of personality disorders, while two-thirds

Table 2 Comparison of the number of personality disorders at the start with the total SCL-90 score pre- and post-treatment

Number of personality disorders at $t − 1$		Total SCL-90 score					
	n	$t − 1$		$t − 2$		t	p
		Mean	SD	Mean	SD		
0	5	172.20	48.90	168.20	78.84	0.15	.891
1	29	240.31	51.39	187.07	60.05	4.27	.000
2	16	255.25	40.39	198.25	70.18	3.61	.003
> 2	6	263.50	44.38	198.50	73.40	3.04	.029

did not meet the SCID-II criteria for a personality disorder after treatment any longer. However, a large part of the sample was not assessed at the end of the treatment. Since this cohort study was not randomised, it is not possible to draw conclusions about the direct effect of the treatment itself. Furthermore, symptom reduction could not be predicted by pre-treatment personality disorder variables. Nevertheless, this pilot study suggests that personality disorders in adolescents can diminish during intensive psychotherapy.

It is of substantial clinical interest to examine whether the positive outcome obtained in the part of the sample that completed measurements at t − 1 and t − 2 was the result of the provided treatment or other factors. Age-related development or the social support of family and friends [35] may partly have been responsible for the decrease in symptoms and personality pathology. Nevertheless, if the treatment affected the outcome, focus should be placed on examining which element of the treatment caused these improvements. A hypothesis is that working in a group with a group psychodynamic approach is especially relevant for adolescents [36]. In combination with MBT [8–10] and the focus on the relationships with group members and therapists, this may have stimulated a positive outcome. Future research directions should focus on the role of treatment groups for adolescents with personality disorders in treatment outcomes.

Moreover, the duration of the partial hospitalisation may be a factor of particular relevance. The treatment lasted relatively long, and effects of time cannot be ruled out without a control group. The effectiveness of approximately 5 months inpatient psychotherapeutic treatment was described as optimal for adults with cluster B personality disorders [37], cluster C personality disorders [38] and with personality disorders not otherwise specified [39], in comparison to longer inpatient psychotherapeutic treatment. Currently, the maximum duration of partial hospitalisation is set at 6 months. Future research should examine whether there is a general optimal duration of hospitalisation for an intensive group psychotherapy programme for adolescents with personality disorders or the variables a personal optimal length depends on.

Considering our results, the question is whether adolescents with personality disorders are more capable of change than adults with similar problems, as our study found larger changes than those observed in most adult studies. Developmental change may have played a role, as it is known that adolescents become more capable of regulating emotions and behaviour over time. Adolescence may be a developmental phase in which opportunities for change in personality pathology are greater, under the right conditions, than in adulthood. Furthermore, clinical impression suggests that joint problem definition between parents and adolescents, willingness to change and parental support, together with a relatively stable and safe home environment, are crucial to the treatment's success. These factors may be of less crucial importance in adults. If parents are not able to reflect on family dynamics and are critical towards treatment offers, the treatment has fewer chances of success. Unfortunately, in this study no data were collected regarding the role of parents. Future research should examine the effect of the role of parents on the treatment outcome in adolescents with personality disorders.

It is necessary to discuss the strengths and limitations of this study. One strength was the inclusion of a high risk adolescent sample with comorbidity that is rarely examined. The first limitation is that only part of the patients that were included in this study could be followed from the start until the end of treatment. Information about the patients we did not follow is scarce. Initially, however, these patients did not differ in number and type of personality disorders. The shorter duration of treatment suggests that this group either profited less from treatment than those who completed it or improved enough so as not wish to continue treatment. In this study, possible causal mechanisms for the premature termination of therapy amongst adolescents with personality disorders remained unclear. The second shortcoming of this study was that the Axis I disorders were left out due to the practical consideration of not overloading patients with assessment instruments. Finally, the third limitation is that, due to the research design, the extent to which treatment played a role in the positive outcome and which parts of the programme may have contributed remains unknown.

Research on the outcome of treatment for adolescents with personality disorders other than borderline personality disorder or a combination of personality disorders is scarce [5]. Examining the specific mechanisms of change in the different treatments for adolescents with personality disorders is thus important. The treatment examined in this pilot study is promising, although essential questions remain unanswered. Replication is necessary in order to determine whether the results were based on coincidence or not.

Authors' contributions

KH performed the data collection and wrote the manuscript; AB contributed to the design of the research project, performed the statistical analyses in the study and revised the manuscript; RV oversaw the research project and reviewed the manuscript. All authors read and approved the final manuscript.

Author details

[1] De Jutters B.V, Centre for Youth Mental Healthcare Haaglanden, The Hague, The Netherlands. [2] Lucertis, Child and Adolescent Psychiatry Rotterdam, Rotterdam, The Netherlands. [3] Department of Child and Adolescent Psychiatry,

Curium-Leiden University Medical Centre, Leiden, The Netherlands. [4] Department of Child and Adolescent Psychiatry, VU University Medical Centre, Amsterdam, The Netherlands.

Acknowledgements
Authors are grateful and would like to thank all adolescents and colleagues who collaborated in this research. The support of Maaike de van der Schueren and Theo Ingenhoven was deeply appreciated.

Competing interests
The authors declare that they have no competing interests.

Funding
This clinical practice study was not supported by a funding or a scholarship.

References
1. Hutsebaut J, Feenstra DJ, Luyten P. Personality disorders in adolescence: label or opportunity? Clin Psychol Sci Pract. 2013;20(4):445–51.
2. Courtney-Seidler EA, Klein D, Miller AL. Borderline personality disorder in adolescents. Clin Psychol Sci Pract. 2013;20(4):425–44.
3. Chanen AM, McCutcheon L. Prevention and early intervention for borderline personality disorder: current status and recent evidence. Br J Psychiatry. 2013;202:s24–9.
4. Biskin RS. Treatment of borderline personality disorders in youth. J Can Acad Child Adolesc Psychiatry (Journal de l'Académie canadienne de psychiatrie de l'enfant et de l'adolescent). 2013;22(3):230–4.
5. Weisz JR, et al. Performance of evidence-based youth psychotherapies compared with usual clinical care: a multilevel meta-analysis. JAMA Psychiatry. 2013;70(7):750–61.
6. Feenstra DJ, et al. The burden of disease among adolescents with personality pathology: quality of life and costs. J Pers Disord. 2012;26(4):593–604.
7. Soeteman DI, et al. The economic burden of personality disorders in mental health care. J Clin Psychiatry. 2008;69:259–65.
8. Bateman A, Fonagy P. Handbook of mentalizing in mental health practice. Arlington: American Psychiatric Publishing Inc; 2012.
9. Bateman A, Fonagy P. Mentalization based treatment for borderline personality disorder: a practical guide. Oxford: Oxford University Press; 2006.
10. Hauber K. Mentaliseren en de kwetsbare adolescent. Kinder jeugd psychotherapie. 2010;37:45–58.
11. Fonagy P, Luyten P, Strathearn L. Borderline personality disorder, mentalization, and the neurobiology of attachment. Infant Ment Health J. 2011;32(1):47–69.
12. Feenstra DJ, et al. Prevalence and comorbidity of axis I and Axis II disorders among treatment refractory adolescents admitted for specialized psychotherapy. J Pers Disord. 2011;25(6):842–50.
13. Tyrer P, Reed GM, Crawford MJ. Classification, assessment, prevalence, and effect of personality disorder. Lancet. 2015;385:717–26.
14. NICE. Borderline personality disorder. The NICE guidelines on treatment and management, in young people with borderline personality disorder. Leicester: British Psychological Society; 2009. p. 346–77.
15. Kaltiala-Heino R, Eronen M. Ethical issues in child and adolescent forensic psychiatry: a review. J Forensic Psychiatry Psychol. 2015;26(6):759–80.
16. Mehlum L, et al. Dialectical behavior therapy for adolescents with repeated suicidal and self-harming behavior: a randomized trial. J Am Acad Child Adolesc Psychiatry. 2014;53(10):1082–91.
17. Rathus JH, Miller AL. Dialectical behaviour therapy adapted for suicidal adolescents. Suicide Life Threat Behav. 2002;32:146–57.
18. Chanen AM, et al. Early intervention for adolescents with borderline personality disorder: quasi-experimental comparison with treatment as usual. Aust N. Z. J Psychiatry. 2009;43(5):397–408.
19. Rossouw TI, Fonagy P. Mentalization-based treatment for self-harm in adolescents: a randomized controlled trial. J Am Acad Child Adolesc Psychiatry. 2012;51(12):1304–13.
20. Feenstra DJ, et al. Predictors of treatment outcome of inpatient psychotherapy for adolescents with personality pathology. Personal Ment Health. 2014;8(2):102–14.
21. Rothwell PM. Treating individuals—external validity of randomised controlled trials: "To whom do the results of this trial apply? Lancet. 2005;365:82–93.
22. Des Jarlais DC, Lyles C, Crepaz N. Improving the reporting quality of non-randomized evaluations of behavioral and public health interventions: the TREND statement. Am J Public Health. 2004;94:361–6.
23. de Haan AM, et al. A meta-analytic review on treatment dropout in child and adolescent outpatient mental health care. Clin Psychol Rev. 2013;33(5):698–711.
24. Swift JK, Greenberg RP. A treatment by disorder meta-analysis of dropout from psychotherapy. J Psychother Integr. 2014;24(3):193–207.
25. Duijsens IJ, Eurelings-Bontekoe EHM, Diekstra RFW. The VKP, a self-report instrument for DSM-III-R and CD-10 personality disorders: construction and psychometric properties. Personality Individ Differ. 1996;20(2):171–82.
26. Arrindell WA, Ettema JHM. SCL-90: Manual for a multidimensional psychopathology indicator. 2nd ed. Amsterdam: Pearson; 2003.
27. Derogatis LR, Lipman RS, Covi L. SCL-90: an outpatient psychiatric rating scaled preliminary report. Psychopharmacol Bull. 1973;9:13–22.
28. Spitzer RL, et al. User's guide for the structured clinical interview for DSM-III-R: SCID. Arlington: American Psychiatric Association; 1990.
29. Verheul R, Van der Brink W, Spinhoven P. Richtlijnen voor klinische diagnostiek van DSM-IV-persoonlijkheidsstoornissen. Tijdschrift voor Psychiatrie. 2000;42:409–22.
30. Dingemans P, Sno H. Meetinstrumenten bij persoonlijkheidsstoornissen. Tijdschrift voor Psychiatrie. 2004;46:705–9.
31. Segal DL, Hersen M, Van Hasselt VB. Reliability of the SCID: an evaluative review. Compr Psychiatry. 1994;35:316–27.
32. Weertman A, Arntz A, Kerkhofs MLM. SCID II; Gestructureerd Klinisch Interview voor DSM-IV As-II Persoonlijkheidsstoornissen. Amsterdam: Amsterdam Harcourt Test Publishers; 2000.
33. Eurec. http://www.eurecnet.org/information/netherlands.html. 2017. Accessed 10 Aug 2017.
34. IBM Corp. IBM SPSS statistics for windows. Armonk: IBM Corp; 2011.
35. van Harmelen A-L, et al. Friendships and family support reduce subsequent depressive symptoms in at-risk adolescents. PLoS ONE. 2016;11(5):e0153715.
36. Yalom ID, Leszcz M. The theory and practice of group psychotherapy. 5th ed. New York: Basic Books; 2005. p. 668.
37. Bartak A, et al. Effectiveness of outpatient, day hospital, and inpatient psychotherapeutic treatment for patients with cluster B personality disorders. Psychother Psychosom. 2010;80(1):28–38.
38. Bartak A, et al. Effectiveness of different modalities of psychotherapeutic treatment for patients with cluster C personality disorders: results of a large prospective multicentre study. Psychother Psychosom. 2009;79(1):20–30.
39. Horn EK, et al. Effectiveness of psychotherapy in personality disorders not otherwise specified: a comparison of different treatment modalities. Clin Psychol Psychother. 2015;22:426–42.

14

Impediments and catalysts to task-shifting psychotherapeutic interventions for adolescents with PTSD: perspectives of multi-stakeholders

Tanya van de Water[1], Jaco Rossouw[1,3*], Elna Yadin[2] and Soraya Seedat[1]

Abstract

Background: This qualitative study was nested within a randomized controlled trial (RCT) where two psychotherapeutic interventions (supportive counselling and prolonged exposure for adolescents) were provided by supervised nurses (who served as 'nurse counsellors') to adolescents with PTSD in school settings. This paper describes the perspectives of nurse counsellors (NCs) and school liaisons (SLs). SLs were teachers or administrative personnel at the schools who coordinated the study visits of participants with the NCs. We focus on the impediments and catalysts to and recommendations for treatment implementation.

Methods: NCs (n = 3) and SLs (n = 3) who participated in the RCT during 2014 were purposively recruited by telephone and participated in face-to-face semi-structured in-depth interviews that were recorded and doubly transcribed. Thematic content analysis was applied using Atlas.ti software to identify emerging themes. This paper describes the impediments and catalysts to provide psychotherapy by task-shifting in a community setting across three sub-themes: personal, community, and collaborative care.

Results: Although nurses were initially resistant to supervision it was central to personally coping with complex interventions, managing traumatic content, and working apart from a multi-disciplinary team. Delivering the interventions in the community presented multiple logistical impediments (e.g. transport, communication, venue suitability) which required creative solutions. In light of resource shortages, networking is central to effective delivery and uptake of the interventions. Collaboration between government departments of health and education may have a major impact on providing school-based psychotherapy through task-shifting.

Conclusions: Impediments to implementation are not insurmountable. This article provides recommendations to maximize the success of task-shifting interventions should they be rolled out.

Keywords: Task-shifting, South Africa, Adolescents, Nurses, School, PTSD, Barriers, Facilitators

Background

Task-shifting is the rational redistribution of tasks among health teams and involves the appropriate transfer of specific tasks from specialists to those with abbreviated training [1]. Because of resource shortages, this approach

---
*Correspondence: jacorossouw@hotmail.co.za
[3] Faculty of Medicine and Health Sciences, Stellenbosch University, PO Box 241, Cape Town 8000, South Africa
Full list of author information is available at the end of the article

has risen in popularity in the treatment of various health problems including tuberculosis [2–4], HIV [5–7], midwifery [8, 9], and mental health [10–14]. Task-shifting has been used to treat PTSD: (i) in adult refugees placed in Uganda by applying narrative exposure therapy and trauma counselling [15], (ii) adult survivors of systematic violence in Thailand and Iraq using Common Elements Treatment Approach (CETA) [16], (iii) adult survivors of torture in Iraq using Cognitive Processing Therapy and CETA in community settings [17], and (iv) in orphaned and vulnerable children in Zambian community settings using trauma focused cognitive behaviour therapy (TF-CBT) [18]. These studies did not report on the in depth experiences of the non-specialist health workers who provided the task-shifted interventions.

Other studies report that task-shifting implementation can be hindered by professional and institutional resistance (e.g. seeing task-shifting as competition), lack of regulatory frameworks, limited funding, concerns about the quality of care (e.g. not acting in close consultation with specialist) [15], interruptions, lack of privacy, and costs of ongoing expert training and supervision [12]. The efficacy of task-shifting is dependent on training, supervision, support and teamwork, regardless of field [8, 14, 16]. Practical training is the most effective way to train new skills and to reduce the anxiety of undertaking complex new responsibilities [8, 12]. For example, community mental health workers and stakeholders in Ghana highlighted the need to review task-shifting roles, training, and supervision arrangements to ensure quality of care [19].

Objectives
No existing studies exclusively provide qualitative descriptions of the barriers, facilitators, and recommendations for implementation of task-shifting in a community based setting from the perspectives of non-specialist health workers. We sought to explore the impediments and catalysts to and recommendations for the implementation of psychotherapeutically informed task-shifting interventions, through the lenses of NCs and SLs. Their perspectives are important when considering rapid scale-up of these evidence-based interventions in community settings.

Methods
Framework
We undertook a nested, qualitative study evaluating the experiences of stakeholders who participated in a randomized controlled trial (RCT) [20]. We used a biomedically influenced empiricist framework, which places emphasis on biomedical causal mechanisms, evidence-based practices and measurable outcomes. Both first and second authors are practicing clinical psychologists from an upper-middle class background and, as such, the data was not approached in a value-free manner. Instead, the authors utilized their knowledge obtained through clinical practice. In order to neutralize the researchers' inherent investment in the success of the task-shifting paradigm, an empiricist framework was adopted. The authors were concerned with uncovering the truth and presenting it through empirical means [21], believing knowledge to be hard, real, and acquirable. Thus a systematic methodology that relied on control was employed in data analysis.

RCT sampling
For the above mentioned RCT [22], registered nurses studying towards a diploma in advanced psychiatry were trained (5 days of theoretical and practical application) in prolonged exposure therapy for adolescents (PE-A) [25–25] and supportive counselling (SC) [26].

In 2014, six nurses volunteered to participate in the study as an opportunity to add variety to their course prescribed practical hours. All six met the inclusion criteria (doing an advanced nursing certificate in psychiatry and having their own transport) and received the training. NCs were allocated to treatment and participant through block randomization. As such, NCs were randomly assigned to PE-A and SC cases. The nurses received weekly group supervision with the trainer (second author is a male psychologist, experienced PE-A and SC therapist and supervisor, study PI) where they discussed video recordings of both PE-A and SC cases.

The interventions were provided at participating schools, except during school holidays when sessions were moved to the Stellenbosch University campus. To facilitate these meetings, each school nominated a staff member (e.g. teacher, secretary) to act as liaison between the school, NC, and adolescent counselee.

Fifty-three adolescents from four schools volunteered for the RCT during 2014, 12 of whom consented and met inclusion criteria (13–18 years old, PTSD diagnosis by independent evaluator). There were four active SLs during 2014.

Nested study sampling
Data was collected in 2015 where all of the stakeholders who had been in the trial in 2014 [NCs (n = 6), SLs (n = 4), adolescent participants (n = 12)], were telephonically invited to participate in the qualitative study [22]. All were invited regardless of treatment arm or completion status in an attempt to draw on a broad range of experiences. Participants were informed that their feedback could provide valuable insights on improving the interventions and that their feedback, participation, or withdrawal would not affect their status in the RCT.

The first author, a clinical psychologist new to the study, conducted in person semi-structured interviews with the SLs (discussion schedule Appendix A), NCs (discussion schedule Appendix B), and adolescents (results provided elsewhere). The discussion schedule was used as a flexible tool to guide exploration of stakeholder experiences to inform the research team about the acceptability, feasibility, and impact [29–29] of the task-shifting interventions. Interviews ranged between 30 and 90 min. SLs and NCs were specifically questioned about their experiences of providing or coordinating treatment at school, perceived impediments to implementation, and recommendations for future intervention delivery. Interviews took place at Stellenbosch University Campus or at the representative school, as best suited to participants. One interview took place via video Skype.

Participants
The six eligible NCs and four SLs were female. Three NCs declined participation on account of time constraints and one SL was unreachable. Table 1 provides a summary of background information for the NCs who consented (identified by pseudonyms starting with N) and the SLs (identified by pseudonyms starting with T since most were teachers). Unfortunately the age of participants was not collected during the interview.

Analysis
The first author and a research assistant doubly transcribed the audio recordings to enhance accuracy, particularly in view of the dual language of the recordings (English and Afrikaans). Afrikaans transcripts were translated into English. Due to resource constraints, only nurse transcripts were member checked for the accuracy of transcription. The analysis process followed five steps:

The first two authors independently read through all the transcripts of all the stakeholders and identified 36 coding units.

Following discussion between authors 1 and 2, the 36 coding units were collapsed into six overarching themes.

The first author used Atlas.ti software to code the data into coding units and identified themes.

The second author re-read the transcripts and included any contradictory and/or outstanding data.

Upon further analysis and discussion, themes were re-named and re-grouped based on overlap that emerged among the three stakeholder groups (adolescents, NCs, SLs).

i. Adolescent experiences of accessing treatment (described elsewhere)
ii. Adolescent and NC perspectives of treatment efficacy (described elsewhere)

iii. NC and SL identified catalysts and impediments to task-shifting strategy

In this manuscript, we elaborate on NCs and SLs descriptions of the catalysts and impediments (and accompanying recommendations) they encountered during these task-shifting interventions. This narrative is made up of three sub-units: (i) personal care (coping), (ii) community care (logistics of the community setting), and (iii) collaborative care (importance of networking).

Ethics
The study was approved by Stellenbosch University Human Research Ethics Committee (N12/06/031). Participants provided written informed consent for participation in recorded interviews. Transcripts were de-identified and stored in a locked research office with the audio recordings. Participants received a ZAR 50 grocery voucher for their time and transport costs.

Results
The results are presented in three clusters: Personal Care, Community Care, and Collaborative Care.

Personal Care
Impediments
Mastery of the interventions was regarded as *"rather tough"* ('Natasha'). The PE-A treatment manual was complex and nurses often requested verbal explanations as a memory refresher. 'Natalia' felt like she was *"hyperventilating"* the first time she recorded a session for supervision.

Nurses approached the adolescents with grave responsibility. Participants were minors who *"puts his trust in you as the adult"* ('Natalia'). Nurses were required to function independently from the customary setting where they were typically acting as a junior member in a multi-disciplinary team and having *"shared responsibility"* ('Noleen')—where *"you are a supportive person"* ('Natasha'). Nurses wrestled with the notion of *"keep[ing] your professional distance"* ('Natalia') during counselling.

Table 1 Demographics of Participants

Pseudonym	Background
'Natasha' (N1)	White Afrikaans nurse from out of town with 6 years psychiatry experience
'Natalia' (N2)	White Afrikaans nurse with 30 years nursing experience
'Noleen' (N3)	Black Xhosa nurse, working in psychiatric hospital since 2006
'Theresa' (T1)	Afrikaans coloured administrator, basic counselling training at local NGO (*Lifeline*)
'Tina' (T2)	Coloured Afrikaans teacher, youth work experience, desires to study psychology
'Thandi' (T3)	Black Xhosa teacher, no known counselling background

This challenge was amplified by not being prepared *"for what the children would actually tell you"* ('Natasha'), knowing that the child would be returning to a *"dysfunctional system"* ('Noleen'), being *"acutely aware of their circumstances"* ('Natalia'), and feeling guilt about *"leaving them again"* ('Noleen').

> *After I've realized what they've gone through... you want to see them succeed... Like, a mother. You give birth to a child because at the end of the day you want them to be independent ... I think in a study or it was just a neighbour's child or whatever I would have done something. But I was also aware of the professional boundary. Because I was a professional in that space... That sense of wishing to do more and thinking that the child is going to that situation. I was overwhelmed. I was really overwhelmed by that... But you also know that you are not a mom... But it's like, who is going to do this? ('Noleen')*

The struggle was not exclusive to the NCs, but also to the SLs. 'Theresa', now retired, described how challenging it was for her to know that there are children at her school who are going through hard times:

> *When I started there I, yoh, took everything home with me. Everything. Until the school psychologist told me: you cut off! Because one night I was in such a state about a child that I started to shake. And my husband said: you can't carry on like this. You must cut off! Then I said: but how do you sleep if you know that the child might not be safe? So I have had children at my home too, who slept there to be a safe haven. ('Theresa')*

Catalysts

Aside from 30 years of nursing experience which *"teaches you to keep your distance.... [otherwise] every time that I was there I would have cried with that child"* ('Natalia'), supervision helped 'Natasha' to learn to *"not make [what the adolescent tells me] my own... Supervision is really important else you sit with those feelings."* Supervision was also an opportunity to receive peer support and feedback in addition to guidance from an experienced trainer. It extended beyond the practical components of treatment adherence (review of video recordings of sessions) and incorporated support to aid NCs coping with traumatic stories.

The supervisor was easily accessible and attentive to 'Natasha's distress and individually taught her *"how to regulate my breathing and how to manage my own anxiety... that I don't freak out while I am busy with [counselling]."* Additionally, supervision also provided 'Noleen' with the reassurance that adolescents would be

appropriately referred if needed and that fieldworkers *"won't just cross [their] arms and do nothing."*

However, 'Natalia' noted that whilst she appreciated the supervision, she found it challenging to receive the supervision in a group setting. *"I [had] things that I can say but I keep it to myself... I know it is my own fault... Because ... everyone was actually so extroverted"* ('Natalia').

Recommendations

NCs initially resisted supervision as they had no comparable previous experience. 'Natasha' has a hometown supervisor with *"no comprehension of psychiatry"* or the impact it can have on a person when *"you take all these things with you"* ('Natasha'). *"They will just tell you to phone ICAS [Independent Counselling and Advisory Services]. I don't want to... I want to see the person that I am talking to"* ('Natasha'). Receiving face-to-face supervision allowed 'Noleen' to overcome her previous sensitivity to criticism, something she wished she was assisted with during her training as nurse:

> *At the end sometimes I wouldn't like that if my recording is stopped before time because I want ... [the supervisor] to hear the whole thing, not just a bit ... For the first time in 6 years working in a therapeutic ward, I am not ashamed ... to have people observing me behind the mirror because, I feel because I received the supervision. I am able to communicate ... in a right way.*

Having witnessed the benefits of supervision in their personal development, they emphasized that nurses would be less resistant to supervision if it was incorporated throughout their nursing training – making it a norm rather than an exception.

Community Care
Transport
Impediments

NCs experienced the process of traveling to the schools in unfamiliar areas as *"the most negative thing"* ('Natalia') and *"a nightmare"* ('Natasha'). For 'Natalia' *'a big negative thing [was the] distance... because this is not an area where I live."* 'Natasha' described her concern of driving to a school in a crime-riddled area: *"I stand out like a sore finger... This little car with the white woman into [this neighbourhood] .... I was rather anxious about that... I didn't know if I would come out alive on the other side."*

Catalysts

Although the driving was very stressful, it was also highly appreciated. 'Natalia' found it helpful to see the adolescents' circumstances to understand her counselee better. Furthermore, 'Tina' (NC) was really pleased about the service delivery, including providing transport if the sessions were conducted at the university campus.

Recommendations

NCs recommended that counselling continue to be provided in school settings, highlighting that they would *"feel safer"* ('Natasha') if a fieldworker showed them a safe route the first time. 'Natalia' recommended that nurses be sent to the schools in areas that they were familiar with or that schools be allocated to counsellors according to the distance from their homes.

Communication
Impediments

Recruitment took place during school assemblies or Life Orientation lessons which are compulsory school lessons dedicated to self- and career- development. Although those classes were smaller, it *"was still not intimate enough ... Children are smart. They can read body language"* ('Tina'). The teachers' criticism of the task-shifting interventions was that they did not receive feedback on the participants' progress. They highlighted the urgency of providing continued interventions or suitable alternatives (e.g. referrals and follow-ups).

Catalysts

Teachers concurred that the Life Orientation classes were more intimate and thus more effective for recruitment. Other efforts to maximize privacy included refraining from talking to the adolescents *"about their problem; what they experienced... because I am sitting with a full classroom when the child comes in here... I don't want others to hear"* ('Tina').

Recommendations

'Thandi' recommended including parents in the recruitment process to *"explain how the counselling would help their children"* as adolescents *"are even afraid to tell them."* In accordance with the need for holistic interventions, teachers urged waiver of age related criteria: *"We would really appreciate it if the project would cover them as well as long as they are part of this High School community"* ('Thandi'). In fact, there is a *"very large need [to include primary schools]. Because that child comes with that problem from primary school"* ('Tina').

Having one person coordinating all the referrals of potential participants was found to be helpful since at least one person at the school had *"an understanding of what it is that we are coming to do ... [and made an] effort for you to get the venue and get the children together"* ('Noleen'). Feedback could be provided to this coordinator through a short report enabling the school to follow

up and refer adolescents post-trial and assist the school to assess *"the success of whatever happened"* ('Thandi').

Coordination of sessions
Impediments

At some schools, NCs could *"liaise with the teacher"* whilst at other schools *"there is not even anyone if the child is emotional... [to] ask that at least they can just look in for her"* ('Noleen'). 'Thandi' sometimes forgot *"it's Friday... and then maybe find out at the last hour that the hall is being used. Then, yoh!"* NCs admitted that it was frustrating when venues were unprepared because it made them look *"unprofessional"* ('Natalia') or like they didn't follow *"certain processes"* ('Noleen'). Nevertheless, SLs experienced the NCs as *"very understanding. They would be patient and allow me to do whatever is needed to be done at that moment"* ('Thandi').

Although 'Thandi' made the library hall (and corners of the hall for multiple sessions at the same time) available, *"we do not have enough rooms."* NCs, SLs, and the first author's field notes emphasise that the school venues were not the most suited for therapy. Sessions were characterised by interruptions such as *"a knock at the door... the telephone that rings every time"* ('Theresa'), lack of private space, and noise (construction and traffic noise). Whilst this was alleviated by fieldworkers collecting participants for their therapy appointments to take place at university, it added to the burden of time- and resource constraints.

Catalysts

'Natalia' described herself as one of the *"lucky ones"* because she got the same venue every time which enabled her to acclimatise. Nevertheless, she preferred counselling at the *"quiet"* university when the school setting was unavailable (e.g. school holidays). SLs made use of creative strategies to ensure that participants attended counselling sessions. During term time, *"we didn't tell them what time the [counsellors] are going to come"* ('Theresa') because else they would skip school that day. During exam times 'Theresa' would remind both the student and supervising teacher, to ensure that the participant was at the appropriate venue once the bell had rung. 'Tina' tried to prepare a day ahead to keep everything organized. These preparations were made amidst teaching responsibilities and included securing approval from the principal, coordinating a venue, receiving the fieldworker or counsellor, and accompanying them to the venue.

Recommendations

Coordination efforts worked best for teachers and fieldworkers using WhatsApp ('Theresa').

Collaborative care
Impediments

Throughout the interviews it became clear that community members did not have access to psychologists, or suitably trained nurses, teachers, or community resources; which had been highlighted in previous research [32–32]. In 'Noleen's' experience people are *"chase[d] away"* at private and public institutions because nurses do not get *"intensive psychiatric skills"* during their four-year training resulting in" *a lot of damage ... being done ... to people by nurses who don't have the skills"*. Teachers are also limited in their scope—*"you can't do the work of psychologist. You can cause major damage"* ('Tina'). 'Thandi's school once facilitated a forum where students could talk about their problems. Despite honest and emotional sharing, *"it ended there. We couldn't help those kids."* 'Thandi' reported that pressures to complete the curriculum, assessments, administrative tasks, and manage the sheer number of students in a class *"gets so frustrating... You don't even have a chance to ask if there is a problem or something."* External stressors also affected nurses' capacity to engage in the project. Part of *"having my own load"* ('Noleen') included academic pressures, studying away from home, and not having their own transport. This pressure is exacerbated due to lack of staff, for example in 'Natasha's home town they *"don't have a Multidisciplinary Team (MDT). It's just me ... You are the psychiatrist... You are the psychologist... You are the social worker. You are the whole team. So you do everything."*

As the department of education does not provide funding for psychologists to visit the school weekly, 'Theresa' asserts the importance of collaboration with community resources. Teachers expressed frustration at the lack of teamwork. Positive initiatives fail, for example, *Power Child* is no longer offered at 'Thandi's school because staff are unwilling *"to take the responsibility... Once you come up with an idea it is your baby"* ('Tina'). Similarly, although 'Noleen' was convinced about the value of prolonged exposure therapy, she *"won't be able to do it at work ... I don't have the power to convince my team that [it] is something that can help the patient."*

NCs and SLs expressed frustration that *"sometimes people work against you"* ('Noleen'), *"breaking down where I am trying to build ... your hands are tied behind your back... you feel like you are against the wall"* ('Tina'). 'Noleen' described one particularly distressing experience where she was trying to provide counselling to a participant:

> I didn't have space and I was given someone else's space. And then he came. He demanded to use his space ... This child who had been absent to school. He wants his office to work... It's like, he is not even interested why this child has not been coming to school, or if

maybe I am trying to do something that is going to help the child ... I would feel like, you know, I am failing this child... I was thinking a lot of things the child might think: why should I carry on with this thing because even the teachers they don't even see any value in what is going on.

Catalysts

In contrast, there are times where *"[staff] realizes that there is a need... and they are willing to help as far as they can even if it is only to supervise your class; then they have done something"* ('Tina'). Throughout the interviews teachers provided rich evidence of resourceful networking (Table 2) to identify opportunities for their students.

Recommendations

Nurses and teachers concurred that although teachers could acquire necessary skills, it may be easier to train nurses. 'Theresa' said: *"You need somebody from the community to run it. You can't have a teacher run it."* Teachers have *"their own responsibilities"* ('Noleen') and their psychology studies are not *"that in depth"* ('Thandi'). In contrast, nurses have *"an understanding already of psychiatry"* ('Noleen') and acquiring counselling training can make them central to the successful identification and *"hold[ing]"* of persons with emotional problems ('Noleen') resulting in *"less need for medication"* ('Natasha').

Furthermore, 'Noleen' recommended that teachers understand the project and see it as part of their job (not something additional), perhaps through collaboration between government departments of health and education. She added that even if all the nurses at the various community clinics do not have the necessary skills, it would be helpful for at least one staff member to have some counselling skills to *"identify what are the emotional problems, mental health problems, and all of that, and then intervene when it's necessary"* ('Noleen').

Discussion

Based on these qualitative descriptions of the experiences of nurse counsellors delivering psychotherapeutic interventions under supervision and the perspectives of liaisons at the schools where most of the interventions were offered, it appears that providing treatment within the community was well received in spite of the many impediments mentioned. In fact, SLs expressed a strong urging that children not be excluded from the interventions going forward due to age-related criteria.

Personal care

The underlying maternal nature of the SLs and NCs struggles are evident. In a country where the number

Table 2 Community resources accessed by the schools

Resource	Description and success
School staff	'Tina' and 'Theresa' received counselling training at a youth centre and *Lifeline* respectively, but both were too busy to implement their skills. *"It's not only a parental responsibility, the child spends a lot of time at school so the school needs to take up some responsibility and take care of the children"* ('Thandi')
Student development centre	'Thandi' explained that the school makes venues available during lunch time and after school for community programs. Although initially stigmatized, now students *"bring a friend"* ('Tina'). At these centres, students can bring their social, learning, and emotional problems, or even use it as a study venue ('Theresa')
Lay counsellor	A community lay person does workshops at 'Theresa's' school. A clergy member initially worked for free to *"liaise with social workers and psychologists to collect the child's whole background so that they can deal with it"* ('Tina'). This volunteer now *"has a small office, tiny, and she earns a salary... student governing body"* ('Tina')
Community organizations	*African Tycoon* and *Power Child* *"offer computer literacy, computer training, sport ... a plate of a full meal"* ('Thandi') while *Read and Write Solutions* takes parents from the community to visit schools to help the children to read and do math. *Molo Songololo* had powerful impact in the community where one graduated student is now in Amsterdam working for *LoveLife* and another is a chef while *We Can* teaches students *"how to start your own business"* ('Theresa')
University	'Theresa' reported collaboration with local universities sending remedial student teachers and staff serving at the *Bathuthuzele Care Centre*
Social worker	'Theresa' telephonically consults a social worker where to refer students (e.g. NGOs). *"There is one social worker ... [She] is ... busy... Has got her own work schedule... Parents just don't have time to consult"* ('Thandi')

of child-headed households is high (54,000 households) and the majority of children do not live with both parents (66%) or either of their parents (20%) [33], children often lack the *"adult"* ('Natalia') and *"supportive person"* ('Natasha') they need. It is not surprising that the adolescents so freely shared their experiences and put their trust in the adults who showed an interest, as was also indicated in previous research [34]. This highlights the importance of providing teachers and nurses with the necessary support and training in order to assist them with keeping professional boundaries. Although initially resistant to supervision, it was central to the success of the intervention and provided an excellent vehicle to support the NCs while functioning away from the MDT. It may be advisable to include a one on one individual supervision session to navigate personality differences and counteract missing valuable feedback. Whilst valuable, supervision during training may not be feasible due to resource constraints at training institutions [30, 35]. NCs reports of anxiety initiating the delivery of the interventions highlights the importance of ensuring that intervention manuals are as simple as possible. When employing task-shifting, enough time should be allocated to training not only to ensure successful delivery of the intervention, but build confidence in the service providers [8, 12].

Community care

Logistical limitations included transport, communication, and securing suitable times and venues for sessions. NCs took pride in their work and felt frustrated when the logistical arrangements were not done as professionally as they would have liked. In providing community based care, service providers will have to become more

flexible to allow for sustainable service delivery. One way to help them accept these practical challenges (e.g. getting lost, miscommunication, appointments being late or not kept, trouble securing venues), could be to reduce their fear of being reprimanded for not following the red-tape associated with the service. Supervision and support could help service providers to navigate their anxiety of being perceived as unprofessional or ill-prepared. With Cape Town being labelled as the most congested city in South Africa in 2016 (http://www.tomtom.com), it is not surprising that the nurses found driving to and from the schools daunting. Whilst not necessarily mentioned by the participants, allocating counsellors according to the distance from their home will also make the intervention more cost- and time-effective.

Collaborative care

SLs were master networkers able to identify a myriad of resources available to their students despite acute resource shortages in mental health care in South Africa. Both SLs and NCs were optimistic about the task-shifting interventions and recommended training more nurses. Unfortunately, imperfect collaboration will remain a potential barrier to successful scale-up unless there is greater teamwork between government departments of health and education.

Conclusion

This study adds to the small body of literature describing the experiences of the non-specialist health workers providing task-shifting mental health care. This study is unique in the way it not only addresses the experience of the NCs, but also the SLs who acted as a link between the intervention and the adolescents in a community based setting.

Limitations include the lack of individual follow up interviews restricting opportunities to clarify content and guarantee data saturation. In addition, stakeholders who declined participation may have provided stronger criticism of the RCT.

Policy makers and clinicians should heed the following practical recommendations for scale-up:

I. Provide counselling training to nurses as part of the undergraduate training program and incorporate supervision in the process. Identify suitable nurses and distribute them throughout communities to act as liaisons.

II. Assign at least one staff member at each school and guarantee time off for effective coordination, referral and feedback. A quiet, private venue should be made available.

III. Continuation of treatment at schools beyond the RCT. Nurses will need support with transport. Teachers and coordinators can communicate most effectively using a mobile phone application such as WhatsApp.

Our findings provide support for the capability of task-shifting psychotherapeutic interventions for PTSD in a school setting while affirming the importance of supervision [12]. Future studies should include follow up interviews to ensure data saturation. We also recommend optimising the use of existing resources and the potential of nurses to receive training in these two interventions.

Abbreviations

RCT: randomized controlled trail; PTSD: posttraumatic stress disorder; PE-A: prolonged exposure therapy for adolescents; SC: supportive counselling; NC: nurse counsellor; SL: school liaison; MDT: multi-disciplinary team.

Authors' contributions

SS conceptualized and funded the project. TVDW designed the project, did data collection and analysis. JR contributed to the funding and data analysis. EY made major contributions in the writing of the manuscript. All authors read and approved the final manuscript.

Author details

[1] Department of Psychiatry, Stellenbosch University, Cape Town, South Africa. [2] Department of Psychiatry, University of Pennsylvania, Philadelphia, PA, USA. [3] Faculty of Medicine and Health Sciences, Stellenbosch University, PO Box 241, Cape Town 8000, South Africa.

Acknowledgements

Our appreciation to Tracy Jacobs for her assistance with the transcriptions. We are indebted to Berte van der Watt and Donald Skinner for sharing their expertise on qualitative research.

Competing interests

The authors do not have an affiliation with or financial interest in any organization that might pose a competing interests.

Funding

This project is funded in part by Stellenbosch University Rural Medical Education Partnership Initiative (SURMEPI) and the South African Research Chair Initiative—PTSD (DST/NRF Tier 1 level Research Chair). The funding body had no role in the design of the study, the analysis and interpretation of data, or the writing of the manuscript.

References

1. WHO. Task shifting to tackle health worker shortages. Geneva: World Health Organization; 2007 p. 1–12. (HIV/AIDS Programme). Report No.: WHO/HSS/2007.03.
2. Mafigiri DK, McGrath JW, Whalen CC. Task shifting for tuberculosis control: a qualitative study of community-based directly observed therapy in urban Uganda. Glob Public Health. 2012;7(3):270–84.
3. Patel MR, Yotebieng M, Behets F, Vanden Driessche K, Nana M, Van Rie A. Outcomes of integrated treatment for tuberculosis and HIV in children at the primary health care level. Int J Tuberc Lung Dis. 2013;17(9):1206–11.
4. Semakula-Katende NS, Andronikou S, Lucas S. Digital platform for improving non-radiologists' and radiologists' interpretation of chest radiographs for suspected tuberculosis—a method for supporting task-shifting in developing countries. Pediatr Radiol. 2016;46:1384–91.
5. Chibanda D, Verhey R, Munetsi E, Cowan FM, Lund C. Using a theory driven approach to develop and evaluate a complex mental health intervention: The friendship bench project in Zimbabwe. Int J Ment Health Syst. 2016;10(1). https://www.scopus.com/inward/record.uri?eid=2-s2.0-84963743920&partnerID=40&md5=61c6ba23726be3ab3e86722e63d62085.
6. Emdin CA, Chong NJ, Millson PE. Non-physician clinician provided HIV treatment results in equivalent outcomes as physician-provided care: a meta-analysis. J Int AIDS Soc. 2013;16(1):1–10.
7. Green A, de Azevedo V, Patten G, Davies MA, Ibeto M, Cox V. Clinical mentorship of nurse initiated antiretroviral therapy in Khayelitsha, South Africa: a quality of care assessment. PLoS ONE. 2014;9(6):e98389.
8. Colvin CJ, de Heer J, Winterton L, Mellenkamp M, Glenton C, Noyes J, et al. A systematic review of qualitative evidence on barriers and facilitators to the implementation of task-shifting in midwifery services. Midwifery. 2013;29(10):1211–21.
9. Floyd BO, Brunk N. Utilizing task shifting to increase access to maternal and infant health interventions: a case study of midwives for Haiti. J Midwifery Womens Health. 2016;61(1):103–11.
10. Lund C, Schneider M, Davies T, Nyatsanza M, Honikman S, Bhana A, et al. Task sharing of a psychological intervention for maternal depression in Khayelitsha, South Africa: study protocol for a randomized controlled trial. Trials. 2014;15:457.
11. Patel V. Task shifting: a practical strategy for scaling up mental health care in developing countries. South Afr J Psychiatry. 2008;14(3):108.
12. Singla DR, Kohrt BA, Murray LK, Anand A, Chorpita BF, Patel V. Psychological treatments for the world: lessons from low- and middle-income Countries. Annu Rev Clin Psychol. 2017;13(1).
13. van Ginneken N, Tharyan P, Lewin S, Rao GN, Meera SM, Pian J, et al. Non-specialist health worker interventions for the care of mental, neurological and substance-abuse disorders in low- and middle-income countries. Cochrane Database Syst Rev. 2013;11:CD009149.
14. Weinmann S, Koesters M. Mental health service provision in low and middle-income countries: recent developments. Curr Opin Psychiatry. 2016;29(4):270–5.
15. Neuner F, Onyut PL, Ertl V, Odenwald M, Schauer E, Elbert T. Treatment of posttraumatic stress disorder by trained lay counselors in an african refugee settlement: a randomized controlled trial. J Consult Clin Psychol. 2008;76(4):686–94.
16. Murray LK, Dorsey S, Haroz E, Lee C, Alsiary MM, Haydary A, et al. A common elements treatment approach for adult mental health problems in low- and middle-income Countries. Cogn Behav Pract. 2014;21(2):111–23.
17. Weiss WM, Murray LK, Zangana GAS, Mahmooth Z, Kaysen D, Dorsey S, et al. Community-based mental health treatments for survivors of torture and militant attacks in Southern Iraq: a randomized control trial. Bmc Psychiatry. 2015;15:249.

18. Murray LK, Familiar I, Skavenski S, Jere E, Cohen J, Imasiku M, et al. An evaluation of trauma focused cognitive behavioral therapy for children in Zambia. Child Abuse Negl. 2013;37(12):1175–85.

19. Agyapong V, McAuliffe E, Farren C. Improving Ghana's mental health care through task shifting—psychiatrists and health policy directors views. Eur Psychiatry. 2016;33:S607–8.

20. Rossouw J, Yadin E, Alexander D, Seedat S. Study protocol of prolonged exposure treatment for posttraumatic stress disorder and supportive counselling in adolescents: a third world, task shifting, community-based sample, including experiences of stakeholders. In review.

21. Henning E, van Rensburg W, Smit B. Finding your way in qualitative research. Van Schaik; 2004.

22. Rossouw J, Yadin E, Alexander D, Mbanga I, Jacobs T, Seedat S. A pilot and feasibility randomised controlled study of prolonged exposure treatment and supportive counselling for post-traumatic stress disorder in adolescents: a third world, task-shifting, community-based sample. Trials. 2016;17(1):548.

23. Foa EB. Prolonged exposure therapy: past, present, and future. Depress Anxiety. 2011;28(12):1043–7.

24. Foa EB, Kozak MJ. Emotional processing of fear: exposure to corrective information. Psychol Bull. 1986;99(1):20–35.

25. Foa EB, Gillihan SJ, Bryant RA. Challenges and successes in dissemination of evidence-based treatments for posttraumatic stress lessons learned from prolonged exposure therapy for PTSD. Psychol Sci Public Interest. 2013;14(2):65–111.

26. Foa EB, McLean CP, Capaldi S, Rosenfield D. Prolonged exposure vs supportive counseling for sexual abuse-related PTSD in adolescent girls: a randomized clinical trial. JAMA. 2013;310(24):2650–7.

27. Cook JM, Schnurr PP, Foa EB. Bridging the gap between posttraumatic stress disorder research and clinical practice: the example of exposure therapy. Psychother Theory Res Pract Train. 2004;41(4):374–87.

28. Mendenhall E, De Silva MJ, Hanlon C, Petersen I, Shidhaye R, Jordans M, et al. Acceptability and feasibility of using non-specialist health workers to deliver mental health care: stakeholder perceptions from the PRIME district sites in Ethiopia, India, Nepal, South Africa, and Uganda. Soc Sci Med. 2014;118:33–42.

29. Nyatsanza M, Schneider M, Davies T, Lund C. Filling the treatment gap: developing a task sharing counselling intervention for perinatal depression in Khayelitsha, South Africa. BMC Psychiatry. 2016;16(1). https://www.scopus.com/inward/record.uri?eid=2-s2.0-84973390057&partnerID=40&md5=41a26fddd550c89f54ebfa09fe717dbf.

30. Liu G, Jack H, Piette A, Mangezi W, Machando D, Rwafa C, et al. Mental health training for health workers in Africa: a systematic review. Lancet Psychiatry. 2016;3(1):65–76.

31. Willcox ML, Peersman W, Daou P, Diakité C, Bajunirwe F, Mubangizi V, et al. Human resources for primary health care in sub-Saharan Africa: progress or stagnation? Hum Resour Health. 2015;13(1):76.

32. Rabie T, Coetzee SK, Klopper HC. The nature of community health care centre practice environments in a province in South Africa. Afr J Nurs Midwifery. 2016;18(2):27–41.

33. Delany A, Jehoma S, Lake L. South African Child Gauge 2016. Cape Town: Children's Institute, UCT. https://www.childrencount.org.za/uploads/SA_ChildGauge_Poster_2016.pdf.

34. van de Water T, Rossouw J, van der Watt ASJ, Yadin E, Seedat S. Adolescents' experience of stigma when accessing a school-based PTSD intervention. Qual Health Res Rev. **(under review)**.

35. Armstrong SJ, Rispel LC. Social accountability and nursing education in South Africa. Glob Health Action. 2015;8(s4):27879.

15

Quality of life, delinquency and psychosocial functioning of adolescents in secure residential care: testing two assumptions of the Good Lives Model

C. S. Barendregt[1*], A. M. Van der Laan[1], I. L. Bongers[2,3] and Ch. Van Nieuwenhuizen[2,3]

Abstract

Background: In this study, two assumptions derived from the Good Lives Model were examined: whether subjective Quality of Life is related to delinquent behaviour and psychosocial problems, and whether adolescents with adequate coping skills are less likely to commit delinquent behaviour or show psychosocial problems.

Method: To this end, data of 95 adolescents with severe psychiatric problems who participated in a four-wave longitudinal study were examined. Subjective Quality of Life was assessed with the ten domains of the Lancashire Quality of Life Profile and coping skills with the Utrecht Coping List for Adolescents.

Results: Results showed that adolescents who reported a lower Quality of Life on the health domain had more psychosocial problems at follow-up. No relationship was found between Quality of Life and delinquent behaviour. In addition, active and passive coping were associated with delinquent behaviour and psychosocial functioning at follow-up.

Conclusions: Based on the results of this longitudinal study, the strongest support was found for the second assumption derived from the Good Lives Model. Adolescents with adequate coping skills are less likely to commit delinquent behaviour and have fewer psychosocial problems at follow-up. The current study provides support for the use of strength-based elements in the treatment programmes for adolescents in secure residential care.

Background

It is well established that criminogenic risks, such as age at first offense and number of prior convictions, predict later offending behaviour [1, 2]. As a consequence (juvenile) offender rehabilitation has primarily been focused on mapping and managing risks in the lives of delinquent adolescents. Herein, the Risk-Need-Responsivity (RNR) Model has for years been regarded as the standard approach in offender rehabilitation and therefore the most widely used rehabilitation theory [3]. The main underlying assumption of a risk management approach

such as the RNR-Model, is that every individual that has offended in the past carries a risk for future reoffending [3]. By adhering to three main RNR principles (i.e., the risk principle, the need principle, and the responsivity principle) during treatment, this risk of reoffending can be decreased. The risk perspective in offender rehabilitation has been criticised for a number of reasons. First, it has been argued that the one-sided view of risk management does not allow for a more positive way of living and there is a lack of interest for positive indicators that might change behaviour [4]. Second, within the risk perspective in offender rehabilitation, a predominant 'one size fits all' mentality is apparent, with little attention for individual needs, skills and abilities [5]. In line with this, the risk perspective has also been criticised for its failure to motivate and engage offenders in their rehabilitation process

*Correspondence: c.s.barendregt@minvenj.nl
[1] Research and Documentation Centre (WODC) of the Dutch Ministry of Justice and Security, PO Box 20301, 2500 EH The Hague, The Netherlands
Full list of author information is available at the end of the article

[5]. In recent years, a shift has taken place from a risk-oriented view of offender rehabilitation towards a more strength-based rehabilitation view in which individuals' needs, abilities and skills take a central role [3, 6]. Instead of looking at offenders as an accumulation of risks, they are seen as individuals who want to give meaning to their lives like any other person [6].

Alternative rehabilitation theories, such as the Good Lives Model, have been proposed and have been labelled 'strength-based' or 'restorative' approaches in working with individuals who have offended [3, 5]. This shift in offender rehabilitation can (at least partly) be attributed to several other findings. First, a large proportion of youngsters reoffended after they had received treatment in secure residential care [7–9]. This finding suggests that there is considerable scope for improvement in working with delinquent adolescents [3]. Second, there is a growing number of studies that identify factors other than risk factors that are associated with successful interventions and rehabilitation programmes, for example, subjective well-being and employment [e.g., [10–12]. Finally, especially for adolescents and young adult offenders, strength-based rehabilitation can be helpful guiding them in becoming healthy-functioning and productive adults [13].

The Good Lives Model operates according to a strength-based or restorative perspective in which the underlying processes of healthy functioning are the primary objects of treatment instead of those that underlie dysfunctional behaviour. Why and how adolescents desist from their criminal careers cannot be explained by risk factors alone. Other factors, such as meeting individual needs, improving Quality of Life (QoL), and developing coping skills might also be related to decreasing the risk of reoffending [6]. The Good Lives Model can be seen as a holistic approach that combines both the management of risk with the promotion of an offender's well-being [4, 14]. According to the Good Lives Model, treatment should focus on the potential of an offender rather than emphasizing their incapacities and risk factors. From this holistic perspective, treatment is not only directed at decreasing the risk for reoffending but also to increasing an individuals' psychosocial well-being. In addition, individuals should be engaged in productive activities in which they can learn and enhance skills, such as coping skills, that might help them in achieving their life goals. When individuals get the opportunity to create good and fulfilling lives for themselves, their individual risk of reoffending will decrease [4, 5]. Accordingly, a good and fulfilling life can be created by securing meaningful needs (i.e., primary human needs). The Good Lives Model proposes 11 groups of needs: (1) life, (2) knowledge, (3) excellence in work, (4) excellence in play, (5) excellence in agency, (6) inner peace, (7) relatedness, (8) community, (9) spirituality, (10) happiness, and (11) creativity [4, 6, 14]. It is assumed that each human being seeks these needs to some degree throughout their lives, although individual differences might exist. Fulfilling these needs in a socially acceptable manner will lead to an increase in an individuals' subjective QoL and might also decrease the likelihood of reoffending.

Compared to the abundance of empirical studies that have been conducted with regard to risk factors in offender rehabilitation, relatively few studies have focused on the long term effects of securing needs, thereby increasing an individuals' subjective QoL, and strengthening skills during treatment. In this paper, the focus will be on two concepts that both play a significant role in the Good Lives Model, namely subjective QoL and coping. Although the Good Lives Model acknowledges the importance of risk reduction, it also has a strong focus on the enhancement of an offender's well-being or QoL. In daily practice, the enhancement of an individual's QoL translates into identifying individuals' priority needs in life and devising a good lives plan during treatment. This good lives plan consists of internal and external skills, abilities and resources that will contribute to the success of the plan, thereby increasing an individuals' subjective QoL. Subjective QoL is a multidimensional concept and focuses on a person's overall sense of well-being and satisfaction with life [15–17]. Among adults, a higher subjective QoL is associated with better emotional adjustment after discharge from a secure care facility [10]. Low subjective QoL, on the other hand, might increase the likelihood of delinquent behaviour [10, 18, 19]. Thus, according to the Good Lives Model, it can be assumed that the fulfilment of individual needs as described in a personalized good lives plan, increases a person's subjective QoL, while also attending to risk factors, and thereby decreasing the chance of reoffending.

Coping can be seen as an internal resource or ability an individual can be equipped with in order to realize the goals set in his or her good lives plan. After identifying and prioritizing the primary human needs, a next step in the treatment process is to fulfil those needs in a socially acceptable manner. Once individuals are lacking proper skills or capabilities, they might use delinquent behaviour to secure the needs described in their good lives plan. Coping, in general, refers to the cognitive and emotional-behavioural strategies individuals use in response to stress [20], and is found to be related to the well-being of incarcerated adolescents [21]. From a Good Lives Model's point of view, adequate coping skills can help individuals deal with problems and stress that individuals might experience in trying to fulfill their needs. In addition, adequate coping skills can help institutionalized offenders to adjust to the restricted environment of secure residential care. An active coping strategy is, for example, exercising while self-imposed social isolation is an example of a passive coping strategy [22]. Research has shown that poor coping strategies predict behavioural and emotional problems, such as problems with alcohol, depressive symptoms, and delinquent behaviour [23, 24]. More specifically, passive coping in adolescents is associated with adjustment problems [25] and depressive symptoms [24], and predicts poor well-being among adolescent detainees [26]. Thus, from a Good Lives Model perspective, the assumption is that using inadequate coping strategies might hinder the success of an individuals' good lives plan and might increase the chance of reoffending.

The aim of this study is to test the following two assumptions derived from the Good Lives Model: (1) a higher subjective QoL in secure residential care is related to less reported delinquent behaviour and psychosocial problems at follow-up, and (2) having adequate coping skills in secure residential care, such as active coping, is related to less reported delinquent behaviour and psychosocial problems at follow-up. Both assumptions are connected since having adequate coping skills can also enable adolescents to fulfil their primary human needs and therefore increase their subjective QoL.

Methods
Setting
Participants were recruited from ten secure residential care facilities throughout the Netherlands that varied in terms of security level. Adolescents could be admitted to youth forensic psychiatric hospitals, child and adolescent psychiatric hospitals, orthopsychiatric institutions or youth detention centres. Throughout this paper, we use the term 'secure residential care' to refer to these institutions. Secure residential care refers to the most intensive or restrictive type of youth care in the Netherlands. Care, guidance and treatment are offered in a secure environment. Although adolescents from different treatment facilities were included, they shared comparable problems in multiple life domains such as experiencing problems with their living situation and having difficulties managing their finances, as well as a high prevalence of psychiatric disorders.

Participants
The sample consisted of 95 Dutch male adolescents with severe psychiatric problems and problems in multiple life domains (e.g., raised in a single parent family). All adolescents were admitted to secure residential care. Respondents' overall mean age at admission to secure residential care was 16.1 years ($SD = 1.0$). At the time of the first assessment their mean age was 16.7 years ($SD = .9$).

Adolescents were eligible for participation if they were 16, 17 or 18 years of age, and if time of admission would be longer than 3 months. Of the 95 adolescents, 52 adolescents (54.7%) were sentenced under Dutch juvenile civil law and 43 adolescents (45.3%) were sentenced under Dutch juvenile criminal law. One of the measures under the Dutch juvenile civil law is the family supervision measure. This supervision measure is applied when the development of an adolescent is at risk and their parents or other caretakers are not able to help. These adolescents display severe behavioural problems and often lack motivation for voluntary treatment. The Dutch juvenile criminal law encompasses the treatment and rehabilitation of adolescents who have committed a serious criminal offense. Adolescents sentenced under the Dutch juvenile criminal law either have a regular detention sentence or a mandatory treatment order. Furthermore, 79 adolescents (83.2%) indicated that they used drugs at least once during their lives. The most common psychiatric disorder was a disruptive behaviour disorder (DBD: $n = 58$; 61.1%). Adolescents were also diagnosed with a range of other presenting issues including autism spectrum disorder (ASD: $n = 29$; 30.5%), attention deficit hyperactivity disorder (ADHD: $n = 24$; 25.3%), reactive attachment disorder (RAD: $n = 14$; 14.7%) and intellectual disability (ID: $n = 17$; 17.9%). In addition, it was known that 23 adolescents (24.2%) had debts during the Time 1 assessment and 57 adolescents (60.0%) indicated that their parents were divorced. More than half of the adolescents ($n = 51$; 53.7%) had failed a grade in school at least once.

Measures
Predictor variables
The Dutch Youth version of the Lancashire Quality of Life Profile (LQoLP) was used to measure subjective QoL [27–29]. This semi-structured interview was conducted at Time 1, which was during stay in a secure residential care facility. The LQoLP consists of objective and subjective indicators of QoL and measures the adolescent's satisfaction with different QoL domains. For the subjective QoL estimates, the domains 'social participation' (6 items), 'health' (7 items), 'family relations' (6 items), 'living situation' (4 items), 'safety' (5 items), and 'finances' (4 items) were assessed using a 7-point Likert scale, ranging from '1 = could not be worse' to '7 = could not be better'. The domains 'positive esteem' (5 items) and 'negative esteem' (5 items) were measured by means of a modified version of the Self-esteem Scale [30], while the domains 'framework' (10 items) and 'fulfilment' (13 items) were assessed using a 3-point Likert scale. The 'framework' subscale measured the degree to which an adolescent could envision having a meaningful perspective in his

life, and the 'fulfilment' subscale measured whether the adolescents also had a set of life goals. Both scales were measured by the Life Regard Index [31]. The following transformation was applied in order to compare the mean scale scores of the domains with a 3-point response category to those with a 7-point response category: $M' = (M: 3) \times 7$ [M' = transformed mean score; M = raw mean scale score]. Psychometric properties of the LQoLP have been demonstrated to be good [27, 32, 33].

To measure coping, the Utrecht Coping List for Adolescents (UCL-A) was used [34]. This questionnaire had to be filled in by the adolescents themselves during the Time 1 assessment in secure residential care. The UCL-A consists of seven scales: 'active problem solving' (7 items), 'distraction' (8 items), 'avoidance' (8 items), 'social support seeking' (6 items), 'depressive reaction' (7 items), 'expressing emotions' (3 items), and 'comforting thoughts' (5 items). All items were scored on a 4-point Likert scale, ranging from '1 = seldom or never', '2 = sometimes', '3 = often', and '4 = very often', with higher scores indicating more frequent use of a coping strategy. Active coping consists of the mean scores of the scales 'confrontation' and 'seeking social support', and passive coping consists of the mean scores of the scales 'avoidance' and 'depressive reactions' [35].

The Structured Assessment of Violence Risk in Youth (SAVRY) [36] was used to measure the risk and protective factors. The SAVRY is a risk assessment instrument designed to assist clinicians in evaluating risk for violence in adolescents. If a SAVRY was not conducted by a clinician, it was filled in by the researchers for the purpose of this study. The SAVRY was administered around the Time 1 assessment, when adolescents were admitted to a secure residential care facility. The SAVRY consists of 24 risk items and 6 protective items. The risk items are divided over three risk domains: 'historical' (10 items), 'social/contextual' (6 items), and 'individual' (8 items). The historical items are static in nature, while the social/contextual and individual items are dynamic. The risk items were scored '0 = low', '1 = moderate', or '2 = high', and the protective items were scored '0 = absent' or '2 = present'. A total risk score was calculated by summing the scores of the historical, social/contextual, and individual domains and a protective score was calculated by summing the protective items. A higher score on the risk and protective items indicated the presence of more risks and/or protective factors.

Outcome variables

The Youth Delinquency Survey was used to measure self-reported delinquency at follow-up (Time 4) [37]. This survey is produced by the Research and Documentation Centre (WODC) of the Dutch Ministry of Justice

and Security. Self-reported delinquency was measured by means of Computer Assisted Self Interviewing (CASI), whereby adolescents were asked if and how often they had committed a number of offenses over the previous 12 months. The delinquency score is a multiplication of the number of serious and non-serious delinquent behaviour and the frequency of the delinquent behaviour in the past year. Non-serious delinquent behaviour (e.g., 'vehicle vandalism' and 'shoplifting of goods to the value of less than 10 euro's') was scored 1, whereas serious delinquent behaviour (e.g., 'burglary' and 'use of violence in order to commit theft') was scored 3. In addition, the frequency of the delinquent behaviour in the past year was scored as follows. Non-serious offenses committed 1–4 times were scored 1, and offenses committed 5 times or more were scored 2. Serious offenses committed 1 time were scored 1, offenses committed 2–4 times were scored 2, offenses committed 5–10 times were scored 3, and offenses committed 11 times or more were scored 4.

The Strengths and Difficulties Questionnaire (SDQ) was used to measure the psychosocial problems at follow-up (Time 4) [38–40]. For the administration of the SDQ, the CASI method was also used. The SDQ consists of 25 items that can be allocated to five subscales: 'emotional symptoms', 'conduct problems', 'hyperactivity-inattention', 'peer problems', and 'pro-social behaviour. Each item has to be scored on a 3-point scale with '0 = not true', '1 = somewhat true', and '2 = certainly true'. A total difficulties score can be calculated by summing the scores of the subscales emotional symptoms, conduct problems, hyperactivity-inattention, and peer problems. In the current study, only the total difficulties score was used, with higher scores on this scale indicating more problems in psychosocial functioning.

Descriptive information on the predictor and outcome variables are shown in Table 1.

Procedure

The current study was part of a prospective longitudinal study with four waves of data (i.e., Time 1, Time 2, Time 3, and Time 4). Prior to the start of the study, the Medical Ethics Committee for Mental Health Institutions in the Netherlands (Ref. No: NL29932.097.09 CCMO) and the Ministry of Justice and Security gave their approval. Inclusion criteria were (1) male, (2) adolescents who remained institutionalized for a minimum period of 3 months after the Time 1 assessment and, (3) finished primary school in the Netherlands or had sufficient Dutch language skills. There were no specific exclusion criteria. However, adolescents had to be able to participate during the assessment. For example, being floridly psychotic at the time of the assessment would lead to exclusion from the study.

Table 1 Descriptive information on predictor and outcome variables ($n = 95$)

Variables	M	SD	Range	α
Risk and protective factors				
Total risk score	17.83	5.3	5–33	
Protective score	7.83	2.2	2–12	
Predictor variables (Time 1)				
Coping				
Active coping	14.73	3.4	7.5–24.5	.84
Passive coping	14.16	3.0	8.0–23.0	.76
Subjective QoL domains				
Living situation	3.45	1.2	1.0–6.0	
Social participation	5.24	.7	3.0–6.7	
Finances	4.02	1.5	1.0–7.0	
Health	5.36	.7	3.0–6.6	
Family relations	5.83	1.0	2.2–7.0	
Safety	5.76	.7	3.6–7.0	
Positive esteem	6.61	.6	4.2–7.0	
Negative esteem	6.32	1.0	3.3–7.0	
Fulfilment	5.71	1.0	3.1–7.0	
Framework	6.35	.7	3.7–7.0	
Outcome variables (Time 4)				
Delinquency	19.20	30.9	0–137	
Psychosocial problems	10.49	5.9	1.0–27.0	

QoL quality of life

A total of 228 adolescents in secure residential care were approached to participate in the study. Of these, 40 adolescents refused to participate or their parents did not sign informed consent, and 16 adolescents were unable to participate because they transferred to other institutions or were discharged before the first assessment. The total response rate at Time 1 was 75.4% ($N = 172$). Of these 172 participants, 95 (55.2%) also conducted the follow-up assessment. To investigate the potential impact of attrition, we tested for differences between participants who completed the first assessment and the follow-up assessment ($n = 95$) and participants who dropped out after the first assessment ($n = 77$). Adolescents who completed the first assessment and the follow-up assessment were more often diagnosed with an autism spectrum disorder (ASD) and with a reactive attachment disorder (RAD) (respectively: $\chi^2 (1) = 4.289, p < .05; \chi^2 (1) = 7.428, p < .01$). There were no other significant differences found between the participants and the dropouts.

For all adolescents, clinicians as well as group workers estimated whether an adolescent could be asked to participate in the study. Once professionals had agreed, an adolescent was approached for participation and informed about the content of the study by the researchers. In addition, adolescents received an information leaflet that contained relevant information regarding the study, disclosed in understandable language. Adolescents were told no repercussions would follow upon refusing participation in the study. After verbal and written explanation of the study was given, a written informed consent was obtained from each adolescent who agreed to participate. For participants under the age of 18, parents were also asked for written informed consent.

In the current study only juveniles with both the first assessment (Time 1) and the follow-up assessment (Time 4) were analysed. The Time 1 assessment was at age 16, 17 or 18 and all adolescents were admitted to secure residential care during this assessment. Mean duration of stay in a secure residential care facility at the Time 1 assessment was 7.5 months ($SD = 7.7$). The follow-up assessment (Time 4) was planned 12 months after discharge from a secure residential care facility. Adolescents who were discharged were either living independently, moved back in with their parents or still received some sort of support or assistance with their living circumstances. Due to prolonged treatment some adolescents remained institutionalized during the course of the study. For those adolescents who remained institutionalized, the follow-up assessment was planned during their continued stay in secure residential care. Time in months between the Time 1 assessment and the follow-up assessment did vary ($M = 19.6$ months, $SD = 4.8$, range 10–32 months). This variation was dependent on the duration of juveniles' stay in secure residential care. For those juveniles who remained institutionalized, the follow-up assessment (Time 4) was carefully planned in order for the time in months between the Time 1 assessment and the follow-up assessment to be equal for the *admitted* and *discharged* juveniles (respectively $M = 18.2$ months, $SD = 4.6$; $M = 20.4$ months, $SD = 4.7$).

Data analysis

First, Pearson correlations of the predictors and outcomes measures were calculated. Predictor variables that showed non-significant associations with the outcome measures were removed from further analysis. Level of significance was set at $p < .05$. Second, stepwise linear multiple regression analyses were performed. A total risk score and a total protective score were continuously entered in the linear regression analyses. To predict delinquency and psychosocial problems at follow-up four models were estimated, and for each model the predictors were entered in one block. Model 1 included whether juveniles were admitted or discharged from secure residential care at the Time 4 follow-up assessment. This variable was included since differences were found between these groups. Admitted adolescents were significantly older at admission to secure residential care $[F(93) = 2.180, p < .05]$, were more often admitted under the Dutch juvenile criminal law $[\chi^2 (1) = 31.381, p < .001]$, had a higher total risk score $[F(93) = .068, p < .01]$, and were more often diagnosed with conduct disorder $[\chi^2 (1) = 5.450, p < .05]$, and intellectual disability $(\chi^2 (1) = 8.718, p < .01)$. Model 2 added the total risk score and the protective score of the SAVRY. Model 3 added active and passive coping as predictors. In Model 4, the subjective QoL domains were added to the model. Multicollinearity between the independent variables was not a problem since the VIF values were below 5 and tolerance was above .2. The plots showed that the assumptions for linearity and homoscedasticity were not violated. SPSS version 19.0 was used to perform the analyses.

Results

Correlation analysis

First, in order to identify the variables for use in the predictive model, we looked at correlations between the predictor variables (i.e., active and passive coping and the QoL domains) and the outcome variables (i.e., self-reported delinquency and psychosocial problems). Table 2 shows these bivariate correlations between the dependent and independent variables. Only those predictors that were significantly $(p < .05)$ correlated with the outcome measures delinquent behaviour and psychosocial problems at follow-up were used in further analyses. Only active coping $(r = -.25, p < .01)$ at the Time 1 assessment was significantly correlated with delinquency

at follow-up (Time 4). Therefore, both passive coping and all of the subjective QoL domains were excluded from any further analyses with regard to the outcome measure delinquency. With regard to the second outcome measure, psychosocial problems at follow-up, passive coping $(r = .37, p < .01)$ and the subjective QoL domains social participation $(r = -.22, p < .05)$, health $(r = -.28, p < .01)$ and fulfilment $(r = -.25, p < .05)$ showed a significant correlation. Therefore, active coping and all nonsignificant subjective QoL domains were excluded from any further analyses with regard to the outcome measure psychosocial problems.

Delinquency

A second step in the analyses was to test how well the predictor variables were able to predict the outcome variable by means of a stepwise linear regression analysis. Thus, we studied how much variance in the outcome variable delinquency could be explained by active coping. Due to the variety in time of discharge at the Time 4 assessment, we included a dummy variable in every first model. In addition, to account for the disadvantaged backgrounds of the adolescents, a total risk score and a protective score were added to every second model. Finally, active coping was added in the third model. In the first model, being admitted or discharged from secure residential care at follow-up did not explain any variance in delinquency at follow-up [see Table 3: Model 1: $R^2 = .001$, adjusted $R^2 = -.010$, $F(1,93) = .057, p = .811$]. In the second model, adding

Table 2 Correlations between risks, coping, subjective QoL domains and self-reported delinquency and psychosocial problems ($N = 95$)

Variables	1	2	3	4	5	6	7	8	9	10	11	12	13	14	15
Total risk score	–														
Protective score	.32**	–													
Active coping	– .02	– .11	–												
Passive coping	– .11	– .04	.21*	–											
Living situation	– .01	.10	– .05	– .20*	–										
Social participation	– .16	– .09	.04	– .16	.31**	–									
Health	– .02	– .02	.08	– .13	– .04	.26*	–								
Finances	.15	.04	– .03	– .14	.08	.25*	.17	–							
Family relations	.11	– .16	– .08	– .44**	.15	.13	.05	.19	–						
Safety	.10	– .09	– .16	– .24*	– .11	.05	.16	.26*	.25*	–					
Positive esteem	– .01	– .01	– .06	– .22*	.06	– .05	.21*	.15	.06	.25*	–				
Negative esteem	.18	.13	– .20	– .44**	.12	– .03	.17	.10	.28**	.22*	.45**	–			
Fulfilment	.07	– .10	.09	– .37**	.28**	.40**	.20*	.19	.45**	.31**	.32**	.45**	–		
Framework	– .05	– .15	.32**	– .13	.08	.10	.03	– .02	.04	.20	.31**	.21*	.47**	–	
Delinquency	.17	.08	– .25*	– .03	– .10	– .12	– .08	.05	– .03	.16	.02	.11	– .06	.01	–
Psychosocial problems	.13	.08	.09	.37**	– .17	– .22*	– .28**	– .03	– .18	– .05	– .16	– .15	– .25*	– .10	.40**

$* p < .05, ** p < .01$

Table 3 Linear regression to predict delinquency ($N = 95$)

Variable	Model 1			Model 2			Model 3		
	B	SE	β	B	SE	β	B	SE	β
Discharged	− 1.57	6.54	− .03	− 5.78	6.89	− .09	− 4.99	6.73	− .08
Total risk score				1.14	.67	.20	1.14	.66	.19
Protective score				.31	1.53	.02	− .07	1.50	− .01
Active coping							− 2.18	.92	− .24*
Adjusted R^2		− .01			.01			.05	
ΔR^2					.02			.04	

B unstandardized coefficients, SE standard error, β standardized coefficients

* $p < .05$

risk and protective factors explained .5% of the variance in delinquency at follow-up [Model 2: $R^2 = .037$, adjusted $R^2 = .005$, $F(3,91) = 1.173$, $p = .324$]; this model however was not significant. In model 3, adding active coping as a predictor to the model explained 5.4% of the variance in delinquency at follow-up [Model 3: $R^2 = .094$ adjusted $R^2 = .054$, $F(4,90) = 2.337$, $p = .061$]. In this final model, active coping was a significant predictor of delinquency at follow-up (β = − .240, $p < .05$). The use of active coping was related to a decrease in self-reported delinquent behaviour at follow-up.

Psychosocial problems

As a third and final step we tested how much variance in the outcome measure psychosocial problems can be explained by passive coping and three of the subjective QoL domains. Again, we accounted for whether adolescents were discharged or not in the first model, and for risk and protective factors in the second model. Then, passive coping was added in the third model and the QoL domains social participation, health and fulfilment in the

fourth model. In the first model, being admitted or discharged from secure residential care at follow-up did not explain any variance in psychosocial problems at follow-up [see Table 4: Model 1: $R^2 = .010$, adjusted $R^2 = − .001$, $F(1,93) = .893$, $p = .347$]. In the second model, adding risk and protective factors also did not explain any variance in psychosocial problems at follow-up [Model 2: $R^2 = .022$, adjusted $R^2 = − .011$, $F(3,91) = .673$, $p = .571$]. Adding passive coping to the third model explained 13.7% of the variance in psychosocial problems at follow-up [Model 3: $R^2 = .173$, adjusted $R^2 = .137$, $F(4,90) = 4.718$, $p < .05$]. In model 4, adding the subjective QoL domains social participation, health, and fulfilment to the model, explained 16.9% of the variance in psychosocial problems at follow-up [Model 4: $R^2 = .231$, adjusted $R^2 = .169$, $F(7,87) = 3.724$, $p < .05$]. In this final model, passive coping was a significant predictor of psychosocial problems at follow-up (β = .329, $p < .05$). This indicates that adolescents who use more passive coping strategies in their problem solving, reported more psychosocial problems at follow-up. Additionally, the subjective QoL domain

Table 4 Linear regression to predict psychosocial problems ($N = 95$)

Variable	Model 1			Model 2			Model 3			Model 4		
	B	SE	β	B	SE	β	B	SE	β	B	SE	β
Discharged	1.18	1.25	.10	.77	1.33	.06	.86	1.23	.07	.74	1.22	.06
Total risk score				.10	.13	.09	.15	.12	.13	.14	.12	.13
Protective score				.13	.30	.05	.14	.27	.05	.10	.27	.04
Passive coping							.79	.19	.39***	.66	.21	.33**
Social participation										− .46	.90	− .06
Health										− 1.61	.80	− .20*
Fulfilment										− .43	.69	− .07
Adjusted R^2		− .00			− .01			.14			.17	
ΔR^2					.01			.15			.03	

B unstandardized coefficients, SE standard error, β standardized coefficients

* $p < .05$, ** $p < .01$, *** $p < .001$

health was also a significant predictor of psychosocial problems at follow-up ($\beta = -.198$, $p < .05$). Adolescents who were more satisfied with their health during their stay in secure residential care reported less psychosocial problems at follow-up.

Discussion

The aim of the present study was to test two assumptions derived from the Good Lives Model. First, it is assumed that a higher subjective QoL in secure residential care facility is related to less self-reported delinquency and psychosocial problems after discharge from the secure residential care facility. The current findings show that none of the subjective QoL domains were associated with delinquency. With regard to psychosocial functioning, the subjective QoL domain health was a significant predictor. Adolescents who reported a lower QoL on the health domain during their stay in a secure residential care facility had more psychosocial problems at follow-up. Second, it is assumed that having adequate coping skills during stay in a secure residential care facility, such as active coping, is related to less self-reported delinquency and psychosocial problems after having left the facility. The results of the current study support this assumption. Adolescents who used active coping strategies when facing a stressful or problematic situation while institutionalized reported less delinquent behaviour once they had left the facility.

The Good Lives Model places strong emphasis on the process of engaging individuals in their treatment by focusing on life goals and needs that are important to them. As a result, adolescents create a 'good life' for themselves, which is characterized by a sense of purpose, autonomy and a high QoL [3]. It is hypothesized that, due to increased feelings of agency and a higher QoL, adolescents are motivated to live a different kind of life and this will also help prevent them from re-offending [5]. However, the findings of the present study do not support this assumption, indicating that increasing the subjective QoL of adolescents who were institutionalized did not directly relate to a decrease in delinquency after they were discharged. A previous study among a sample of adult forensic psychiatric outpatients did find support for this assumption [10]. Adult forensic psychiatric outpatients who were more satisfied with their health reported less violent and general offenses. This difference in results might be due to the difference in the studied population and the context in which they resided during the time of the study. Whereas the current study examined adolescents that were admitted to a secure residential care facility and were treated for their emotional and behavioural problems, Bouman and colleagues studied adult forensic psychiatric outpatients, who did not receive treatment in

a secured setting. Thus, it may be that the secure nature of the facility influenced the results of the current study. A second difference between both studies that might explain the difference in findings is that the current study included adolescents while Bouman and colleagues included adults. Adults and adolescents might differ in the weightings that they give to their primary human needs (i.e., their QoL domains). Specific needs that adults generally find very important might not be perceived as that important by adolescents and as a result also not strongly relate to delinquent behaviour or psychosocial well-being.

With regard to the second outcome variable psychosocial functioning we found a relationship with the subjective QoL domain health. This finding is comparable to other researchers that have studied these concepts in the general population [41]. Adolescents who reported to be more satisfied with their health during their stay in a secure residential care facility (e.g., being satisfied with their medicine use and their mental health), reported lower levels of psychosocial problems after they were discharged from that secure residential care facility. This finding remained even after controlling for the presence of risk factors and the use of active and passive coping strategies. Thus, once adolescents are more satisfied with their health during institutionalization, the likelihood that they will experience psychosocial problems after they leave the facility will decrease, regardless of the presence of risks or type of coping strategies used during their admittance.

Consistent with our expectations, adolescents who used adequate coping strategies during their admission in a secure residential care facility reported less delinquent behaviour and fewer psychosocial problems after they were discharged from that facility. These relationships were found regardless of whether adolescents had a disadvantaged background as indicated by the presence of multiple risk factors. According to the Good Lives Model, adolescents that are lacking adequate skills in order to secure needs that are meaningful to them will attempt to achieve these needs by (re-)offending [3]. The results of the present study support this assumption and are in line with the results of other studies [21, 23, 42]. Adolescents using active coping strategies (e.g., actively trying to sort out a problematic or stressful situation or seek social support with friends or family) during their stay in secure residential care reported less delinquent behaviour after they left the secured facility. Teaching adolescents the use of active coping skills during their institutionalization might decrease the chance that they will show delinquent behaviour again after their discharge. In addition, adolescents who used passive coping strategies, such as avoiding the problem or showing a depressive response when facing a problem or stressful situation, reported higher levels of psychosocial problems after leaving the facility. Previous studies also showed that the use of passive coping was associated with negative outcomes among adolescent prisoners, such as a reduced well-being [26] and increased psychological stress [43]. Our findings support the assumption derived from the Good Lives Model that a lack of adequate coping strategies is predictive of delinquent behaviour and psychosocial problems at follow-up, even after controlling for the presence of risk and protective factors.

The current study has a number of limitations that should be considered when interpreting the results. First, only self-report measures were used to assess delinquent behaviour and psychosocial functioning at follow-up. Although we considered both the severity of the offenses, as well as the number of offenses that were committed, it remains possible that the findings reported here under represent official registration data. Second, the current study is part of a longitudinal study with four waves of data. Adolescents were approached every 6 months to assess their subjective QoL during their stay in a secure residential care facility and also 12 months after discharge. The current study only used data from participants who completed the first assessment and the follow-up assessment. This way, only data was used of 95 of the 172 included adolescents. Attrition analysis revealed that these adolescents were more often diagnosed with an autism spectrum disorder (ASD) and with a reactive attachment disorder (RAD), which might cause results to be less generalizable.

Conclusions

Subjective QoL and coping are important components of the Good Lives Model framework and are assumed to play a role in the onset and maintenance of delinquent behaviour and psychosocial problems [4, 6]. Strength-based approaches are increasingly used in the treatment of adolescents in secure residential care and might be an important complement to the prevailing risk perspective. By solely focusing on criminogenic risks as main treatment targets, other factors, such as subjective QoL and coping are neglected. The current study showed that adolescents who reported a lower QoL on the health domain had more psychosocial problems at follow-up. No relationship was found however, between QoL and delinquency. Based on the results of the current study, the strongest support was found for the second assumption derived from the Good Lives Model: adolescents with adequate coping skills report less delinquent behaviour and fewer psychosocial problems. Adolescents lacking adequate coping skills were more likely to experience adjustment problems upon returning to society.

Adolescents who used active coping during their stay in secure residential care reported lower levels of delinquent behaviour at follow-up, while adolescents who used passive coping during their stay in secure residential care reported higher levels of psychosocial problems at follow-up. To conclude, we could not confirm the first assumption derived from the Good Lives Model in our sample of adolescents with severe psychiatric problems. However, results of this study provide support for the second assumption and therefore underline the importance of developing and strengthening adequate coping skills in the treatment of adolescents with severe psychiatric problems.

Authors' contributions
All authors have contributed to the preparation of the manuscript. All authors read and approved the final manuscript.

Author details
[1] Research and Documentation Centre (WODC) of the Dutch Ministry of Justice and Security, PO Box 20301, 2500 EH The Hague, The Netherlands. [2] GGzE Center for Child & Adolescent Psychiatry, PO Box 909 (DP 8001), 5600 AX Eindhoven, The Netherlands. [3] Scientific Center for Care & Welfare (Tranzo), Tilburg University, PO Box 90153, 5000 LE Tilburg, The Netherlands.

Acknowledgements
We are grateful to all participating institutions for their cooperation in this project and for the adolescents who were willing to participate. In addition, the authors thank Lenneke Vugs M.Sc. for her help in the data coordination and data collection. We also wish to thank all the research interns for their help in the data collection.

Competing interests
The authors declare that they have no competing interests.

Funding
This study was funded by The Netherlands Organization for Health Research and Development (ZonMw): 157.003.004. The funding body did not have any role in the design of the study and collection, analysis, and interpretation of data, nor in writing the manuscript.

References

1. Farrington DP. Developmental and life-course criminology: key theoretical and empirical issues—the 2002 Sutherland award address. Criminology. 2003;41(2):221–55.
2. Stouthamer-Loeber M, Loeber R, Wei E, Farrington DP, Wikstrom POH. Risk and promotive effects in the explanation of persistent serious delinquency in boys. J Consult Clin Psychol. 2002;70(1):111–23.
3. Fortune C-A, Ward T, Willis GM. The rehabilitation of offenders: reducing risk and promoting better lives. Psychiatry Psychol Law. 2012;19(5):646–61.
4. Ward T, Gannon TA. Rehabilitation, etiology, and self-regulation: the comprehensive Good Lives Model of treatment for sexual offenders. Aggress Violent Behav. 2006;11(1):77–94.
5. Ward T, Marshall WL. Good lives, aetiology and the rehabilitation of sex offenders: a bridging theory. J Sex Aggress. 2004;10(2):153–69.
6. Purvis M, Ward T, Willis G. The Good Lives Model in practice: offence pathways and case management. European Journal of Probation. 2011;3(2):4–28.
7. Letourneau EJ, Armstrong KS. Recidivism rates for registered and nonregistered juvenile sexual offenders. Sex Abuse. 2008;20(4):393–408.
8. Mulder E, Vermunt J, Brand E, Bullens R, Van Marle H. Recidivism in subgroups of serious juvenile offenders: different profiles, different risks? Crim Behav Mental Health. 2012;22(2):122–35.
9. Van Marle HJC, Hempel IS, Buck NML. Young serious and vulnerable offenders in the Netherlands: a cohort follow-up study after completion of a PIJ (detention) order. Crim Behav Mental Health. 2010;20(5):349–60.
10. Bouman YHA, Schene AH, De Ruiter C. Subjective well-being and recidivism in forensic psychiatric outpatients. Int J Forensic Mental Health. 2009;8:225–34.
11. Bahr SJ, Harris L, Fisher JK, Harker Armstrong A. Successful reentry: what differentiates successful and unsuccessful parolees? Int J Offender Ther Comp Criminol. 2010;54(5):667–92.
12. Tripodi SJ, Kim JS, Bender K. Is employment associated with reduced recidivism? The complex relationship between employment and crime. Int J Offender Ther Comp Criminol. 2010;54(5):706–20.
13. Steinberg L, Chung HL, Little M. Re-entry of young offenders from the justice system: a developmental perspective. Youth Violence Juv J. 2004;2(1):21–38.
14. Ward T. The management of risk and the design of good lives. Aust Psychol. 2002;37(3):172–9.
15. Lehman AF. Measures of quality of life among persons with severe and persistent mental disorders. Soc Psychiatry Psych Epidemiol. 1996;31(2):78–88.
16. Lehman AF. The well-being of chronic mental patients. Arch General Psychiatry. 1983;40:369–73.
17. Reininghaus U, McCabe R, Burns T, Croudace T, Priebe S. The validity of subjective quality of life measures in psychotic patients with severe psychopathology and cognitive deficits: an item response model analysis. Qual Life Res. 2012;21(2):237–46.
18. Draine J, Solomon P. Comparison of seriously mentally ill case management clients with and without arrest histories. J Psychiatry Law. 1992;20(3):335–49.
19. Draine J, Solomon P. Jail recidivism and the intensity of case management services among homeless persons with mental illness leaving jail. J Psychiatry Law. 1994;22:245–61.
20. Compas BE, Connor-Smith JK, Saltzman H, Thomsen AH, Wadsworth ME. Coping with stress during childhood and adolescence: problems, progress, and potential in theory and research. Psychol Bull. 2001;127(1):87–127.
21. Gullone E, Jones T, Cummins R. Coping styles and prison experience as predictors of psychological well-being in male prisoners. Psychiatry Psychol Law. 2000;7(1):170–81.
22. Ashkar PJ, Kenny DT. Views from the inside—young offenders' subjective experiences of incarceration. Int J Offender Ther Comp Criminol. 2008;52(5):584–97.
23. Mulder E, Brand E, Bullens R, Van Marle H. Risk factors for overall recidivism and severity of recidivism in serious juvenile offenders. Int J Offender Ther Comp Criminol. 2011;55(1):118–35.
24. Windle M, Windle RC. Coping strategies, drinking motives, and stressful life events among middle adolescents: associations with emotional and behavioral problems and with academic functioning. J Abnorm Psychol. 1996;105(4):551–60.
25. Ebata AT, Moos RH. Coping and adjustment in distressed and healthy adolescents. J Appl Dev Psychol. 1991;12:33–54.
26. Brown SL, Ireland CA. Coping style and distress in newly incarcerated male adolescents. J Adolesc Health. 2006;38(6):656–61.
27. Van Nieuwenhuizen C, Schene AH, Koeter MWJ, Huxley PJ. The Lancashire quality of life profile: modification and psychometric evaluation. Soc Psychiatry Psych Epidemiol. 2001;36(1):36–44.
28. Van Nieuwenhuizen C, Schene AH, Koeter MWJ. Quality of life in forensic psychiatry: an unreclaimed territory? Int Rev Psychiatry. 2002;14(3):198–202.
29. Harder AT, Knorth EJ, Kalverboer ME. Transition secured? A follow-up study of adolescents who have left secure residential care. Child Youth Serv Rev. 2011;33(12):2482–8.
30. Rosenberg M. Society and the adolescent self-image. Princeton: Princeton University Press; 1965.
31. Debats DL, Van der Lubbe PM, Wezeman FRA. On the psychometric properties of the life regard index (lri)—a measure of meaningful life—an evaluation in 3 independent samples based on the Dutch version. Pers Indiv Differ. 1993;14(2):337–45.
32. Van Nieuwenhuizen C, Schene A, Boevink W, Wolf J. The Lancashire quality of life profile: first experiences in the Netherlands. Commun Mental Health J. 1998;34(5):513–24.
33. Oliver JPJ, Huxley PJ, Priebe S, Kaiser W. Measuring the quality of life of severely mentally ill people using the Lancashire quality of life profile. Soc Psychiatry Psych Epidemiol. 1997;32(2):76–83.
34. Bijstra JO, Bosma HA, Jackson S. The relationship between social skills and psychosocial functioning in early adolescence. Pers Indiv Differ. 1994;16(5):767–76.
35. Meijer SA, Sinnema G, Bijstra JO, Mellenbergh GJ, Wolters WHG. Coping styles and locus of control as predictors for psychological adjustment of adolescents with a chronic illness. Soc Sci Med. 2002;54(9):1453–61.
36. Borum R, Bartel P, Forth A. Manual for the structured assessment of violence risk in youth (SAVRY), consultation edition, version 1. Tampa: University of South Florida; 2002.
37. Van der Laan AM, Blom M, Kleemans ER. Exploring long-term and short-term risk factors for serious delinquency. Eur J Criminol. 2009;6(5):419–38.
38. Goodman R. The strengths and difficulties questionnaire: a research note. J Child Psychol Psychiatry. 1997;38(5):581–6.
39. Goodman R. The extended version of the strengths and difficulties questionnaire as a guide to child psychiatric caseness and consequent burden. J Child Psychol Psychiatry. 1999;40(5):791–9.
40. Goodman R. Psychometric properties of the strengths and difficulties questionnaire. J Am Acad Child Psychiatry. 2001;40(11):1337–45.
41. Bartels M, Cacioppo JT, van Beijsterveldt TCEM, Boomsma DI. Exploring the association between well-being and psychopathology in adolescents. Behav Genet. 2013;43(3):177–90.
42. Shulman EP, Cauffman E. Coping while incarcerated: a study of male juvenile offenders. J Res Adolesc. 2011;21(4):818–26.
43. Ireland JL, Boustead R, Ireland CA. Coping style and psychological health among adolescent prisoners: a study of young and juvenile offenders. J Adolesc. 2005;28(3):411–23.

16

Intense/obsessional interests in children with gender dysphoria: a cross-validation study using the Teacher's Report Form

Kenneth J. Zucker[1*], A. Natisha Nabbijohn[2], Alanna Santarossa[2], Hayley Wood[3], Susan J. Bradley[1], Joanna Matthews[2] and Doug P. VanderLaan[2,4]

Abstract

Objective: This study assessed whether children clinically referred for gender dysphoria (GD) show symptoms that overlap with Autism Spectrum Disorder (ASD). Circumscribed preoccupations/intense interests and repetitive behaviors were considered as overlapping symptoms expressed in both GD and ASD.

Methods: To assess these constructs, we examined Items 9 and 66 on the Teacher's Report Form (TRF), which measure obsessions and compulsions, respectively.

Results: For Item 9, gender-referred children (n = 386) were significantly elevated compared to the referred (n = 965) and non-referred children (n = 965) from the TRF standardization sample. For Item 66, gender-referred children were elevated in comparison to the non-referred children, but not the referred children.

Conclusions: These findings provided cross-validation of a previous study in which the same patterns were found using the Child Behavior Checklist (Vanderlaan et al. in J Sex Res 52:213–19, 2015). We discuss possible developmental pathways between GD and ASD, including a consideration of the principle of equifinality.

Keywords: Gender dysphoria, Autism Spectrum Disorder, Teacher's Report Form, Equifinality, DSM-5

Background

Children with a DSM-5 diagnosis of gender dysphoria (GD) [Gender Identity Disorder of Childhood in DSM-III and III-R and Gender Identity Disorder (GID) in DSM-IV] have a marked incongruence between the gender they have been assigned to at birth and their experienced/expressed gender [1].[1] The DSM-5 indicators for the diagnosis, as in DSM-III and DSM-IV, include an array of sex-typed behaviors (e.g., toy and activity interests, dress-up play, roles in fantasy play, etc.) that often signal a strong identification with the other gender. Over three decades ago, Coates [2] reported the clinical impression that at least some boys with GD appeared to show an intense, if not obsessional, interest in gender-related themes, as manifested in their surface behaviors and in fantasy play, and in their responses during projective testing such as the Rorschach [3] (for a recent clinical example, see Saketopoulou [4]. It is unclear, however, whether these patterns of behavior are simply an "inverted" instance of the intense gender-related interests and behaviors seen in typically-developing children [5, 6] or represent something that is qualitatively distinct or, at least, at the extreme end of a quantitative spectrum.

One relatively recent line of research, stimulated by a series of clinical case reports and one internet-recruited sample (of children, adolescents, and adults), has pointed to a possible link between GD and Autism Spectrum Disorder (ASD) or at least traits of ASD [7–19]. Using a structured diagnostic interview schedule, dimensional

*Correspondence: ken.zucker@utoronto.ca
[1] Department of Psychiatry, University of Toronto, Toronto, ON M5T 1R8, Canada
Full list of author information is available at the end of the article

[1] We will use primarily GD to reflect the current DSM-5 diagnostic label, but use GID when it is historically accurate to do so (e.g., regarding the clinical diagnosis of the participants in this study).

measures, or chart review, several studies have reported, compared to normative samples, an overrepresentation of either ASD or ASD traits among clinic-referred children and/or adolescents [20–23] or adults [24, 25] with a diagnosis of GID/GD (for an internet-recruited sample, see also Kristensen and Broome [26] (for reviews, see Glidden et al. [27], Strang et al. [28], van der Miesen et al. [29], and van Schalkwyk et al. [30]).

One potential explanation for the putative link between GD and ASD is the intense focus on, or an obsessional interest in, specific activities [31, 32]. Such interests relate to the DSM-5 ASD criterion pertaining to highly restricted and fixated interests. For example, it is conceivable that children with ASD who form intense and focused attention to cross-sex objects or activities may then begin to express other characteristics of GD (e.g., see Strang et al. [33]). Conversely, GD may give rise to such interests and obsessions, leading to a clinical presentation consistent with ASD. In order to appraise these two proposed pathways, however, the first step would be to determine empirically if, in fact, children with GD manifest an elevated pattern of intense interests and obsessions.

To our knowledge, only two studies have focused on a possible elevation in obsessional/repetitive interests and behaviors in GD children using dimensional metrics. Skagerberg et al. [23] used the Social Responsiveness Scale (SRS) in a mixed sample of 166 children and adolescents and found an elevation on the "Autistic Mannerisms" subscale completed by the parents [now labeled "Restricted Interests and Repetitive Behaviors" (RIRB) on the SRS-2] [34] compared to a normative sample. However, two methodological issues call for some caution in appraising the results. First, the participation rate was only 46%, which may represent a threat to the internal validity of the sample [35]. Second, a clinic-referred comparison group, consisting of children/adolescents referred for other clinical problems, was not included. Thus, it is not clear if the elevation on the Autistic Mannerisms subscale is specific to children/adolescents referred for gender dysphoria or characteristic of clinic-referred children/adolescents in general.

Taking advantage of a large "archival" data set, VanderLaan et al. [36] analyzed two items on the Child Behavior Checklist (CBCL) [37] pertaining to obsessionality and repetitive behavior: Item 9 ("Can't get his/her mind off certain thoughts; obsessions") and Item 66 ("Repeats certain acts over and over; compulsions") in a sample of 534 children referred clinically for gender identity concerns, 419 siblings, and 1201 referred and 1201 non-referred children from the CBCL standardization sample [37],

with an age range of 3–12 years.[2] For both items, parental responses were dichotomized as either present ("Somewhat or sometimes true"/"Very true or often true") or absent ("Not true"). In their study, the parental participation rate was over 90% for the gender-referred sample.

For Item 9, the percentage of mothers of the gender-referred children who endorsed it (62.4%) was significantly greater than that of their siblings (22.2%) and significantly greater than the ratings of the mothers of both the referred (48.7%) and non-referred (21.9%) children from the CBCL standardization sample (odds ratios, with a 95% CI ranged from 1.66 to 10.96). The percentage of mothers of the referred children who endorsed it was also significantly greater than the ratings for the siblings and of the non-referred children. For Item 66, the percentage of mothers of the gender-referred children who endorsed it (25.3%) was significantly greater than that of their siblings (8.2%) and the ratings of the non-referred children (5.4%) (odds ratios ranged from 3.04 to 6.77), but not of the referred children (24.9%), who also had higher endorsement ratings than the siblings of the gender-referred children and of the non-referred children. Thus, in this study, there was evidence for both specificity and non-specificity for these two behaviors: On the one hand, both the gender-referred children and the referred children were elevated on both items compared to the siblings and non-referred children (non-specificity); on the other hand, a greater percentage of the gender-referred children than the referred children were elevated on Item 9, evidence for at least partial specificity.

For the gender-referred children and their siblings, it was also possible to code qualitatively the reasons that the mothers endorsed these two items. A two-option coding scheme classified the reasons as either gender-related (e.g., "Cinderella" for Item 9) or non-gender-related (e.g., "killing"). For Item 9, VanderLaan et al. [36] found that gender-related themes were significantly more common for the gender-referred boys than that of the male siblings, but the difference between the gender-referred girls and that of the female siblings was not significant (possibly due to low power because of the smaller sample size). For Item 66, there was no significant difference in

---

[2] In developmental clinical psychology and psychiatry, the CBCL [37] is one of the most widely used parent-report measures of behavioral and emotional problems in children and adolescents. It contains a total of 118 items, each of which is rated on a 0–2 point scale for frequency of occurrence. Factor analysis has identified both broad-band (Internalizing, Externalizing) and eight narrow-band dimensions of behavioral and emotional disturbance (e.g., "Anxious/Depressed," "Aggressive Behavior." Items 9 and 66 load on the "Thought Problems" narrow-band scale, which is part of a suite of three narrow-band dimensions that do not load on either the Internalizing or Externalizing broad-band dimensions. On average, completion of the CBCL takes about 15–17 min [37, p. 14].

gender-related themes for the gender-referred children and their siblings.

The purpose of the present study was to cross-validate the VanderLaan et al. [36] findings for these two items using teacher ratings on the Teacher's Report Form [38] to see if teachers would also report elevations in gender-referred children when compared to both referred and non-referred children in the TRF standardization sample [39].[3]

Methods
Participants
Between 1986 and 2013, TRFs were obtained for 386 children (304 boys; 82 girls) who were referred to, and then assessed in, a specialty gender identity service for children, housed within a child psychiatry program at an academic health science center. The children had a mean age of 7.77 years (SD = 2.41). All of the children met DSM-III, DSM-IV or DSM-5 criteria for GID/GD or were subthreshold for the diagnosis (e.g., Gender Identity Disorder NOS). During this time period, TRFs were not available for an additional 145 gender-referred children. The main reasons for this were: the parents did not want the teacher to complete the TRF (because of concerns about privacy/confidentiality); a TRF was mailed to the teacher/school, but it was not returned; the child was too young for the TRF to be administered (e.g., not yet in school); the child was being home-schooled; or, the family chose not to complete the assessment so the TRF was not sent to the teacher.[4]

For comparative purposes, we used the TRF referred (498 boys; 467 girls) and non-referred (498 boys; 467 girls) standardization samples for children ages 6–12 years from Achenbach and Rescorla [39]. As reported by Achenbach and Rescorla, the referred sample was obtained from various mental health and special educational settings, primarily in the U.S., heterogeneous with regard to DSM diagnoses. The non-referred sample was obtained from the 1999 National Survey of Children, Youths, and Adults conducted between February 1999 and January 2000. Parents who completed the CBCL were asked for permission to mail a TRF to one of their child's teachers, who received $10 in compensation

for participation. Children were included in the non-referred sample if they had not received professional help for behavioral, emotional, substance use, or developmental problems in the preceding 12 months [39, pp. 75–76]. The referred and non-referred samples were matched for gender, age, socioeconomic status, and ethnicity [39, pp. 75–76, p. 109].

Measures
For both Items 9 and 66, teacher responses were dichotomized where 0 = 0 and 1 or 2 = 1. Using the parental data from our previous study for the gender-referred sample [36], we calculated mother–teacher and father–teacher correlations for both items using the continuous 0 to 2 coding system. For the gender-referred children, we recorded the comments provided by the teacher if the items were scored either as a 1 ("somewhat or sometimes true") or 2 ("very true or often true") and then used our previously-developed two-category qualitative coding scheme by classifying the teacher descriptions as either gender-related or non-gender-related. Examples of gender-related themes for Item 9 were "Obsessed with female actions, colors, activities," "preoccupied with dressing up at house center," and "Spiderman." Examples of non-gender-related themes were "frequently day dreams," "… food," and "revengeful thoughts." Corresponding gender-related theme examples for Item 66 were "Dresses up like a female" and "Drawing females" and non-gender-related themes were "paces" and "repeated cracking knees and elbows." Two authors (ANN, JM) independently coded both items as either gender-related or non-gender-related. For Item 9 (n = 129), the kappa was .87 ($p < .001$); for Item 66 (n = 47), the kappa was .95 ($p < .001$). Unfortunately, it was not possible to code for qualitative comments in the referred and non-referred standardization samples because they were not available in the raw data file provided to us by Achenbach.

The present study constituted a reanalysis of data from previous research projects for which there was ethics approval from the [Centre for Addiction and Mental Health] Research Ethics Board. This research was conducted in accordance with the Declaration of Helsinki.

Results
Preliminary analyses
We first compared the gender-referred children for whom a TRF was completed vs. those for whom it was not (including the cases in which the TRF version for preschoolers was used). As expected, children for whom the TRF was completed were, on average, significantly older than those children for whom it was not, $t(529) = 7.02$, $p < .001$. There was no significant difference for year of assessment. Children for whom a TRF

---

[3] The TRF [38] is similar in design and format to that of the CBCL. There are 25 items on the TRF that are more appropriate for the school setting (e.g., "Dislikes school") and these items replace 25 items on the CBCL. Factor analysis has identified the same broad-band and narrow-band dimensions of behavioral and emotional disturbance as on the CBCL. The behavioral and emotional problem items on the TRF can be completed, on average, in about 10 min [38, p. 11].

[4] Our clinic began administering the TRF in 1986, when it was first published [40]. For preschoolers, the Caregiver-Teacher Report Form for Ages 1-1/2–5 was administered once it became available [41]; unfortunately, this version of the TRF does not contain the two items analyzed in this study.

was completed had a significantly lower Full-Scale IQ (M, 101.1 vs. 108.4), came from a somewhat lower social class background (M, 42.1 vs. 46.8; absolute range 8–66) [42], and had higher Internalizing (M, 62.1 vs. 56.8) and Externalizing (M, 61.5 vs. 54.4) T scores on the CBCL (all $p < .001$). With age co-varied, these differences remained statistically significant, with the exception of social class.[5]

Teacher ratings for Items 9 and 66
Table 1 shows the dichotomized teacher ratings for Items 9 and 66 (in percent) for the gender-referred children, the referred children, and the non-referred children, stratified by sex. For both the boys and the girls, the overall chi square test was statistically significant for both Items 9 and 66: Item 9 for boys, $\chi^2(2) = 90.61$, $p < .00001$; for girls, $\chi^2(2) = 42.86$, $p < .00001$; Item 66 for boys, $\chi^2(2) = 42.21$, $p < .00001$; for girls, $\chi^2(2) = 16.28$, $p = .00029$. To decompose the overall effect, three paired contrasts were conducted for both items: gender-referred vs. referred children from the standardization sample, gender-referred vs. non-referred children from the standardization sample, and referred vs. non-referred children from the standardization sample, by sex (Table 1).

For Item 9, for the boys, it can be seen that teachers were significantly more likely to endorse this item with a rating of either a 1 or a 2 for both the gender-referred and referred samples when compared to the non-referred sample. It can also be seen that teachers were significantly more likely to endorse this item for the gender-referred boys than for the referred boys. For the girls, the findings were similar.

For Item 66, for the boys, it can be seen that teachers were significantly more likely to endorse this item with a rating of either a 1 or a 2 for both the gender-referred and referred samples when compared to the non-referred sample, but the comparison between the gender-referred boys and the referred boys in the standardization sample was not significant. For the girls, the findings were similar.

Correlational analyses
In the gender-referred sample (collapsed across sex), we calculated the correlation between the continuous ratings for Items 9 and 66 for the TRF and the CBCL [36]. For Item 9, the mother-teacher correlation was .28 (n = 337, $p < .001$) and the father-teacher correlation was .23 (n = 248, $p < .001$). For Item 66, the mother-teacher correlation was .17 (n = 345, $p = .002$) and the father–teacher correlation was .11 (n = 255, $p = .091$). We also calculated the correlation between the continuous ratings for Items 9 and 66 and age (collapsed across sex), which were .11

$(p = .029)$ and .00 (ns), respectively. For the referred sample, the correlations were .05 (ns) and −.07 ($p = .033$), respectively. For the non-referred sample, the correlations were −.01 and .02, respectively (both ns).[6] Thus, age effects were either non-existent or extremely small.

Qualitative analysis
For the qualitative analyses, teachers provided written comments for 84.3% (n = 129/153) of the gender-referred sample for whom Item 9 was rated as a 1 or a 2 and for 74.6% (n = 47/63) of the sample for who Item 66 was rated as a 1 or a 2 (see Table 1). For Item 9, 47.2% of the comments for boy were coded as gender-related compared to 30.4% for girls, a non-significant difference, $\chi^2(1) = 1.52$. For Item 66, the corresponding percentages were 32.4 and 0%, respectively, which was also not significant, $\chi^2(1) < 1$.

Discussion
An emerging clinical and research literature has suggested a co-occurrence between GD and ASD (or ASD traits). VanderLaan et al. [36] had hypothesized that this link might be due, at least in part, to an elevated presence of intense/obsessional interests that involve gender-related behaviors. In their study, parents of gender-referred children endorsed CBCL Item 9 more frequently than they did for siblings and by parents in both referred and non-referred children from the CBCL standardization sample. This finding was, therefore, consistent with the proposition that the basis of the GD-ASD link is the tendency of gender-referred children to present clinically in a manner that corresponds to the ASD criterion pertaining to highly restricted and fixated interests. In this regard, it is important to note that this item corresponds very closely to two items on the SRS-2 that load on the RIRB subscale (Items 26: "Thinks or talks about the same thing over and over" and Item 31: "Can't get his or her mind off something once he or she starts thinking about it"). The results for Item 66 also suggested that the ASD diagnostic criterion pertaining to repetitive behaviors and routines might also be relevant to GD in children. For this item, parental ratings were also elevated compared to siblings and non-referred children, but not when compared to referred children, so there was less support for a specificity effect. In relation to the SRS-2, this item bears some similarity to RIRB subscale Item 4: "When under stress...shows rigid or inflexible patterns of behavior..." In a comparative perspective, however, it could be argued that intense/obsessional interests (Item

---

[5] These analyses are available from the corresponding author upon request.

[6] It was not possible to calculate mother–teacher correlations for Items 9 and 66 in the standardization samples because the raw data for the CBCL and TRF were in separate SPSS files.

Table 1 Teacher ratings of TRF Items 9 and 66 as a function of group and sex

Ratings of obsessions (Item 9)

Groups	0		1 or 2		$\chi^2(1)$	p	OR (95% CI)
	n	%	n	%			
Boys							
Gender-referred vs.	172	58.3	123	41.7			
Referred	332	66.7	166	33.3	5.23	.022	1.43 (1.06–1.92)
Non-referred	433	86.9	65	13.1	82.45	< .001	4.76 (3.36–6.75)
Referred vs. non-referred					56.36	< .001	3.33 (2.41–4.58)
Girls							
Gender-referred vs.	49	62.0	30	38.0			
Referred	356	76.2	111	23.8	6.39	.011	1.96 (1.18–3.24)
Non-referred	414	88.7	53	11.3	35.12	< .001	4.78 (2.78–8.18)
Referred vs. non-referred					24.03	< .001	2.43 (1.70–3.47)

Ratings of compulsions (Item 66)

Groups	0		1 or 2		$\chi^2(1)$	p	OR (95% CI)
	n	%	n	%			
Boys							
Gender-referred vs.	247	81.2	55	18.2			
Referred	415	83.3	83	16.7	< 1	ns	1.11 (.76–1.62)
Non-referred	473	95.0	25	5.0	34.90	< .001	4.21 (2.56–6.92)
Referred vs. non-referred					33.74	< .001	3.78 (2.37–6.03)
Girls							
Gender-referred vs.	72	90.0	8	10.0			
Referred	421	90.1	46	9.9	< 1	ns	1.01 (.46–2.24)
Non-referred	451	96.6	16	3.4	5.56	.018	4.90 (1.99–12.07)
Referred vs. non-referred					14.52	< .001	3.07 (1.71–5.52)

Referred and non-referred raw data from Achenbach and Rescorla [39] provided by Achenbach in an SPSS file

9) provide a stronger basis than repetitive behaviors/routines (Item 66) for the link between GD and ASD.

Using the TRF, the present study provided a cross-validation of the CBCL findings [36]. For Item 9, the gender-referred children had significantly higher ratings than both the referred and non-referred children in the standardization sample but, for Item 66, the ratings were significantly higher only when compared to the non-referred children. Although the percentage of gender-referred children for which Items 9 and 66 were endorsed by teachers was lower than the percentage for which the items were endorsed by parents in VanderLaan et al. [36], the same was true for the referred and non-referred children. Also as in VanderLaan et al., gender-related themes were identified on both Items 9 and 66 for boys and, on Item 9, for girls as well. For example, on Item 9 for boys, 47% of the descriptors pertained to gender-related themes, which was similar to the percentage of 54% that mothers provided. Thus, the pattern across the two informants (parents, teachers) was very similar.

If there is, indeed, an empirical basis for the role of gender-related obsessionality that contributes to the GD-ASD link, the possible developmental pathways need to be formulated. As noted earlier, one idea is that ASD sometimes leads to intense interests in cross-sex objects or activities, giving rise to a clinical presentation of GD. Thus, on this basis, one would predict that GD children would also exhibit additional features of ASD. In the study by Skagerberg et al. [23], this appeared to be the case: although Skagerberg et al. did not provide formal statistical tests, our own analysis of their data showed that, compared to a normative sample, children and adolescents with GD had significantly higher ratings on all of the other subscales of the SRS, not just the one pertaining to restricted interests and repetitive behaviors.[7]

---

[7] We conducted t tests on the data provided in Table 2 in Skagerberg et al. [23]. These analyses are available from the corresponding author upon request.

The Skagerberg et al. [23] data would appear to challenge another developmental pathway proposed by VanderLaan et al. [36]. If restricted and intense cross-sex interests are simply a manifestation of GD, the ASD "flavor" might be only subclinical or even superficial, because the intensity of the interests is only a marker of the GD and not an underlying ASD. If such were the case, then few, if any, additional ASD features should accompany intense cross-sex interests. But this was clearly not the case in the Skagerberg et al. data set.

From Skagerberg et al. [23] and other systematic studies of GD samples (noted earlier), it is clear that there are many children with GD who would not be diagnosed with an ASD or would even be in the clinical range on dimensional measures of ASD traits, as, for example, on the SRS. Recognition of this variability is consistent with the principle of equifinality [43]. ASD or ASD traits, including the presence of intense and restricted interests, may lead to gender dysphoria, but for those GD children without ASD or ASD traits the presence of intense and restricted interests may be caused by other underlying processes. This would, of course, be consistent with multifactorial models of gender dysphoria, in which the relative contribution of risk factors will vary in their relative weight from one child to the next [44]. Along similar lines, it should also be noted that there are now several studies which document an elevation in ASD traits, as measured by the SRS, in children referred for a variety of clinical problems [45–49], not just in children referred for GD, which clearly points to a pattern of non-specificity.

This non-specificity effect is a clear indication that the hypothesized GD-ASD link requires a more nuanced examination. One such strategy would be to design formal tests of equifinality in which GD children are divided into two subgroups: those with ASD or ASD traits and those without. One could then examine whether or not the two subgroups differ in other important ways. In one study, VanderLaan et al. [50] reported in a sample of children with GD that those with higher ASD traits and a higher score on a dimensional measure of gender-variant behavior had a higher birth weight. VanderLaan et al. [50] noted that high birth weight has been identified as a risk factor for ASD and that it is also associated with lower prenatal levels of testosterone in males and with masculinized somatic features, such as a greater anogenital distance, in females. This finding is consistent with one study that reported an association between the degree of demasculinizing endocrine disruptor chemicals in maternal blood and ASD traits in children [51]. In another study, Shumer et al. [52] found that mothers (but not fathers) in the Nurses' Health Study II and the Growing Up Today Study 1 who had higher self-reported SRS scores rated their children as higher in gender-variant behaviors, suggesting

some type of underlying biological liability, perhaps along the maternal line, for both variables. These two studies lend some support for further tests of the equifinality principle with regard to the GD-ASD link.

Limitations

There are four limitations to the current study that should be noted. First, we assessed the focal variables of obsessional interests and repetitive behaviors using only single items from the TRF and our primary analysis was based on a dichotomous (present vs. absent) metric. Although both our prior CBCL analysis and the current TRF analysis were quite successful in detecting significant between-groups effects, we recognize that dimensional measures, such as the SRS, would be psychometrically superior as this line of research continues. However, given the current intense interest in the GD-ASD link in the literature, it was our view that the use of a large "archival" data set (i.e., using a sample of children going back several decades) would add to this contemporary discourse. Second, although we were able to obtain TRFs on 73% of the entire sample of gender-referred children assessed between 1986 and 2013, we were not able to use the TRF data that were available for preschoolers because the relevant items are not on this version. Thus, future research should use the SRS so that the restricted interests and repetitive behaviors construct can be evaluated during the developmental period in which GD is often first expressed [1]. Third, it should be considered whether or not parents and teachers who endorsed Items 9 and 66 and provide gender-related themes were "over-reacting" because the child's gendered behavior was atypical or if the ratings represent bona fide evidence of obsessionality and compulsivity. On this point, one could test this by looking at children whose parents describe them as being preoccupied with gender-typical behaviors, as in the Halim et al. [6] study of the "pink frilly dresses" phenomenon in young girls and to see if they too would be more likely to endorse these items when compared to girls who are not seen as overly preoccupied with gender normative behaviors. Lastly, it should be emphasized that our data speak more to the potential presence of ASD traits than to the categorical ASD diagnosis.

We recognize that our data only speak to one aspect of an ASD but not other core elementss, such as marked impairment in social communication and social interaction. Thus, we in no way wish to argue that elevations in obsessional interests/behaviors per se are sufficient in making any kind of definitive conclusion about ASD. However, it is important to note that our data are consistent with one study that analyzed CBCL and TRF items that discriminated children with an ASD diagnosis from clinic-referred children classified as having an internalizing disorder, an externalizing disorder, no diagnosis, and children from the general population [53]. So et al. [53] found that 10 CBCL/TRF items were significantly higher in the ASD group than the other four groups: Items 9 and 66 were two of these items, with between-groups odds ratios ranging from 1.25 to 2.08 for the 10 CBCL items and 1.17–1.55 for the 10 TRF items. Given these findings, it is our view that Items 9 and 66, at least in children, may be more suggestive of ASD traits than traits suggestive of an Obsessive–Compulsive Disorder because natural history data suggest that OCD onsets at a much later age than ASD [1].

To date, the GD-ASD literature in children has been largely limited to case reports. Other than our own work [36, 49], only the Skagerberg et al. [23] study used a dimensional assessment measure to assess putative ASD traits and only one study, which used a selective sub-sample of children and adolescents referred for gender dysphoria, employed a structured diagnostic interview schedule to ascertain an autism diagnosis [20]. Going forward, researchers in this specialty area will need to decide if there would be benefits in using more formal diagnostic methods, such as the Autism Diagnostic Observation Schedule [54], to ascertain the percentage of children referred for gender dysphoria who would meet criteria for the diagnosis.

Conclusion

Our TRF study provides a cross-validation of our previous CBCL study of an elevation in intense interests/obsessional traits among children referred for gender dysphoria as compared to both referred and non-referred children in the standardization sample and, to a lesser extent, with regard to repetitive behaviors. These findings, therefore, give some support to the idea that there may be a link between gender dysphoria and ASD traits. However, the emerging literature that suggests a non-specific pattern of elevations in ASD traits among clinic-referred children in general calls for a more focused examination of why such a link may be present among at least some children with a DSM diagnosis of gender dysphoria.

Abbreviations

ASD: Autism Spectrum Disorder; CBCL: Child Behavior Checklist; DSM: Diagnostic and Statistical Manual of Mental Disorders; GD: gender dysphoria; GID: Gender Identity Disorder; SRS: Social Responsiveness Scale; TRF: Teacher's Report Form.

Authors' contributions

KJZ, HW, SJB, and DPV were responsible for the conceptual basis of the study and its design. KJZ, ANN, AS, and DPV were involved in the data analysis and interpretation. JM contributed to data coding. The manuscript was prepared by KJZ with assistance from all coauthors. All authors read and approved the final manuscript.

Author details

[1] Department of Psychiatry, University of Toronto, Toronto, ON M5T 1R8, Canada. [2] Department of Psychology, University of Toronto Mississauga, Mississauga, ON, Canada. [3] Psychological Services, Toronto District School Board, Toronto, ON, Canada. [4] Underserved Populations Research Program, Child, Youth and Family Division, Centre for Addiction and Mental Health, Toronto, ON, Canada.

Acknowledgements
Not applicable.

Competing interests
The authors declare that they have no competing interests.

Funding
DPV was supported by a Canadian Institutes of Health Research Postdoctoral Fellowship, the Centre for Addiction and Mental Health, and the University of Toronto Mississauga. AS and ANN were supported by University of Toronto Excellence Awards funded by the Social Sciences and Humanities Research Council of Canada.

References

1. American Psychiatric Association. Diagnostic and statistical manual of mental disorders. 5th ed. Arlington: American Psychiatric Press; 2013.
2. Coates S. Extreme boyhood femininity: overview and new research findings. In: DeFries Z, Friedman RC, Corn R, editors. Sexuality: new perspectives. Westport: Greenwood Publishing; 1985. p. 101–24.
3. Tuber S, Coates S. Interpersonal phenomena in the Rorschachs of extremely feminine boys. Psychoanal Psychol. 1985;2:251–65.
4. Saketopoulou A. Mourning the body as bedrock: developmental considerations in treating transsexual patients analytically. Int J Psychoanal. 2014;62:773–806.
5. DeLoache JS, Simcock G, Macari S. Planes, trains, automobiles—and tea sets: extremely intense interests in very young children. Dev Psychol. 2007;43:1579–86.
6. Halim ML, Ruble DN, Lurye LE, Greulich FK, Zosuls KM, Tamis-Lemonda CS. Pink frilly dresses and the avoidance of all things "girly": children's appearance rigidity and cognitive theories of gender development. Dev Psychol. 2014;50:1091–101.
7. Galucci G, Hackerman F, Schmidt CW. Gender identity disorder in an adult male with Asperger's syndrome. Sex Disabil. 2005;23:35–40.
8. Jacobs LA, Rachlin K, Erickson-Schroth L, Janssen A. Gender dysphoria and co-occurring autism spectrum disorders: review, case examples, and treatment considerations. LGBT Health. 2014;1:277–82.
9. Kalafarski EG. Gender identity development in individuals with autism. Unpublished Master of Social Work degree, Smith College School for Social Work, Northampton; 2010.
10. Kraemer B, Delsignore A, Gundelfinger R, Schnyder U, Hepp U. Comorbidity of Asperger syndrome and gender identity disorder. Eur Child Adolesc Psychiatry. 2005;14:292–6.
11. Landén M, Rasmussen P. Gender identity disorder in a girl with autism—a case report. Eur Child Adolesc Psychiatry. 1997;6:170–3.
12. Lemaire M, Thomazeau B, Bonnet-Brilhault F. Gender identity disorder and autism spectrum disorder in a 23-year-old female. Arch Sex Behav. 2014;43:395–8.
13. Mukkades NM. Gender identity problems in autistic children. Child Care Health Dev. 2002;28:529–32.
14. Parkinson J. Gender dysphoria in Asperger's syndrome: a caution. Australas Psychiatry. 2014;22:84–5.
15. Perera H, Gadambanathan T, Weerasiri S. Gender identity disorder presenting in a girl with Asperger's disorder and obsessive compulsive disorder. Ceylon Med J. 2003;48:57–8.
16. Tateno M, Ikeda H, Saito T. Gender dysphoria in pervasive developmental disorders. Seishin Shinkeigaku Zasshi. 2011;113:1172–83.

17. Tateno M, Tateno Y, Saito T. Comorbid childhood gender identity disorder in a boy with Asperger syndrome [Letter to the Editor]. Psychiatry Clin Neurosci. 2008;62:238.

18. Tateno M, Teo AR, Tateno Y. Eleven year follow-up of a boy with Asperger syndrome and comorbid gender identity disorder of childhood. Psychiatry Clin Neurosci. 2015;69:658.

19. Williams PG, Allard AM, Sears L. Case study: cross-gender preoccupations with two male children with autism. J Autism Dev Disord. 1996;26:635–42.

20. de Vries ALC, Noens IL, Cohen-Kettenis PT, van Berckelaer-Onnes IA, Doreleifers TA. Autism spectrum disorders in gender dysphoric children and adolescents. J Autism Dev Disord. 2010;40:930–6.

21. Di Ceglie D, Skagerberg E, Baron-Cohen S, Auyeung B. Empathising and systemising in adolescents with gender dysphoria. Opticon. 2014;12(16):6. doi:10.5334/opt.bo.

22. Shumer DE, Reisner SL, Edwards-Leeper L, Tishelman A. Evaluation of Asperger syndrome in youth presenting to a gender dysphoria clinic. LGBT Health. 2016;3:387–90.

23. Skagerberg E, Di Ceglie D, Carmichael P. Autistic features in children and adolescents with gender dysphoria. J Autism Dev Disord. 2015;45:2628–32.

24. Jones RM, Wheelwright S, Farrell K, Martin E, Green R, Di Ceglie D, Baron-Cohen S. Female-to-male transsexual people and autistic traits. J Autism Dev Disord. 2012;42:301–6.

25. Pasterski V, Gilligan L, Curtis R. Traits of autism spectrum disorders in adults with gender dysphoria. Arch Sex Behav. 2014;43:387–93.

26. Kristensen ZE, Broome MR. Autistic traits in an internet sample of gender variant UK adults. Int J Transgenderism. 2015;16:234–45.

27. Glidden D, Bouman WP, Jones BA, Arcelus J. Gender dysphoria and autism spectrum disorder: a systematic review of the literature. Sex Med Rev. 2016;4:3–14.

28. Strang JF, Meagher H, Kenworthy L, de Vries ALC, Menvielle E, Leibowitz S, et al. Initial clinical guidelines for co-occurring autism spectrum disorder and gender dysphoria or incongruence in adolescents. J Clin Child Adolesc Psychol. 2016. doi:10.1080/15374416.2016.1228462.

29. van der Miesen AIR, Hurley H, de Vries ALC. Gender dysphoria and autism spectrum disorder: a narrative review. Int Rev Psychiatry. 2016;28:70–80.

30. van Schalkwyk GI, Klingensmith K, Volkmar FR. Gender identity and autism spectrum disorders. Yale J Biol Med. 2015;88:81–3.

31. Baron-Cohen S, Wheelwright S. 'Obsessions' in children with autism or Asperger syndrome: content analysis in terms of core domains of cognition. Br J Psychiatry. 1999;175:484–90.

32. Klin A, Danovitch JH, Merz AB, Volkmar FR. Circumscribed interests in higher functioning individuals with autism spectrum disorders: an exploratory study. Res Prac Pers Sev Disabil. 2007;32:89–100.

33. Strang JF, Kenworthy L, Dominska A, Sokoloff J, Kenealy LE, Berl M, et al. Increased gender variance in autism spectrum disorders and attention deficit hyperactivity disorder. Arch Sex Behav. 2014;43:1525–33.

34. Constantino JN, Gruber CP. Social responsiveness scale. 2nd ed. (SRS-2). Torrance: Western Psychological Services; 2012.

35. Campbell DT, Stanley JC. Experimental and quasi-experimental designs for research. Chicago: Rand McNally & Company; 1969.

36. Vanderlaan DP, Postema L, Wood H, Singh D, Fantus S, Hyun J, et al. Do children with gender dysphoria have intense/obsessional interests? J Sex Res. 2015;52:213–9.

37. Achenbach TM. Manual for the child behavior checklist/4-18 and 1991 profile. Burlington: University of Vermont Department of Psychiatry; 1991.

38. Achenbach TM. Manual for the teacher's report form and 1991 profile. Burlington: University of Vermont Department of Psychiatry; 1991.

39. Achenbach TM, Rescorla LA. Manual for the ASEBA school-age forms & profiles. Burlington: University of Vermont, Research Center for Children, Youth, and Families; 2001.

40. Achenbach TM, Edelbrock C. Manual for the teacher's report form and teacher version of the child behavior profile. Burlington: University of Vermont Department of Psychiatry; 1986.

41. Achenbach TM, Rescorla LA. Manual for the ASEBA preschool forms and profiles. Burlington: University of Vermont, Research Center for Children, Youth, and Families; 2000.

42. Hollingshead AB. Four-factor index of social status. Unpublished manuscript, Department of Sociology, Yale University, New Haven; 1975.

43. Cicchetti D, Rogosch FA. Equifinality and multifinality in developmental psychopathology [Editorial]. Dev Psychopathol. 1996;8:597–600.

44. Zucker KJ, Wood H, Singh D, Bradley SJ. A developmental, biopsychosocial model for the treatment of children with gender identity disorder. J Homosex. 2012;59:369–97.

45. Hus V, Bishop S, Gotham S, Huerta M, Lord C. Factors influencing scores on the social responsiveness scale. J Child Psychol Psychiatry. 2013;54:216–24.

46. Cholemkery H, Kitzerow J, Rohrmann S, Freitag CM. Validity of the Social Responsiveness Scale to differentiate between autism spectrum disorders and disruptive behavior disorders. Eur Child Adolesc Psychiatry. 2014;23:81–93.

47. Cholemkery H, Mojica L, Rohrmann S, Gensthaler A, Freitag CM. Can autism spectrum disorders and social anxiety disorders be differentiated by the Social Responsiveness Scale in children and adolescents? J Autism Dev Disord. 2014;44:1168–82.

48. Griffiths DL, Farrell LJ, Waters AM, White SW. ASD traits among youth with obsessive-compulsive disorder. Child Psychiatry Hum Dev. 2017. doi:10.1007/s10578-017-0714-3.

49. Zucker KJ, Leef JH, Wood H, Hughes KH, Wasserman L, VanderLaan DP. LinkedIn? On the relation between gender dysphoria and traits of autism spectrum disorder in children. Paper presented at the meeting of the International Academy of Sex Research, Toronto; 2015.

50. VanderLaan DP, Leef JH, Wood H, Hughes K, Zucker KJ. Autism spectrum disorder risk factors and autistic traits in gender dysphoric children. J Autism Dev Disord. 2015;45:1742–50.

51. Nowack N, Wittsiepe J, Kasper-Sonnenberg M, Wilhelm M, Schölmreich A. Influence of low-level prenatal exposure to PCDD/Fs and PCBs on empathizing, systematizing and autistic traits: results from the Duisburg Birth Cohort Study. PLoS ONE. 2015;10(6):e0129906. doi:10.1371/journal.pone.0129906.

52. Shumer DE, Roberts AL, Reisner SL, Lyall K, Austin SB. Autistic traits in mothers and children associated with child's gender nonconformity. J Autism Dev Disord. 2015;45:1489–94.

53. So P, Greaves-Lord K, van der Ende J, Verhulst PC, Rescorla L, de Nijs PFA. Using the child behavior checklist and the teacher's report form for identification of children with autism spectrum disorders. Autism. 2012;15:595–607.

54. Lord C, Rutter M, DiLavore PC, Risi S, Gotham K, Bishop SL, et al. Autism diagnostic observation schedule. In: 2nd ed: ADOS-2. Oxford: Pearson Assessment; 2012.

17

Supervision trajectories of male juvenile offenders: growth mixture modeling on SAVRY risk assessments

Ed L. B. Hilterman[1,2,3]* , Ilja L. Bongers[1,2], Tonia L. Nicholls[4,5] and Chijs van Nieuwenhuizen[1,2]

Abstract

Background: Structured risk/need assessment tools are increasingly used to orientate risk reduction strategies with juvenile offenders. The assumption is that the risk/need items on these tools are sufficiently sensitive to measure changes in the individual, family and/or contextual characteristics of juvenile offenders. However, there is very little research demonstrating the capacity of these tools to measure changes in juvenile offenders. Congruent with the developmental and life-course criminology theories (DLC) the objective of this study is to explore the existence of heterogeneous trajectories of juvenile offenders across the juvenile justice system as measured through five empirical risk/need areas based on the Structured Assessment of Violence Risk in Youth (SAVRY), one of the most widely applied risk assessment tools for juveniles.

Methods: This longitudinal study included 5205 male juvenile offenders who transitioned through the Catalan juvenile justice system between 2006 and 2014. During intervention they received at least two, and a maximum of seven, consecutive SAVRY risk/need assessments over an 18-month period. The heterogeneity of latent class trajectories was explored through growth mixture modeling (GMM). The trajectory class membership was linked to covariates through multinomial logistic regression analyses.

Results: Through GMM three to four heterogeneous trajectories, with high quality of separation, were identified in each of the risk/need areas. The trajectories with low risk/needs (45–77% of the sample) remained low and presented a very limited increase in risk/needs during the 18-month period. The high risk/need trajectories (20–37% of the sample) showed a limited decrease or no change. Between 5 and 13% of the sample had large reductions in their risk/needs levels, and approximately 5% showed a large increase in risk/needs.

Conclusions: In line with the DLC theories this study shows that trajectories on criminogenic risk/needs can be heterogeneous and indicate distinct rates of change over time. The results of this study also may suggest a limited sensibility to measure change over time of SAVRY's risk and protective items. Suggestions to improve the sensitivity of measuring change over time, such as shorter time frames or future-oriented time frames for the scoring of the items, are offered.

Keywords: Dynamic risk factors, Juvenile offenders, Growth mixture modeling, Risk assessment, Risk/need trajectories, SAVRY

Background

Juvenile offenders have been characterized as 'moving targets' [1]. This refers to the short-term behavioural

*Correspondence: ehilterman@justamesura.com
[3] Justa Mesura, Consultancy & Applied Research, Barcelona, Spain
Full list of author information is available at the end of the article

change juvenile offenders can exhibit, and reflects the particular importance of dynamic criminogenic needs for the orientation of risk reduction strategies with adolescents. Especially in violence risk assessment with juvenile offenders these criminogenic needs gained importance in the shift from a prediction-oriented model to a need-oriented model. Validated risk and need assessment tools played an important role in this change [2]. According to the need-oriented model, risk and need assessment tools are used to guide risk reduction strategies that target specific criminogenic needs that are relevant in individual cases [3]. The underlying assumption is that the targeted risk and need factors have the capacity to change and that these variables, as defined on risk assessment measures, are sensitive to change over time.

Adolescent offending trajectories can change under the influence of emotional processes [4], intimate relations, neighbourhood and community processes, and life-events related to family, education or work [5]. As a result of these processes and life-events changes in offending trajectories during adolescence are common [5] and can have distinct implications such as desisting, escalating, and persisting trajectories [6]. Also the involvement in the juvenile justice system can have effects on desistence or persistence in delinquent behaviour. Juvenile justice programs are intended to reduce juvenile delinquency. However, these programs often are unavailable or poor in quality [7] or do not sufficiently address the criminogenic needs of the juveniles [8]. Illustrating these problems, Viljoen et al. found that treatment received by juvenile offenders was not associated with change in their risk/needs [9]. It is important to match treatment to the individual's risk/needs, after a comprehensive risk/need assessment [10].

The Structured Assessment of Violence Risk in Youth (SAVRY) [11] is one of the most widely used risk and need assessment tools for juvenile offenders. Unfortunately, there is very little known about the extent to which SAVRY is capable of measuring the changes that juvenile offenders experience during adolescence. In a retrospective study in Canada, Viljoen et al. [12] found that approximately one-third part of the sample of 163 juvenile sex offenders, who attended a residential cognitive-behavioural program, showed a decrease in their average scores on the SAVRY dynamic risk items and 8% had an increase on the average scores of the protective items. In a longitudinal study with male ($n = 107$) and female ($n = 49$) juvenile offenders, Viljoen et al. [13] reported that SAVRY reassessments during the probation period were no more predictive than the initial assessment at the start of the probation, suggesting that the average change in risk/needs between the two moments in time had no influence on the predictive validity of the risk assessment. In another Canadian study of 146 juvenile offenders (69.2% male) on probation, Viljoen et al. [9] found that the SAVRY mean-level change scores (baseline scores minus follow-up scores) of the risk and protective items showed limited internal sensitivity to change (i.e., change over time).

These studies were based on the assumption that change trajectories are homogeneous and reflect linear change within the population of interest. However, if change trajectories are not homogeneous but heterogeneous and consist of distinct change trajectories, for example one group with decreasing risk scores and another with increasing scores, the averaging change scores across subgroups could disguise changes, falsely indicating there is no transition over time. The identification of heterogeneous trajectories of change over time is congruent with the developmental and life-course criminology theories (DLC) [14]. According to the DLC theories, the assessment of developmental trajectories of risk and protective factors through longitudinal research can assist in the understanding of within-individual changes over time [15].

Following the DLC theories on the heterogeneity of developmental trajectories, the current study explored the existence of heterogeneous trajectories measured by risk and protective items of male juvenile offenders assessed on SAVRY [11]. The principal research question of this study was: Are there distinct developmental trajectories of male juvenile offenders across the juvenile justice system measured through five empirical risk/need domains based on SAVRY items? Our second question examined whether antecedents (e.g., prior violent and non-violent offenses, previously detained), demographics (e.g., age) and characteristics of the transition through the juvenile justice services could differentiate between any trajectories that emerged.

Methods
Sample
The multiyear sample consisted of 5205 male juvenile offenders for whom at least two SAVRY risk assessments were completed by professionals of the Catalonian juvenile justice system, in the period from January 2, 2006 until September 10, 2014. At the time of the first SAVRY assessment the juveniles had an average age of approximately 17 years ($M = 17.64$; $SD = 1.40$). When they were charged for their first offense, their mean age was 15.72 years ($SD = 1.13$). The majority of the sample was of Spanish origin ($n = 2883$, 55.4%); the remainder were of European ($n = 191$, 3.7%), African ($n = 1065$, 20.5%), South American ($n = 989$, 19.0%) or Asian ($n = 77$, 1.5%) origin. The mean total score of the first SAVRY assessment was 16.08 ($SD = 9.24$), with a range from 0 to 45 (theoretical range 0–48). The average total score of the protective factors was 2.71 ($SD = 1.95$), with a range of 0 to 6. Before the first SAVRY assessment, 86.2% ($n = 4489$) of the male juveniles had been charged with at least one violent offense ($M = 4.51$, $SD = 5.10$, $Mdn = 3.00$), and 68.0% ($n = 3541$) with at least one

non-violent offense ($M = 4.05$, $SD = 4.83$, $Mdn = 3.00$). The proportion of juveniles with a history of youth detention was 17.3% ($n = 898$, $M = 2.91$, $SD = 2.64$). Measured on the number of imposed sentences ($N = 13,228$), the average duration of community probation in the research period was approximately 12 months ($M = .97$ year, $Mdn = .74$, $SD = .71$), and the average duration of detention ($N = 7221$) in a youth detention centre was .64 years ($Mdn = .49$, $SD = .69$).

Between 2006 and 2014 a total of 79,223 SAVRY assessments were completed for the sample. Due to the different duration of penal interventions the juveniles had been subject to a variable number of consecutive SAVRY assessments during their juvenile justice intervention. At the start of the intervention all juveniles had at least two consecutive SAVRY risk assessments, 85.23% ($n = 4436$) had three consecutive assessments, 66.67% ($n = 3470$) had four assessments, 50.70% ($n = 2639$) had five assessments, 38.89% ($n = 2024$) had six assessments and 30.41% ($n = 1583$) had seven consecutive SAVRY assessments over the 18 month study period. The total of SAVRY assessment included in this study was 24,562.

Setting

The Catalonian Justice department administers sentences for adults and juveniles in Catalonia, Spain. The juvenile sector is divided into three sections, pre-trial assessment, probation, and custody. The pre-trial assessment section is divided into eight units that work in close collaboration with the office of the public prosecutor. The probation section, with nine juvenile probation units, is responsible for the administration of all community sanctions. *Llibertat vigilada*, or community probation, is the most frequently imposed sanction. The custody section consists of six youth detention centres. Juveniles from the different settings of the juvenile system are not necessarily distinct groups. For instance, after detention in a custodial setting, juveniles always have community probation and juveniles who violate the conditions of the probation can be transferred to a custodial setting. The intervention most often applied during the research period was probation supervision, 10.7% of juveniles were also sentenced to detention. Juvenile justice professionals could apply treatment components like group or individual programs directed towards violent or sexual offenders, mental health problems, drug abuse, and/or family problems (Fig. 1).

Measures

Structured Assessment of Violence Risk in Youth (SAVRY) [11, 16] is a risk assessment tool in the structured professional judgment (SPJ) tradition. The SAVRY contains 24 risk items and 6 protective items. Each risk item is scored on a 3-point scale; low (0), moderate (1) or high risk (2). Protective items are scored present (1) or absent (0) (note—for interpretation purposes protective items have been reverse scored). The final summary risk rating is the product of a clinical reflection on the basis of the information gathered on the particular juvenile and is not based on a sum score. For research purposes, the risk and protective items can be summed up into total scores with a range from 0 to 48, and 0 to 6, respectively.

Results regarding inter-rater reliability (intraclass correlation coefficients (ICC), two way random effects model for absolute agreement and single raters) with SAVRY in the Catalonian juvenile justice system have been published elsewhere and ranged from .93 for the historical items to .57 for the protective items [17]. Intraclass correlations are often interpreted as follows: $< .40 = $ poor; .40 to .59 = fair; .60 to .74 = good; and .75 to 1.00 = excellent [18].

Instead of relying on the conceptual subscales of SAVRY proposed by the authors for the current study we used a gender sensitive order of the SAVRY items as per their categorization into five factors representing specific risk/need areas based on prior research (see Fig. 1) [17]. Three fit indices were used to assess the fit of the factor models: the comparative fit index (CFI), the Tucker–Lewis index (TLI) and a root mean square of approximation (RMSEA), CFI and TLI exceeding .90, indicate acceptable fit, while values close to .95 are recommended [19]. A RMSEA value close to .06 indicates a good fit [19]. In exploratory factor analyses performed in Mplus [20], both models had a good fit (Males: CFI = .96; TLI = .94; RMSEA = .053, 90% CI .051, .055); females: (CFI = .95; TLI = .94; RMSEA = .049, 90% CI [.044, .054]) these were replicated in confirmatory factor analyses with the validation sample (Males: CFI = .94, TLI = .93, RMSEA = .059, 90% CI [.058, .061], females: CFI = .91, TLI = .90, RMSEA = .063, 90% CI [.058, .068]). The five risk/needs areas had good internal consistency for both genders (between .81 and .71 for males and .82–.70 for females). For the growth mixture modeling the SAVRY items of each of the five risk/need areas were summed up and divided through the theoretical range of the scale, which resulted in a score between 0 and 1. The SAVRY assessments were obtained from a database that is part of the electronic information system of the Catalonian Juvenile Justice system (*Sistema d'Informació de Justícia Juvenil*, SIJJ). All data were anonymized to avoid identification of participants.

Criminal history data and the below listed covariates were collected for each individual from the information systems for juvenile and adult offenders of the Catalonian Department of Justice. These official databases include

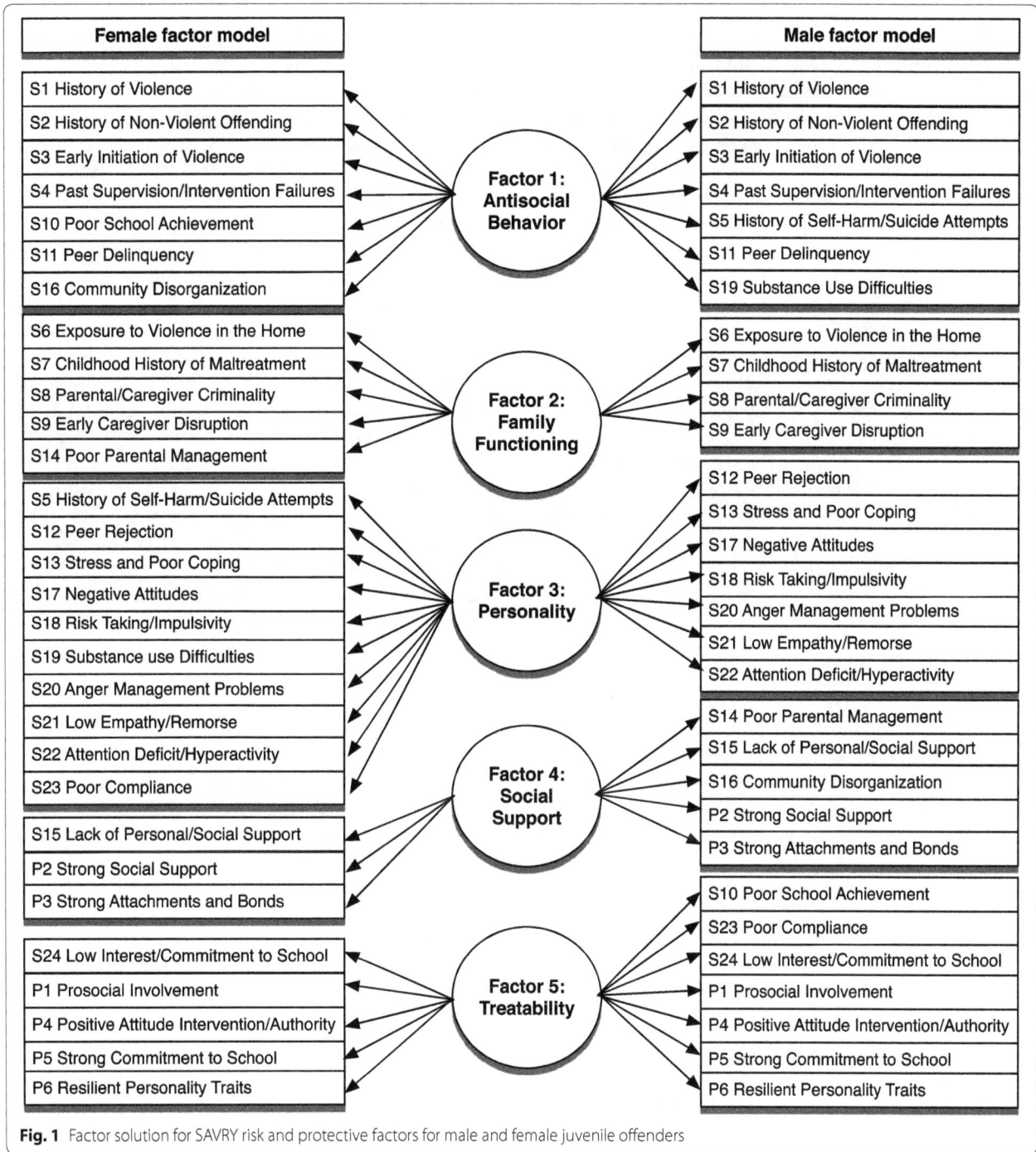

Fig. 1 Factor solution for SAVRY risk and protective factors for male and female juvenile offenders

records of impending prosecutions, convictions, and the process of the execution of sanctions.

Age at first assessment reflects the date of the first SAVRY assessment.

Prior offenses were classified as violent versus non-violent as defined in the SAVRY manual and were measured by the number of criminal charges registered before the

first SAVRY assessment. Because *prior violent offenses and non-violent offenses* were Poisson distributed both variables were recoded into four categories: 0 = zero prior offenses, 1 = first offenders with only one offense preceding the first SAVRY assessment, 2 = 2–9 offenses and 3 = 10 or more prior offenses. The first category, zero prior offenses, was used as the reference category for both variables.

Previous detention was measured as a dichotomous variable, with "0" not previously detained, and "1" having been detained before the first SAVRY risk assessment.

Number of sector changes An increase in the *number of sector changes* between the three sectors of the juvenile justice system is an indication of a problematic passing through the system. Sector changes were measured from the start of the transition through the juvenile justice system, up until the last SAVRY risk/need assessment that was performed. The minimum value was "0", and the maximum value was "3".

Sentence duration During the research period the average duration of community probation, the most frequently imposed sanction, was approximately 12 months ($M = .97$ year, $Mdn = .74$, $SD = .71$). The length of the current sentence (*sentence > 1-year*) was measured as a dichotomized variable with the 1-year average duration as reference ($1 = sentence > 1\text{-}year$, $0 = sentence \leq 1\text{-}year$).

Procedure

According to the protocols that were developed for the implementation of structured risk/need assessments in the Catalonian juvenile justice system, professionals have been using the SAVRY since 2006 for routine risk/need assessments at different points before and during the penal sanction: (a) during pre-trial assessment; (b) at the start of a youth's probation (*llibertat vigilada*) or detention; (c) every 3 months during the probation period or the youth's detention; and (d) at the end of the sentence when the last assessment is performed. Following the method of structured professional judgment, SAVRY risk/need assessment was used to identify relevant goals for the intervention with every individual. From 2006 until 2008 the SAVRY was gradually implemented in the whole Catalonian juvenile justice sector. Before using SAVRY, all professionals (i.e., youth probation officers, group leaders, social workers and psychologists) received 20 h of risk assessment training. After the training, individual supervision was provided. Approximately 1–2 years after the initial training professionals participated in an advanced training to refresh practical and theoretical knowledge. Professionals also received ongoing training on how to target criminogenic needs during intervention.

Statistical analysis

Growth mixture modeling (GMM) in Mplus 7.1 [20] was used to examine the existence of trajectory heterogeneity in the risk and need developmental pathways of juvenile offenders during their intervention in the juvenile justice system. For each possible class GMM estimates the level of the initial status (intercept), linear change over time (linear slope) and nonlinear change over time (quadratic slope) and for each variable the variance and covariance's were estimated. A slope that is significantly different from zero indicates change over time. Change has a linear form when the trajectory is constant across the time points (linear slope) or a nonlinear curvature form (quadratic slope) when the slope describes accelerating or decelerating trajectories.

The number of latent trajectory classes was estimated using three indicators: the Bayesian Information Criterion (BIC), the Lo-Mendell-Rubin adjusted likelihood ratio test and the class size. A model with a lower BIC value performs better in terms of taking into account both fit and parsimony. The BIC was preferred over the adjusted BIC because of its better performance with continuous outcomes [21]. The Lo-Mendell-Rubin adjusted likelihood ratio test (LMR-LRT) compares the fit of the model with one more class to the previously estimated model with one less class. A significant p value of the LMR-LRT indicates that the model with one less class is rejected in favor of the model with one more class. To avoid small classes, models with a class size smaller than 3.0% were rejected as larger classes are preferred to smaller classes which can be less meaningful [21].

The entropy and the average posterior latent class probabilities were used to assess the quality of the trajectory classifications. Both indices have a range between 0 and 1; higher values indicate a better separation between the classes. Entropy values of .80, .60 and .40 indicate high, medium and low class separation [22]. The average latent class probability for each class reflects the highest probability of each individual assigned to a particular class. To avoid incorrect class solutions due to 'local maxima' all models were replicated twice using the seed values from the highest log-likelihood values as described by Asparouhov and Muthen [23]. Through these replications it was confirmed that the models were stable and the model parameters were based on the global solution. Adolescents with shorter sanctions have fewer SAVRY assessments and consequently fewer data points. Elimination of these juveniles from the research would have resulted in the absence of juveniles with shorter sanctions. To include these juveniles with less data points in the analysis, the full-information maximum likelihood (FIML) was used to estimate these missing data points of juveniles whose penal sanctions were shorter than 18 months [24, 25].

The trajectory class membership of the five risk/needs areas was linked to covariates through multinomial logistic regression analyses. To eliminate non-significant variables from the equation the backward stepwise method, with the lowest risk/need trajectory classes as reference categories, was used. For the interpretation of the odds ratio (OR) we followed the criteria suggested by previous research [26] in which an OR with a value between 2 and 3 was considered small, 3–5 medium and above 5 large.

Results

Selection of the latent trajectory classes

For the risk/need areas antisocial behaviour, family functioning and personality the linear model with intercept and linear slope was sufficient to describe the model, the incorporation of the quadratic slope in the model resulted in LMR-LRT values that were not significant. The models of the risk/need areas social support and treatability improved after the incorporation of the quadratic slope into the model. Because of the better fit of the model, for the risk/need areas social support and treatability we reported the model with the incorporation of the quadratic slope, for the remaining risk/need areas the model with the linear slope was reported. For each of the risk/need areas, the optimal number of latent class trajectories was estimated; fit statistics for the five models are summarized in Table 1.

For the risk/need area antisocial behaviour the model with three classes was preferred. Although the BIC continued to decrease and the LMR-LRT was significant for the models with four classes, the four-class model identified a class that was too small (.5%, $n = 28$). The entropy (.80) and average posterior probabilities, .93, .87 and .88, for all three classes indicated a clear separation between the trajectories. For the risk/need area family functioning a three-class model fit the data best, a model with four classes was rejected due to the non-significant LMR-LRT ($p = .16$). The classification indices of the three-class model of family functioning indicated a high quality of separation between classes with an entropy of .89 and average posterior probabilities of .97, .89 and .94, respectively. For the personality risk/need area a model with five classes was rejected by the LMR-LRT in favour of a four-class model, moreover the five-class model had one class that was too small (1.5%, $n = 78$). The entropy of the four-class model was .69, and the average posterior probabilities were .76, 80, .87 and .80 for the classes one to four, indicating a slightly above medium quality of class separation. For the risk/need areas social support and treatability also the quadratic slope was included in the model, this resulted in improved class separation and indicated nonlinear development over time. The four-class model fit the data best for the social support risk/need area; the LMT-LRT rejected the five-class model, which also had one too small class (2.1%, $n = 111$). For treatability, the last risk/need area based on SAVRY, a four-class model was also preferred. Although the BIC value of the five-class model was smaller compared to

Table 1 Model fit indices for growth mixture models

Model	BIC	LMR-LRT	Entropy	Smallest class %/(n)
Antisocial behaviour				
1	− 42,552.08	n/a	n/a	n/a
2	− 43,352.39	p < .001	.91	.039 (202)
3	− 44,042.78	p < .001	.80	.040 (207)
4	− 44,209.88	p = .006	.84	.005 (28)
5	− 44,286.48	p = .33	.83	.006 (29)
Family functioning				
1	− 50,973.55	n/a	n/a	n/a
2	− 52,575.68	p < .001	.87	.209 (1088)
3	− 53,646.03	p < .001	.89	.033 (170)
4	− 54,171.66	p = .16	.87	.027 (140)
5	− 54,506.86	p = .20	.90	.021 (111)
Personality				
1	− 29,962.82	n/a	n/a	n/a
2	− 30,254.27	p < .001	.61	.318 (1653)
3	− 30,519.34	p < .001	.74	.157 (818)
4	− 30,721.70	p < .001	.69	.043 (222)
5	− 30,775.80	p = .081	.70	.015 (78)
Social support				
1	− 24,159.37	n/a	n/a	n/a
2	− 24,714.14	p < .001	.72	.337 (1755)
3	− 25,136.04	p < .001	.80	.029 (151)
4	− 25,733.02	p < .001	.82	.053 (278)
5	− 25,913.54	p = .240	.82	.021 (111)
Treatability				
1	− 18,466.19	n/a	n/a	n/a
2	− 18,845.24	p < .001	.65	.416 (2165)
3	− 18,996.01	p < .001	.67	.090 (468)
4	− 19,470.22	p < .001	.75	.049 (256)
5	− 19,559.41	p = .240	.76	.022 (114)

Entropy and LMR-LRT are not applicable for the 1-class model. The values in italics indicate the selected model

BIC Bayesian Information Criterion, *LMR-LRT* Lo-Mendell-Rubin adjusted likelihood ratio test, *Entropy* average quality of classification

the BIC of the previous model, the difference was small, as was the difference between the entropy values (5-class model = .76, 4-class model = .75). The five-class model contained one class which was under the 3.0% cut-off value for the smallest class (2.2%, $n = 114$). The average posterior probabilities of the four-class model were, .86, .88, .84, and .84, respectively.

The developmental processes of the risk/needs areas

The latent class trajectories of the different risk/need areas are shown in Fig. 2.

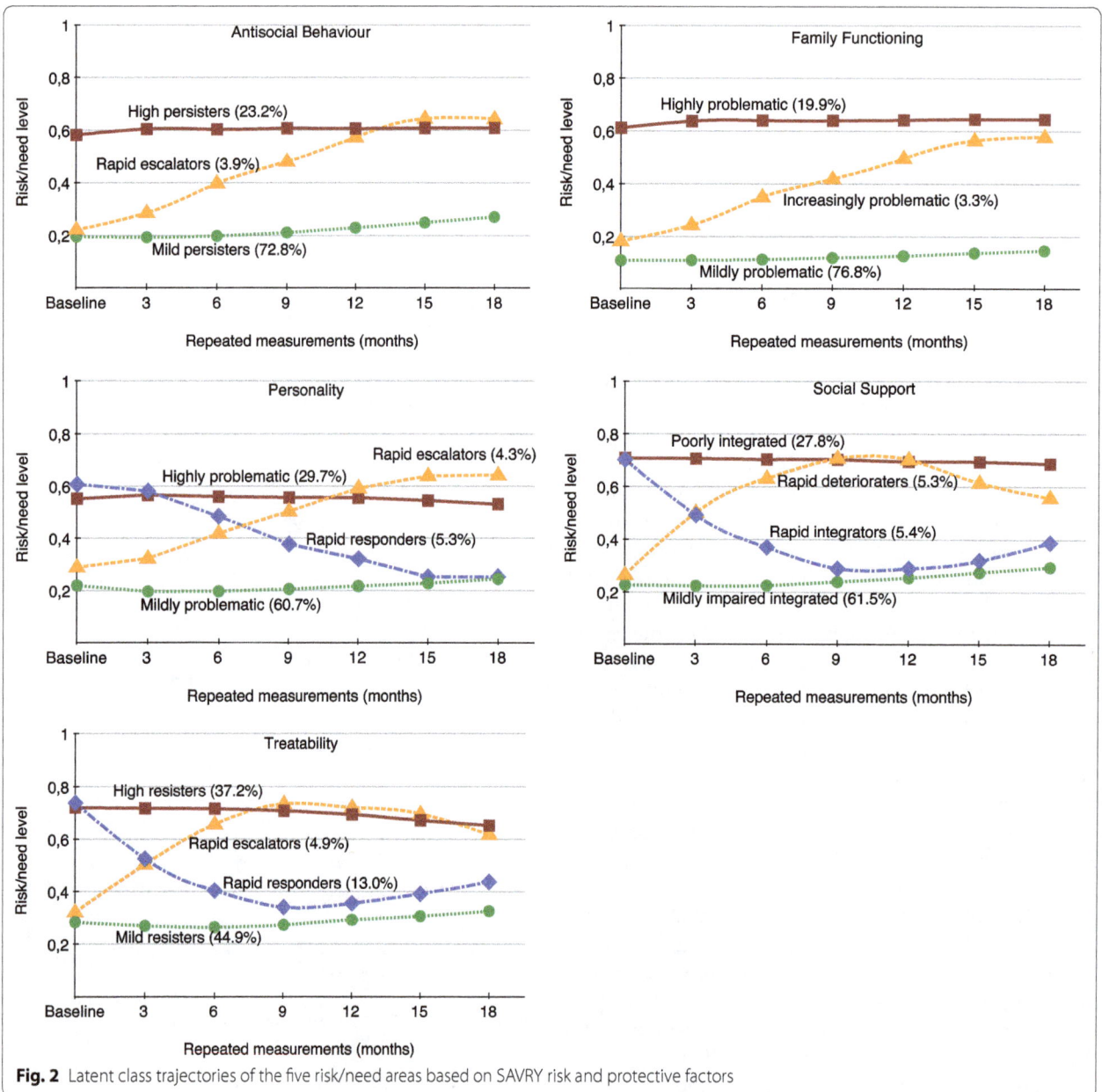

Fig. 2 Latent class trajectories of the five risk/need areas based on SAVRY risk and protective factors

Antisocial behaviour

The largest class (mild persisters, 72.8%, $n = 3788$) was characterized by a low initial status of antisocial behaviour ($\beta_{intercept} = .195$, $p < .001$), which slowly increased during the transition through juvenile justice ($\beta_{linear\ slope} = .002$, $p < .001$; see Fig. 2). The second largest class (High persisters, 23.2%, $n = 1210$) had a high initial status of antisocial behaviour ($\beta_{intercept} = .604$, $p < .001$) and did not change during the study period ($\beta_{linear\ slope} = -.001$, $p > .05$). The smallest group, the rapid escalators (4.0%, $n = 207$) had a low initial status of antisocial behaviour

($\beta_{intercept} = .214$, $p < .001$), and escalated rapidly to a high level ($\beta_{linear\ slope} = .093$, $p < .001$).

Family functioning

The largest group (76.8%, $n = 4000$) was mildly problematic at the starting point ($\beta_{intercept} = .109$, $p < .001$), and during consecutive assessments slightly more problems were detected ($\beta_{linear\ slope} = .001$, $p < .01$). The second largest class (19.9%, $n = 1035$) was observed to be highly problematic at the initial assessment ($\beta_{intercept} = .632$, $p < .001$), and this did not change over time ($\beta_{slope} = .002$, $p > .05$). The smallest group (3.3%, $n = 170$) was increasingly problematic; the initial observation was mildly problematic ($\beta_{\text{intercept}} = .177, p < .001$), but during subsequent assessments significant more problems were observed ($\beta_{\text{linear slope}} = .085, p < .001$).

Personality

The largest class (60.7%, $n = 3162$) was initially characterized by mildly problematic personality traits ($\beta_{\text{intercept}} = .206, p < .001$), which changed minimally over the 18-months period ($\beta_{\text{linear slope}} = -.003, p < .01$). The highly problematic class trajectory had a high starting point (29.7%, $n = 1546$, $\beta_{\text{intercept}} = .596, p < .001$) and exhibited limited improvement during successive assessments ($\beta_{\text{linear slope}} = -.006, p < .001$). The rapid responders (5.3%, $n = 275$), had a high initial status ($\beta_{\text{intercept}} = .648, p < .001$), but improved rapidly during the intervention ($\beta_{\text{linear slope}} = -.087, p < .001$). The rapid escalators (4.3%, $n = 222$) started the trajectory as a mildly problematic group ($\beta_{\text{intercept}} = .269, p < .001$), but rapidly became more problematic ($\beta_{\text{linear slope}} = .076$, $p < .001$).

Social support

The mildly impaired integrators were the largest group (61.5%, $n = 3200$, $\beta_{\text{intercept}} = .227, p < .001$); this group remained stable during the first 6 months of the trajectory ($\beta_{\text{linear slope}} = -.005, p > .05$), and deteriorated slowly during the final 12 months ($\beta_{\text{quadratic slope}} = .002, p < .001$). Almost a third of the sample (27.8%, $n = 1448$) was poorly integrated at baseline ($\beta_{\text{intercept}} = .709, p < .001$), and did not change during subsequent assessments ($\beta_{\text{linear slope}} = .000, p > .05, \beta_{\text{quadratic slope}} = -.001, p > .05$). The rapid integrators had a poor initial status (5.4%, $n = 279$, $\beta_{\text{intercept}} = .697, p < .001$), improved rapidly during the first 12 months ($\beta_{\text{linear slope}} = -.220, p < .001$) but experienced a limited decrease towards the end of the 18-month period ($\beta_{\text{quadratic slope}} = .027, p < .001$). To the contrary, the rapid deterioraters started out as relatively well socially integrated (5.3%, $n = 278$, $\beta_{\text{intercept}} = .275$, $p < .001$), deteriorated rapidly during the initial 9 months ($\beta_{\text{linear slope}} = .254, p < .001$), but then improved slightly towards the end of the trajectory ($\beta_{\text{quadratic slope}} = -.036$, $p < .001$).

Treatability

The largest group, the mild resisters (44.9%, $n = 2337$), exhibited low levels of treatment resistance at baseline ($\beta_{\text{intercept}} = .284, p < .001$), and increased slightly after an initial decrease ($\beta_{\text{linear slope}} = -.016, p < .001, \beta_{\text{quadratic slope}} = .003, p < .001$). The high resisters (37.2%, $n = 1936$, $\beta_{\text{intercept}} = .719, p < .001$) exhibited a high degree of resistance initially but improved somewhat after a short stable period ($\beta_{\text{linear slope}} = .003, p > .05, \beta_{\text{quadratic}}$

slope $= -.003, p < .001$). The rapid responders (13.0%, $n = 676$) started with a high degree of resistance initially ($\beta_{\text{intercept}} = .730, p < .001$), improved rapidly ($\beta_{\text{linear slope}} = -.221, p < .001$), but had a setback after the first 12 months ($\beta_{\text{quadratic slope}} = .029, p < .001$). The rapid escalators (4.9%, $n = 256$) started with low-moderate resistance ($\beta_{\text{intercept}} = .320, p < .001$), escalated rapidly to high resistance ($\beta_{\text{linear slope}} = .227, p < .001$), and improved somewhat in the last part of the intervention ($\beta_{\text{quadratic slope}} = -.030, p < .001$), but never returned to anywhere near baseline.

Association between covariates and latent trajectory class membership

Tables 2 and 3 show the odds ratios and the 95% confidence intervals of the multinomial logistic regression analyses that link the covariates to the latent trajectory class membership of the risk/need areas antisocial behaviour and family functioning (Table 2) and personality, social support and treatability (Table 3). Here we will mainly focus our discussion on medium and large odds ratios.

Antisocial behaviour

All variables in the model were significantly associated with trajectory class membership, which resulted in a significant fit ($\chi^2(20) = 1326.64, p < .001$, Nagelkerke $R^2 = .299$). Under the influence of the other variables, being younger in age increased the odds (OR $= .068$) of being in the rapid escalator trajectory more than in de mild persisters trajectory (for example, compared to a 17 year old juvenile, a 14 year old had a 4.41 higher likelihood ($4.41 = 1/.68$ multiplied by the 3 years difference in age) to be in the rapid escalator class). Juveniles who previously committed ten or more violent and non-violent offenses had a higher likelihood (OR $= 9.10$ for prior violence, OR $= 8.46$ for non-violent offenses) to be in the high persistent trajectory compared to juveniles with no offenses in the mild persistent trajectory. Adolescents who had a lower frequency of prior violent and non-violent offenses (two to nine) this likelihood was approximately three times higher for each of the offense types. For the rapid escalators only ten or more prior violent offenses increased the likelihood (OR $= 4.67$) of being in this rapid ascending trajectory, compared to the mild persisters who did not commit violent offenses. Also an increasing number of changes between sectors of the juvenile justice system, an indication of difficulties during the execution of the sanction, increased the odds of being in the rapid escalator trajectory (OR $= 2.52$ per change). The rapid escalators had a higher average number of changes between the three sectors of the juvenile justice system ($M = 1.43, SD = .88$) compared to the mild

Table 2 Multivariate odds ratios and confidence intervals for predictors of latent trajectory membership for the risk/need areas antisocial behaviour and family functioning (*N* = 5205)

Antisocial behaviour	Latent class trajectories Odds ratios [confidence intervals]	
	Rapid escalators	High persisters
Nagelkerke R^2 .299		
Age at first assessment	.68** [.61, .77]	.99 [.94, 1.05]
Prior violent offenses		
0 (reference category)	1.00	1.00
1	1.12 [.57, 2.61]	1.46* [1.04, 2.05]
2–9	1.77 [.92, 3.40]	3.02** [2.30, 3.98]
≥ 10	4.67** [2.17, 10.05]	9.10** [6.38, 12.99]
Prior non-violent offenses		
0 (reference category)	1.00	1.00
1	1.83* [1.19, 2.82]	1.96** [1.55, 2.47]
2–9	2.18** [1.53, 3.11]	3.18** [2.64, 3.83]
≥ 10	1.11 [.42, 2.92]	8.46** [6.14, 11.66]
Previous detention	1.47 [.84, 2.59]	2.40** [1.83, 3.14]
Number of sector changes	2.52** [2.16, 2.96]	1.49** [1.36, 1.64]
Sentence > 1 year	2.20** [1.46, 3.32]	2.24** [1.88, 2.66]
Family functioning	**Latent class trajectories Odds ratios [confidence intervals]**	
	Increasingly problematic	Highly problematic
Nagelkerke R^2 .067		
Age at first assessment	.83** [.74, .94]	.97 [.92, 1.02]
Prior violent offenses		
0 (reference category)	1.00	1.00
1	2.43* [1.02, 5.76]	.91 [.69, 1.21]
2–9	2.47* [1.12, 5.42]	1.21 [.96, 1.52]
≥ 10	5.35** [2.24, 12.74]	1.98** [1.44, 2.71]
Prior non-violent offenses		
0 (reference category)	1.00	1.00
1	.98 [.59, 1.63]	1.19 [.96, 1.47]
2–9	1.44 [.99, 2.10]	1.41** [1.18, 1.67]
≥ 10	1.87 [.99, 3.55]	2.19** [1.62, 2.96]
Previous detention	1.24 [.73, 2.11]	1.50** [1.16, 1.94]
Number of sector changes	1.55** [1.31–1.85]	1.11* [1.01, 1.22]
Sentence > 1 year	1.75** [1.16, 2.63]	1.36** [1.16, 1.59]

The "mild persisters" trajectory class serves as reference category in the Antisocial behaviour risk/need area, and the "mildly problematic" is the reference category in the Family functioning risk/need area. Previously detained = 1, not previously detained = 0. Duration sentence ≤ 1 year = 0, duration sentence > 1 year = 1

Multinomial logistic regression analyses, with backwards stepwise elimination, was used to link covariates to trajectory class membership

* *p* < .05, ** *p* < .01

persisters (*M* = .44, *SD* = .67) and the high persisters (*M* = .81, *SD* = .90, *F*(2, 5202) = 263.65, *p* < .001).

Family functioning

All covariates had a significant association with trajectory membership and the fit of the model was significant (χ^2(20) = 258.45, *p* < .001, Nagelkerke R^2 = .067).

However, the effect sizes of the odds ratios were generally small. Juveniles who were previously charged with ten or more violent offenses had a high likelihood (OR = 5.35) of being in the increasingly problematic trajectory compared to juveniles with no violent offenses in the mildly problematic trajectory. Compared to the mildly problematic group, also the number of changes between

Table 3 Multivariate odds ratios and confidence intervals for predictors of latent trajectory membership for the risk/ need areas personality, social support and treatability (N = 5205)

Personality	Latent class trajectories Odds ratios [confidence intervals]		
	Rapid responders	Rapid escalators	Highly problematic
Nagelkerke R^2 .158			
Age at first assessment	.85** [.78–.94]	.85** [.76–.95]	.87** [.83, .91]
Prior violent offenses			
0 (reference category)	1.00	1.00	1.00
1	1.99* [1.02, 3.86]	1.83 [.93, 3.62]	1.31* [1.01, 1.69]
2–9	2.69** [1.49, 4.86]	1.93* [1.06, 3.52]	1.68** [1.36, 2.09]
≥ 10	5.84** [2.91, 11.73]	5.04** [2.49, 10.21]	4.00** [2.92, 5.50]
Prior non-violent offenses			
0 (reference category)	1.00	1.00	1.00
1	1.14 [.79, 1.64]	1.40 [.90, 2.16]	1.39** [1.15, 1.68]
2–9	1.11 [.82, 1.49]	1.78** [1.26, 2.52]	1.56** [1.33, 1.82]
≥ 10	1.53 [.88, 2.68]	2.35** [1.29, 4.27]	2.18** [1.61, 2.95]
Previous detention	1.62* [1.03, 2.56]	1.12 [.65, 1.92]	1.77** [1.36, 2.30]
Number of sector changes	1.63** [1.40, 1.90]	2.21** [1.89, 2.58]	1.31** [1.20, 1.44]
Sentence > 1 year	1.97** [1.45, 2.69]	2.21** [1.89, 2.58]	1.66** [1.44, 1.91]

Social support	Latent class trajectories Odds ratios [confidence intervals]		
	Rapid integrators	Rapid deteriorators	Poorly integrated
Nagelkerke R^2 .137			
Age at first assessment	.89* [.81, .98]	.86** [.78, .95]	.96 [.91, 1.00]
Prior violent offenses			
0 (reference category)	1.00	1.00	1.00
1	1.70* [1.00, 2.89]	1.28 [.71, 2.28]	1.13* [.88, 1.46]
2–9	1.61* [1.01, 2.57]	1.62 [.99, 2.66]	1.28* [1.04, 1.58]
≥ 10	1,47 [.75, 2.89]	2.61** [1.39, 4.89]	2.43** [1.79, 3.30]
Prior non-violent offenses			
0 (reference category)	1.00	1.00	1.00
1	1.31 [.91, 1.90]	1.68** [1.17, 2.40]	1.52** [1.24, 1.85]
2–9	1.62** [1.20, 2.19]	1.52** [1.12, 2.06]	2.01** [1.71, 2.36]
≥ 10	2.20** [1.22, 3.97]	1.90* [1.03, 3.49]	3.63** [2.68, 4.91]
Previous detention	2.03** [1.28, 3.23]	1.73* [1.09, 2.76]	1.88** [1.44, 2.46]
Number of sector changes	1.77** [1.51, 2.06]	2.07** [1.79, 2.40]	1.31** [1.19, 1.43]
Sentence > 1 year	1.12 [.85, 1.49]	1.18 [.88, 1.58]	1.80** [1.55, 2.09]

Treatability	Latent class trajectories Odds ratios [confidence intervals]		
	Rapid responders	Rapid escalators	High resisters
Nagelkerke R^2 .133			
Age at first assessment	.86** [.80, .92]	.84** [.74, .90]	.86** [.82, .90]
Prior violent offenses			
0 (reference category)	1.00	1.00	1.00
1	1.47* [1.00, 2.16]	1.31 [.79, 2.19]	.88 [.70, 1.12]
2–9	2.15** [1.54, 2.99]	1.15 [.73, 1.80]	1.09 [.89, 1.32]
≥ 10	2.07** [1.30, 3.31]	2.03* [1.12, 3.68]	1.27 [.93, 1.74]
Prior non-violent offenses			
0 (reference category)	1.00	1.00	1.00

Table 3 continued

Treatability	Latent class trajectories Odds ratios [confidence intervals]		
	Rapid responders	Rapid escalators	High resisters
1	1.43** [1.10, 1.86]	2.01** [1.36, 2.98]	1.71** [1.41, 2.06]
2–9	1.86** [1.50, 2.30]	2.32** [1.66, 3.23]	2.12** [1.81, 2.48]
≥ 10	2.66** [1.73, 4.11]	2.53** [1.32, 4.82]	3.13** [2.26, 4.35]
Previous detention	2.26** [1.57, 3.24]	1.50 [.87, 2.58]	1.88** [1.40, 2.53]
Number of sector changes	1.88** [1.66, 2.12]	1.89** [1.60, 2.24]	1.64** [1.48, 1.80]
Sentence > 1 year	.91 [.75, 1.10]	1.36* [1.00, 1.84]	1.48** [1.29, 1.69]

The "mildly problematic" trajectory class serves as reference category in the personality risk/need area, the "mildly impaired integrators" is the reference category in the Social support risk/need area, and the "mild resisters" is the reference category in the treatability risk/need area

Previously detained = 1, not previously detained = 0. Duration sentence ≤ 1 year = 0, duration sentence > 1 year = 1

Multinomial logistic regression analyses, with backwards stepwise elimination, was used to link covariates to trajectory class membership

* $p < .05$, ** $p < .01$

sectors of the juvenile justice system increased the likelihood of being a member of the increasingly problematic class (OR = 1.55 per change), more so than of being in the highly problematic class (OR = 1.11 per change), although both were significant.

Personality

The model had a good fit ($\chi^2(30) = 752.41$, $p < .001$, Nagelkerke $R^2 = .158$). Although all covariates had a significant association with trajectory membership, the effect sizes of the odds ratios were generally small. Exceptions were the large to medium odds ratios regarding ten or more prior charges for violent offenses and the trajectory membership of the rapid responders, the rapid escalators and the highly problematic trajectories, which were all significantly different from the mildly problematic trajectory. In additional multinomial logistic analyses, with the highly problematic class as the reference group and the mildly problematic class excluded, only the number of sector changes remained significant ($\chi^2(2) = 61.34$, $p < .001$, Nagelkerke $R^2 = .04$, OR = 1.30; CI 95% [1.13, 1.49], for rapid responders, OR = 1.75; 95% CI [1.52, 2.03], for rapid escalators).

Social support

The model had a significant fit ($\chi^2(30) = 650.19$, $p < .001$, Nagelkerke $R^2 = .137$) and all covariates associated significantly with trajectory membership. The effect sizes of the odds ratios were small; the only odds ratio with a medium effect size was the dummy variable ten or more prior non-violent offenses, which increased the likelihood of being in the poorly integrated trajectory, compared to juveniles with no non-violent offenses in the mildly impaired integrators trajectory. In comparison to the reference group, shifting between sectors of the juvenile justice system was a risk factor for the rapid

deterioraters trajectory (OR = 2.07 per change) and rapid integrators trajectory (OR = 1.77 per change) and to a lesser degree for the poorly integrated trajectory (OR = 1.31 per change).

Treatability

All variables of the model were associated with trajectory class membership and contributed to the fit of the model ($\chi^2(30) = 659.80$, $p < .001$, Nagelkerke $R^2 = .133$). Nonetheless, the effect sizes of the odds ratios, albeit significant, were generally small. In comparison to the mild resister subgroup, the high resisters had a moderate higher likelihood to have been charged previously for non-violent offenses (OR = 3.13). Compared to the mild resisters, the number of sector changes in the juvenile justice system increased the likelihood with 1.88 and 1.89, for every change to be in the rapid escalator or rapid responder trajectories, for the high resister trajectory this likelihood was 1.64.

Discussion

The primary aim of this longitudinal study was to examine the existence of heterogeneous latent class trajectories based on the 30 risk and protective items of the SAVRY in a large sample of male juvenile offenders. The identification of risk/need trajectories explores an imperative issue for need-oriented risk management: the capacity of risk/need items to change over time. Research on the changeability of risk/need items of juvenile offenders is scarce but also highly relevant because risk/need assessment tools increasingly inform risk reduction strategies for this population [27]. However, there is very little knowledge about the capacity of these tools to measure change over time and the current study is, as far as we know, the first study to investigate the heterogeneity of trajectories of juvenile offenders on SAVRY risk/need items.

The heterogeneous trajectories that were identified in each of the five risk/need areas of the SAVRY were characterized by the high quality of separation between the trajectories. This indicates that the latent trajectories were distinct from each other. Regarding the principal question of this study it is important to note that the unique patterns of changes in risk/needs of the majority of the identified latent class trajectories showed significant changes over time. In the risk/need area antisocial behaviour, three trajectories were identified, of which two, the mild persisters and the rapid escalators, indicated significant change over time. However, the change in the mild persisters was very minimal at .08 points on a range of 0–1, what would be similar to a 1-point change in SAVRY score (e.g., the change of one risk factor from moderate to high).

Similarly, two of three trajectories of the risk/need area family functioning, the mildly problematic and the increasingly problematic trajectories, showed significant change over time. The change exhibited among juveniles within these two trajectories was unexpected since the items of the family functioning risk/need area are static risk factors. Although unexpected, these results may illustrate that during the adolescent's contact with the juvenile justice system more (often potentially traumatic) events that occurred within the family context can be identified. Notwithstanding the static nature of these items, they can generate important information [28]; in particular for possible trauma informed interventions [29].

In the area of personality, one of the risk/need areas fully composed of dynamic risk and protective factors, all four trajectories showed significant change over time. However, the highly problematic group improved a very minimal .02 points in risk/needs and the mildly problematic group, the largest class with low risk/needs, showed a very limited increase over time (with .03 points). The trajectory of the rapid responders showed an important improvement of .35 points (which coincides with a 5-point change in SAVRY score) in risk/needs over 18 months, but represented only 5.3% of the sample. By contrast, the trajectory of the rapid escalators (4.3%) accelerated in the opposite direction and increased .35 points in risk/needs over the same 18-month period. These results illustrate the heterogeneity of the change patterns in which different groups of adolescents developed in opposite directions over time during the 18-months study time-frame.

Of the four trajectories of the social support risk/need area, the poorly integrated class was the only one that did not show significant change over time. Furthermore,

the increase of .07 points during the 18-months period for the mildly impaired integrators was very limited. Conversely, the trajectory of the rapid integrators had an accelerated reduction in risk/needs (.41 points) during the first 12-months, to increase .09 point in the last 6-months. In comparison, the rapid deterioraters experienced a swift increase in risk/needs of .44 points during the first 9-months, although they did improve somewhat (.15 points) during the remaining 9-months of the trajectory.

In the last risk/need area, treatability, the change over time of the mild resisters (increase of .04 points) and the high resisters (improvement of .07 points) was also minimal. The trajectories of the rapid responders and the rapid escalators illustrated, as the rapid deterioraters and the rapid integrators of the risk/needs area Social support, the possible curvature shape of risk/need trajectories of juvenile offenders. After the baseline assessment the risk/needs trajectory of the rapid escalators group of 4.9% of the sample increased during the first three assessments with .41 points (equivalent to four points on this SAVRY risk/need area), to subsequently decrease with .12 points over the following 9 months. At 13% of the sample, the rapid responders group was the most prevalent class that exhibited a large improvement (.40 points) in risk/needs during the first 9-months; however, this group then slowly increased (.10 points) towards the end of the study period.

In summary, the large classes with high risk/needs did not change over time or showed limited improvement in risk/needs during the 18-month follow-up period. The trajectories with low risk/needs generally remained low and presented a very limited increase in risk/needs. Between 5 and 13% of the juveniles had large reductions in their risk/needs levels; however, approximately 5% of the juveniles had a negative development during the intervention, showing large increases in risk/needs.

Trajectories with extensive change over time in opposite directions were observed in three of the risk/need areas. A visual examination of the graphs in Fig. 2 would suffice to gauge the loss of essential information in all five-risk/need areas if the trajectories were averaged. With the vast majority of research relying on analyses that reflect average sample differences, homogeneous change is assumed and the identification of unique heterogeneous change patterns could be hidden. The heterogeneity of the risk/need trajectories in the current study is consistent with the DLC criminology theories. Similar to the delinquency trajectories [5, 14], the risk/need trajectories of juvenile offenders in the present sample demonstrate that change over time is likely to be heterogeneous.

Our second research question was what characteristics identified from prior research including demographics (age), criminal history (prior violent and non-violent offenses, previously detained), and shifting between sections of the juvenile justice services could differentiate between the risk/needs trajectories. We found that the male juveniles in the low risk/needs trajectories, in comparison with the remainder trajectories, were older in age, and had a low frequency of prior offenses, a lower likelihood of previous detention, shorter current sentences and experienced a very low frequency in sector changes within the juvenile justice system, indicating a smooth transition through the system. The trajectories with high risk/needs and the rapid increasing trajectories were generally the groups of offenders with more prior offenses, longer current sentences and a higher likelihood of multiple sector changes in the juvenile justice system, indicating a problematic transition through the system. The trajectories that presented a large decrease or increase in risk/needs over time were younger in comparison with the high and low risk/need trajectories. However, the decreasing trajectories were generally not very different from the high risk/need and the increasing trajectories. This lack of differences may be explained by the historical nature of the majority of the covariates and that in this study we did not have access to treatment information. Nonetheless, the identified characteristics of the trajectories with low, high and escalating risk/needs are in line with the risk-needs-responsivity (RNR) model [3] in that the most problematic groups were identified with high risk/needs, and the least problematic groups with low risk/needs.

Previous studies have suggested that interventions in juvenile justice services need to be improved and insufficiently target criminogenic needs [7–9]. Unfortunately, in the current study we did not have the data to verify these findings. However, adolescents' capacity to change over short periods of time has been widely documented [1, 5]. Another possibility is that SAVRY may have detected fever changes than actually occurred. This would suggest that the tool is not sufficiently sensitive to measure changes that juvenile offenders experience during their transition through the juvenile justice system. The results of the present study are consistent with the limited number of studies on the measurement of change with SAVRY assessments [9, 12, 13]. This small body of work suggests that SAVRY has difficulties in measuring change in risk/needs of adolescent offenders. Viljoen and colleagues recently suggested several potential strategies to enhance risk assessment tools' sensitivity to change [9]. One of their suggestions was a shorter time frame to assess the items. SAVRY uses time frames that refer "to the latest 6-month period" [11] for the dynamic risk items and "the factor has been active or present over the preceding year" regarding the protective items. In assessing future behaviour the large majority of risk assessment tools orientate the time frames to assess the items backwards, in the direction of the history of a person: the past year or the past 3–6 months. But if the objective is the appraisal of the likelihood of future violent or delinquent behaviour of a person, it might be more logical to orient the time frames of the dynamic items towards the coming period, for example the forthcoming 3–6 months. The SAPROF is the only tool with a time frame oriented towards the future [30]. Results of the SAPROF are promising since it is one of the few adult tools that has shown the ability to measure change over time in risk/needs [31].

Limitations and future directions

Our findings need to be considered in the context of the current study's limitations. First, the use of assessments performed in a naturalistic setting has clear advantages, but using data from daily clinical practice also presents challenges. Previous studies have reported that the use of assessment measures by professionals in the field can result in lower reliability [32, 33]. However, various field studies have shown that SAVRY assessments are completed with sufficient reliability in juvenile justice field settings [17, 34]. Second, our study did not have access to specific information on the nature and quality of the intervention programs provided for the juveniles, nor the intensity of these interventions. Future studies should attempt to obtain information regarding treatment and management that would provide insight into the extent to which the intensity and/or specific features of these interventions are associated with the various risk/need trajectories. Finally, in the present study we focused on the internal sensitivity to change through the identification of risk/need trajectories of juveniles based on their evolution on risk/need areas as they progressed through the juvenile justice system. The association between risk/needs and offending trajectories could contribute importantly to the insight of different developmental paths of juvenile offenders during their adolescence and their course through juvenile justice services and adjust treatment programs for specific subgroups is an important avenue for future research. That line of research could help determine if juveniles in the risk/need trajectories that show large improvements coincide with 'desisters' and the high risk/need groups correspond with life-course persistent offenders, two groups often identified in delinquency trajectories [6].

Risk assessment research has principally been based on cross-sectional research designs and between-individual differences. To validly use risk assessment tools to orient and evaluate risk reduction strategies, more knowledge about the changeability of risk/need items of these tools should become available. Analogue with the DLC theories and the numerous studies on heterogeneous criminal career trajectories, longitudinal research on the development of risk/needs over time could be employed on a broader scale. This type of research could test the heterogeneity of risk/need trajectories, based on items of risk assessment tools and accordingly evaluate their sensitivity to measure within-individual changes over time. It would also be an opportunity to test if future-oriented time frames could improve the sensitivity to measure change over time.

Although SAVRY is a promising tool for risk assessment, recent research suggests it could be insufficiently sensitive to change over time [9, 13]. Since it is one of the most widely used risk assessment tools for adolescents there are large quantities of data available from research and implementation in juvenile justice systems worldwide [35]. It might be worthwhile to explore if this wealth of data, and the valuable experiences of its implementation in juvenile justice systems [36], could be employed to improve SAVRY's sensibility to change over time. A data driven improvement of SAVRY could also stimulate the field towards more effective prevention and risk management.

Conclusions

In line with the developmental and life-course criminology theories this study illustrated that latent class trajectories on the basis of SAVRY risk and protective items can be heterogeneous and indicate distinct rates of change over time. Several of these trajectories revealed different patterns of changes in opposite directions within the same risk/need area, demonstrating the importance of examining change in a manner that does not lose sight of this heterogeneity. Although SAVRY is a promising tool for risk assessment, this study, taken into the light of recent research [9, 13] suggests it could be insufficiently sensitive to change over time.

Authors' contributions
EH was responsible for the study, the design, and the acquisition of the data. EH analysed and interpreted the data in collaboration with IB. EH was a major contributor in writing the manuscript. IB, TN and ChvN were involved in critically revising the work. All authors read and approved the final manuscript.

Author details
[1] GGzE Center for Child & Adolescent Psychiatry, Eindhoven, The Netherlands. [2] Tilburg University, Scientific Center for Care and Welfare (Tranzo), Tilburg, The Netherlands. [3] Justa Mesura, Consultancy & Applied Research, Barcelona, Spain. [4] Department of Psychiatry, University of British Columbia, Vancouver, Canada. [5] BC Mental Health and Substance Use Services, Forensic Psychiatric Services Commission, Coquitlam, Canada.

Acknowledgements
The first author wishes to acknowledge the support of the Centre for Legal studies and Specialized Training of the Generalitat de Catalonia during the implementation phase.

Competing interests
The authors declare that they have no competing interests.

Funding
This study did not receive any funding.

References
1. Grisso T. Evaluating the properties of instruments for screening and risk assessment. In: Grisso T, Vincent G, Seagrave D, editors. Mental Health Screening Assess. Juv. justice. New York: Guildford Press; 2005. p. 71–94.
2. Heilbrun K. Evaluation for risk of violence in adults. New York: Oxford University Press; 2009.
3. Andrews DA, Bonta J. The psychology of criminal conduct. 2nd ed. Cincinnati: Anderson Publishing; 1998.
4. Giordano PC, Schroeder RD, Cernkovich SA. Emotions and crime over the life course: a neo-meadian perspective on criminal continuity and change. Am J Sociol. 2007;112:1603–61. https://doi.org/10.1086/512710.
5. Thornberry TP, Giordano PC, Uggen C, Matsuda M, Masten A, Bulten E, et al. Explanations for offending. In: Loeber R, Farrington DP, editors. From Juv. Delinq. to adult crime Crim. careers, justice policy, Prev. Oxford: Oxford University Press; 2012. p. 47–85. http://oxfordindex.oup.com/view/10.1093/acprof:oso/9780199828166.003.0003?rskey=QE8U0r&result=2.
6. Jennings WG, Reingle JM. On the number and shape of developmental/life-course violence, aggression, and delinquency trajectories: a state-of-the-art review. J Crim Justice. 2012;40:472–89.
7. Haqanee Z, Peterson-Badali M, Skilling T. Making, "What Works" work: Examining probation officers' experiences addressing the criminogenic needs of juvenile offenders. J Offender Rehabil. 2015;54:37–59. https://doi.org/10.1080/10509674.2014.980485.
8. Peterson-Badali M, Skilling T, Haqanee Z. Examining implementation of risk assessment in case management for youth in the justice system. Crim Justice Behav. 2015;42:304. http://rd8hp6du2b.search.serialssolutions.com/?ctx_ver=Z39.88-2004&ctx_enc=info:ofi/enc:UTF-8&rfr_id=info:sid/ProQ:socabsshell&rft_val_fmt=info:ofi/fmt:kev:mtx:journal&rft.genre=article&rft.jtitle=Prison+Journal&rft.atitle=Justice+for+All?+Offenders+w.
9. Viljoen JL, Shaffer CS, Gray AL, Douglas KS. Are adolescent risk assessment tools sensitive to change? A framework and examination of the SAVRY and the YLS/CMI. Law Hum Behav. 2017;41:244–57.
10. Rich P. Forensic case formulation with children and adolescents. In: Sturmey P, MacMurran M, editors. Forensic case formul. Chichester: Wiley; 2011. p. 217–35.
11. Borum R, Bartel P, Forth A. Manual for the structured risk assessment of violence in youth (SAVRY), version 1.1. Tampa: University of South Florida; 2003.
12. Viljoen JL, Gray AL, Shaffer C, Latzman NE, Scalora MJ, Ullman D. Changes in J-SOAP-II and SAVRY scores over the course of residential, cognitive-behavioral treatment for adolescent sexual offending. Sex Abus A J Res Treat. 2015. https://doi.org/10.1177/1079063215595404.
13. Viljoen JL, Gray AL, Shaffer C, Bhanwer A, Tafreshi D, Douglas KS. Does reassessment of risk improve predictions? A framework and examination of the SAVRY and YLS/CMI. Psychol Assess. 2016. https://doi.org/10.1037/pas0000402.
14. Farrington DP. Integrated developmental & life-course theories of offending. New Brunswick: Transaction Publishers; 2005.
15. Loeber R, Slot NW, Stouthamer-Loeber M. A three-dimensional, cumulative developmental model of serious delinquency. In: Wikström P-OH, Sampson RJ, editors. Explan crime. Cambridge: Cambridge University Press; 2006. p. 153–94. http://ebooks.cambridge.org/ref/id/CBO9780511489341A015. Accessed 1 Mar 2017.
16. Vallès MD, Hilterman ELB. SAVRY Manual per a la valoració estructurada de risc de violència en joves [Manual of the Spanish version of the Structured Assessment of Violence Risk in Youth]. Barcelona: Generalitat de Catalunya, Centre d'Estudis Jurídics i Formació Especialitzada; 2006.

17. Hilterman ELB, Bongers I, Nicholls TL, van Nieuwenhuizen C. Identifying gender specific risk/need areas for male and female juvenile offenders: factor analyses with the Structured Assessment of Violence Risk in Youth (SAVRY). Law Hum Behav. 2016;40:82–96.

18. Cicchetti DV., Sparrow SA. Developing criteria for establishing inter-rater reliability of specific items: applications to assessment of adaptive behavior. American Assn on Mental Retardation; 1981. p. 127–37. http://psycnet.apa.org/psycinfo/1982-00095-001. Accessed 24 Apr 2017.

19. Hu L, Bentler PM. Cutoff criteria for fit indexes in covariance structure analysis: Conventional criteria versus new alternatives. Struct Equ Model A Multidiscip J. 1999;6:1–55. https://doi.org/10.1080/10705519909540118.

20. Muthén LK, Muthén BO. Mplus User's Guide. 7th edn. Muthén & Muthén; 2015. http://www.statmodel.com/download/usersguide/MplusUser-GuideVer_7.pdf.

21. Nylund KL, Asparouhov T, Muthén BO. Deciding on the number of classes in latent class analysis and growth mixture modeling: a Monte Carlo simulation study. Struct Equ Model. 2007;14:535–69.

22. Clark SL, Muthén B. Relating latent class analysis results to variables not included in the analysis. 2009. https://www.statmodel.com/download/relatinglca.pdf. Accessed 2 Mar 2017.

23. Asparouhov T, Muthén BO. Using Mplus TECH11 and TECH14 to test the number of latent classes. Mplus Web Notes. 2012. p. 1–17. https://www.statmodel.com/examples/webnotes/webnote14.pdf. Accessed 2 Mar 2017.

24. Little TD, Jorgensen TD, Lang KM, Moore EWG. On the joys of missing data. J Pediatr Psychol. 2014;39:151–62. https://academic.oup.com/jpepsy/article/39/2/151/883719/On-the-Joys-of-Missing-Data. Accessed 2 Apr 2017.

25. Dong Y, Peng C-YJ. Principled missing data methods for researchers. Springerplus. 2013;2:222. https://doi.org/10.1186/2193-1801-2-222.

26. Chen H, Cohen P, Chen S. How big is a big odds ratio? Interpreting the magnitudes of odds ratios in epidemiological studies. Commun Stat Simul Comput. 2010;39:860–4.

27. Wachter A. Statewide risk assessment in juvenile probation. JJGPS StateScan. Pittsburg: National Center for Juvenile Justice; 2015. p. 1–4. http://www.nysap.us/JJGPSStateScanStatewideRiskAssessment-updated-March2015.pdf. Accessed 20 Mar 2017.

28. Fox BH, Perez N, Cass E, Baglivio MT, Epps N. Trauma changes everything: examining the relationship between adverse childhood experiences and serious, violent and chronic juvenile offenders. Child Abus Negl. 2015;46:163–73. https://doi.org/10.1016/j.chiabu.2015.01.011.

29. Ford JD, Kerig PK, Desai N, Feierman J. Psychosocial interventions for traumatized youth in the juvenile justice system: research, evidence base, and clinical/legal challenges. OJJDP J. Juv. Justice. 2016;5:31–49.

30. de Vogel V, de Ruiter C, Bouman Y, de Vries Robbé M. SAPROF. Guidelines for the assessment of protective factors for violence risk. 2nd ed. Utrecht: Van der Hoeven Stichting; 2012.

31. de Vries Robbé M, de Vogel V, Douglas KS, Nijman HLI. Changes in dynamic risk and protective factors for violence during inpatient forensic psychiatric treatment: Predicting reductions in postdischarge community recidivism. Law Hum Behav. 2015;39:53–61. https://doi.org/10.1037/lhb0000089.

32. Boccaccini MT, Turner DB, Murrie DC. Do some evaluators report consistently higher or lower PCL-R scores than others? Findings from a statewide sample of sexually violent predator evaluations. Psychol Public Policy Law. 2008;14:262–83. https://doi.org/10.1037/a0014523.

33. Edens JF, Vincent GM. Juvenile psychopathy: a clinical construct in need of restraint? J. Forensic Psychol Pract. 2008;8:186–97. https://doi.org/10.1080/15228930801964042.

34. Vincent GM, Guy LS, Fusco SL, Gershenson BG. Field reliability of the SAVRY with juvenile probation officers: Implications for training. Law Hum Behav. 2012;36:1–14. https://doi.org/10.1037/h0093974.

35. Borum R, Lodewijks H, Bartel PA, Forth A. Structured Assessment of Violence Risk in Youth (SAVRY). In: Otto RK, Douglas KS, editors. Handbook violence risk Assess. New York: Routledge; 2010. p. 63–80.

36. Vincent GM, Guy LS, Perrault RT, Gershenson B. Risk assessment matters, but only when implemented well: a multisite study in juvenile probation. Law Hum Behav. 2016;40:683–96. https://doi.org/10.1037/lhb0000214.

18

Lost in transition? Perceptions of health care among young people with mental health problems in Germany: a qualitative study

Sabine Loos*, Naina Walia, Thomas Becker and Bernd Puschner

Abstract

Background: The transitioning of young patients from child and adolescent to adult mental health services when indicated often results in the interruption or termination of service. The personal views of young service users on current clinical practice are a valuable contribution that can help to identify service gaps. The purpose of this qualitative study was to explore the perceptions of health care of young people with mental health problems in the transition age range (16–25 years), and to better understand health behaviour, care needs and the reasons for disengaging from care at this point in time.

Methods: Seven group discussions and three interviews were conducted with 29 young people in this age range. Discussions were audio-taped, transcribed verbatim and analysed following the reconstructive approach of R. Bohnsack's documentary method.

Results: An overarching theme and nine subthemes emerged. Participants displayed a pessimistic and disillusioned general attitude towards professional mental health services. The discussions highlighted an overall concern of a lack of compassion and warmth in care. When they come into contact with the system they often experience a high degree of dependency which contradicts their pursuit of autonomy and self-determination in their current life stage. In the discussions, participants referred to a number of unmet needs regarding care provision and strongly emphasised relationship issues. As a response to their care needs not being met, they described their own health behaviour as predominantly passive, with both an internal and external withdrawal from the system.

Conclusions: Research and clinical practice should focus more on developing needs-oriented and autonomy-supporting care practice. This should include both a shift in staff training towards a focus on communicative skills, and the development of skills training for young patients to strengthen competences in health literacy.

Keywords: Mental health service, Youth mental health, Transition, Qualitative research, Health care needs

Background

In recent years, young people aged 16–25 with mental health problems have received increasing attention in research and clinical practice as a vulnerable group with special health care needs. Prevalence rates for mental disorders in this life period are high. For young people in the US, it was found out that 18.7% aged 18–25 years had some form of mental illness, of which 3.9% had a serious mental illness [1]. Similarly, in Germany, the point prevalence of mental illness in 14- to 17-year-olds is 17.8%, with a significant increase of emotional problems over time [2]. The onset age for most persistent mental disorders falls between 12 and 24 years [3]. At the same time, compared to all age groups across the life span, this age group has the lowest rate of access to mental health care [4].

One major reason for the lack of continuity of care is the complexity and the fragmented organisation of mental health services for young people worldwide [5, 6]. In Germany, the official age for transitioning to adult care

---

*Correspondence: sabine.loos@uni-ulm.de
Section Process-Outcome Research, Department of Psychiatry II, Ulm University, Ludwig-Heilmeyer-Str. 2, 89312 Günzburg, Germany

is 18 years, with various exceptions in clinical practice. There is a wide range of special mental health services financed by health insurance companies, community organisations or federal states (e.g. in- and outpatient psychiatric or psychosomatic clinics, outpatient psychiatric clinics or psychotherapies, outreach clinics). A lack of knowledge of where to go for which problems, as well as fewer offers of the low-threshold and less formal services usually preferred by young patients, make it difficult to find the right place to go [7].

Furthermore, differences in care philosophy and working practice between child and adolescent and adult mental health services (CAMHS, AMHS) may hinder effective collaboration [8, 9]. Often clinicians fail to actively refer patients from CAMHS to AMHS, or young people refuse such a referral [10]. Effective programmes to smooth the transition are rare and face logistical and organisational barriers [11, 12]. Personal obstacles for young people receiving adequate mental health care include self-stigma, not recognising symptoms as warning signs, a preference for self-reliant actions, and a lack of mental health literacy [6, 13, 14]. An empathetic, effective, and meaningful practice in mental health service can support youth in building resilience [15].

Qualitative studies provide insight into the subjective experiences of young people and can identify factors which contribute to a successful transition, such as: (i) feeling connected and supported in their relationships to significant others [16–18]; (ii) helpful and reliable connections with health care professionals who are attentive and respectful towards their young patients and who motivate them to continue care [19–21]; (iii) realistic expectations of the care provision provided by AMHS [21]. Moreover, experiences of stigmatising attitudes towards mental illness are a common theme among transitioning youth, which often results in social withdrawal [16, 19]. Practical suggestions for improving and tailoring care from patients' and carers' points of view include a gradual approach to treatment, transfer planning meetings, peer involvement, and elements of social support [22, 23].

In summary, there are some hints for needs-adapted professional care for young people with mental health problems. In addition, young people's implicit motives for discontinuing health service use, their care needs and the determinants of health behaviour could extend our knowledge of how to adapt service culture. To date, group discussions as a qualitative research method have hardly been tested [18], but they are an appropriate method for investigating the views and experiences of youth who share a common social context, and for considering the interactive group process. By using a reconstructive qualitative approach, this study explores the

personal experiences of patients aged 16–25 years with service utilisation. The study's research questions are the following:

(1) What are young patients' perceptions and evaluations of health care during the transition from CAMHS to AMHS? (2) What are their (mental) health care needs? And (3) Which factors influence their health behaviour?

Methods

The study followed a qualitative-explorative and reconstructive approach to gain insight into the action-guiding, common and tacit forms of knowledge of groups on the basis of anecdotes or beliefs [24]. Group discussions are especially appropriate for exploring milieu-specific structures and collective experiences, and are an established method for exploring the attitudes and views of young people [18, 22, 25]. During the research process, however, we were confronted with three potential study candidates who refused to take part in a group discussion for personal reasons. Since they were seen as providing a significant contribution to the study aims and in order to fully explore the field, we decided to give them the opportunity to be personally interviewed. The present paper followed the consolidated criteria for reporting qualitative research (COREQ) checklist [26].

Research team and reflexivity

The research team consisted of three female researchers (SL, NW, and a student assistant, IT, see "Acknowledgements") who were all trained and experienced in conducting qualitative research and group discussions. The research team was not involved in patient care and did not know the participants prior to study inclusion. The researchers explained their personal positions to the team and their interest in the research topic to the participants.

Sampling method

We developed a sampling plan prior to recruitment. Relevant parameters were the current status of participants in the process of transition from CAMHS to AMHS (before or after) and current treatment status (inpatient, outpatient, or currently not in treatment, see Fig. 1). The rationale for case selection was to obtain a maximum level of variation to enhance the external validity of findings. Data saturation was continuously discussed. We adhered to the sampling strategy as much as possible and observed both general and continually emerging themes over the course of the group discussions.

Development of an interview guide

A flexible interview guide with open-ended questions as prompts for discussion was developed in an iterative

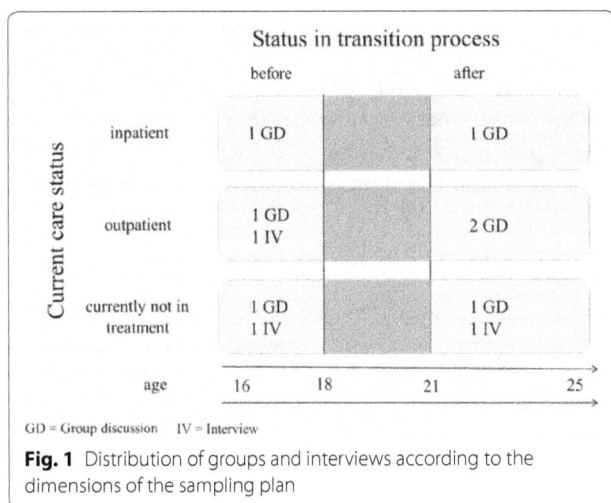

Fig. 1 Distribution of groups and interviews according to the dimensions of the sampling plan

process by the research team. The opening stimulus question was "Tell us about your personal experiences of care for your mental health problems". During discussion, topics (and examples of questions and prompts) were provided. A flexible application of the guide allowed the moderator to individually adapt to the specific dynamics of each individual group discussion. The ideal course of a discussion was intended as follows: [1] warming up [2], main interview phase including queries by the moderator to explore issues raised by participants [3], phase of introducing relevant research topics not yet discussed by the group [4], confrontation phase, where contradictions, impressions or interpretations were addressed by the moderator, and [5] conclusion phase. The interview guide was adapted after pilot-testing in a test group discussion.

Participants and recruitment

Recruitment took place between September 2015 and July 2016 at four study sites in Germany: at the in- and outpatient services of two of Ulm University's Departments of Psychiatry and Psychotherapy, one for children and adolescents (Child and Adolescent Psychiatry and Psychotherapy, Ulm) and the other for adults (Department of Psychiatry II, Clinic for Psychiatry, Psychotherapy and Psychosomatics at the Bezirkskrankenhaus Günzburg); at an outpatient outreach clinic for families, children and adolescents (Psychologische Beratungsstelle Ulm); and at a community mental health clinic for children and adolescents in central Germany (Vitos Klinik Rehberg, Herborn).

Participants were approached via gate-keepers, flyers, and snowballing and gave informed written consent after detailed study information had been provided. If participants were under 18 years old (the age of consent in Germany), informed consent was obtained from both

participants and caregivers. All participants received a voucher of 40 €. The study was approved by Ulm University's Ethics Committee.

Participants were considered eligible if they met the following criteria: [1] aged 16–25 years [2]; at least one personal contact with mental health services prior to the study, either completed or still in progress. Patients with insufficient command of the German language were excluded. After each session, socio-demographic data were obtained using a questionnaire.

Data collection

Group discussions and interviews took place either in a neutral setting at our research division or in settings familiar to the person or group (e.g. inpatient clinic). In case it was not possible to organise a familiar place for the discussion/interview, we invited the participants to our research division. In some groups the study participants knew each other, while in others they did not know each other. The groups were led by a moderator (NW) and an observer (either IT or SL) who took field notes (e.g. on the seating plan, atmosphere, and non-verbal communication). The moderator's tasks during the discussion were to listen to the discussion, to create an information-eliciting atmosphere, and to recognise any common concerns and shared experiences within the group. If verbal communication among participants stopped, the moderator encouraged further discussions by repeating or reframing a question or referring to the interview guide.

Data analysis

The group discussions and interviews were audio-taped and transcribed verbatim. Anonymous code names were given to each participant. Participants were invited to inspect the transcript. Data analysis was based on the reconstructive approach of Bohnsacks' documentary method [27]. A multi-level approach was undertaken by the coders: [1] transcripts were read independently by SL, NW and IT, and the content of each transcript was structured into paragraphs labelled with open, descriptive headings for the themes and sub-themes which were perceived as meaningful [2]. In a mutually consensual process, relevant paragraphs were selected for further analysis due to their interactive intensity and thematic relevance [3]. For each selected paragraph, an independent discourse analysis was conducted to paraphrase and structure the course of discussion [4]. The constant comparison technique was used to compare the meanings of paragraphs within and between groups and interviews to extract group consensus. Alternative interpretations, and the overall impressions and theorisations of the researchers were taken into account [5]. The themes and categories consented to were transferred to an overall coding

Table 1 Sample description (N = 29)

Characteristics	Values
Age, years; M (SD)	20.3 (3.3)
Sex, female; N (%)	19 (65.5)
Educational degree[a]	
Low track[b]; N (%)	10 (34.5)
Middle track[c]; N (%)	7 (24.1)
High track[d]; N (%)	10 (34.4)
No degree; N (%)	1 (3.4)
Duration of illness[e]	
< 2 years; N (%)	0
> 2 years; N (%)	26 (89.7)
Mental health problem (self-report)[f]	
Schizophrenia spectrum; N (%)	3 (10.3)
Affective spectrum; N (%)	9 (31.0)
Anxiety spectrum; N (%)	3 (10.3)
Eating spectrum; N (%)	2 (6.9)
Personality spectrum; N (%)	4 (13.8)
Attention deficit/hyperactivity spectrum; N (%)	3 (10.3)
Unknown; N (%)	3 (10.3)
Current treatment status	
Inpatient; N (%)	10 (34.5)
Outpatient; N (%)	10 (34.5)
Other treatment; N (%)	6 (20.7)
No treatment; N (%)	3 (10.3)

[a] Still at school or completed; missing = 1
[b] Hauptschule
[c] Realschule
[d] (Fach-)Abitur
[e] Missing = 3
[f] Missing = 2

tree which was validated and extended repeatedly. There were regular validation sessions held with an external, multidisciplinary interpretation group to independently discuss preliminary results in light of various professional perspectives. Citations of participant statements were translated into English by SL and approved by the co-authors [28].

Results

Seven group discussions (each with 3–5 participants) and three interviews were conducted, lasting between 59 and 117 min each. A total of 29 participants took part in the study. On average, participants were 20 years old; two-thirds of them were female. Participants' educational background was mixed and their mental health conditions varied (Table 1).

Overall, 43 descriptive and conceptual codes were extracted during analysing process resulting in a hierarchical structure with four levels. Figure 2 shows part of the coding tree as a mind map, a graphical solution including the codes at level 1 and 2. Described codes are grouped in terms of colour according to the three research questions of the study (for the full coding tree, see Additional file 1: Figure S1).

An overarching main theme emerged at level 1 ("dehumanised care"), and nine subthemes were identified at level 2 which are presented in Table 2 as they relate to the study's research questions. The main theme and subthemes are described below.

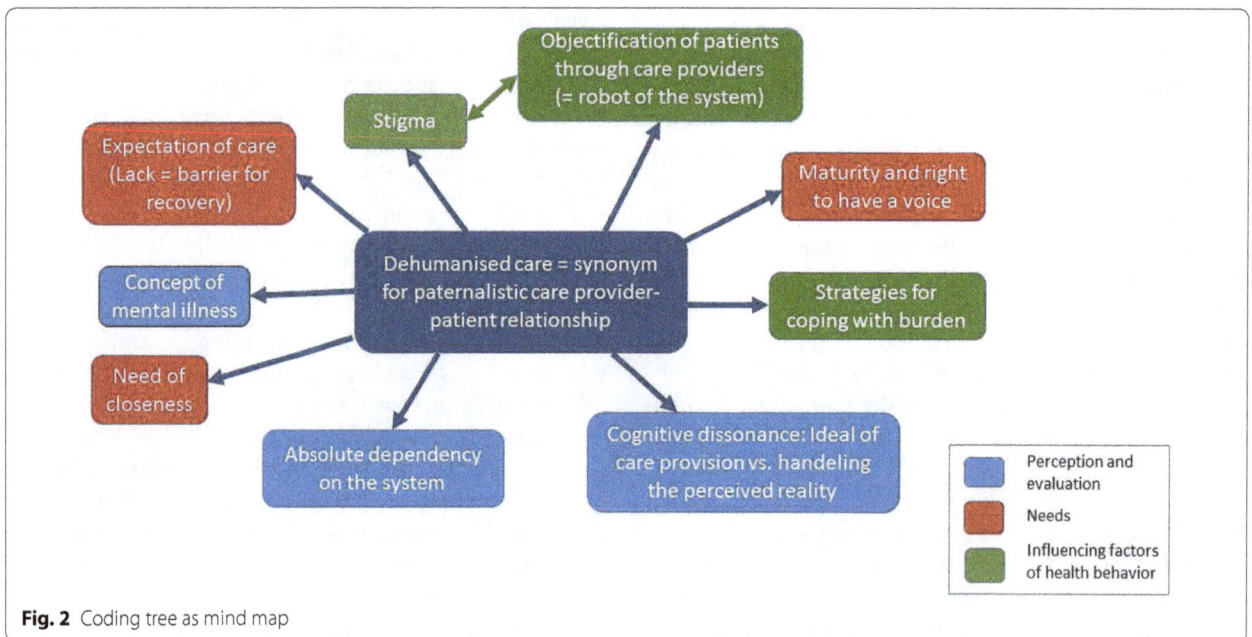

Fig. 2 Coding tree as mind map

Table 2 Summary of research topics and corresponding subthemes at level 2

Research questions	Subthemes (level 2)
Perception and evaluation of care	Absolute dependency on the system Cognitive dissonance (ideal of care vs. reality) Concept of mental illness
Health care needs	Expectations of care Need of closeness Maturity and the right to have a voice
Influencing factors of health behaviour	Stigma Objectification of patients through care providers Strategies for coping with burden

Main theme: dehumanised care

The overall theme identified was "dehumanised care". Young people in the study described a lack of humanity, attentiveness and empathy in the care system, often illustrated by descriptions of personal encounters with care providers which they experienced as paternalistic and authoritarian. They felt that their personal needs and concerns were not addressed. This impression on the part of participants seems to be the main factor shaping their predominantly pessimistic view of the care system. They often felt misunderstood and that their needs especially in crisis situations went unnoticed. Participants often regarded staff as indifferent, obedient to the system, not interested in individual cases, and in thrall to stereotypical thinking where they label and classify patients according to preconceived diagnostic categories. Participants experience diagnosis as an arbitrary act unrelated to the individual and their situation.

Because I still have another life. I also have a life as a human being and not just as a sick person (female, group discussion (GD): inpatient care after the transition process).

One just realises that the ward round is led by people who are not really interested in their work. I do not have the impression that anybody is seriously interested. They are all so apathetic... (female, GD: inpatient care after the transition process).

The doctors quickly get a certain impression of someone. They listen to us but they quickly say (...) you have a little bit of this and much more of that. You know, they are also just humans (...) because in my case—I was recently diagnosed with schizophrenia— I've never been schizophrenic before; and this was a mistake made by a doctor who wrote that down incorrectly; and I think ok, I am here because of

depression and now I have schizophrenia... (male, GD: outpatient care after the transition process).

Research question 1: perception and evaluation of health care

Young people regarded themselves as dependent on the care system, a fact that conflicted with their pursuit of autonomy and self-determination in their current life stage ("absolute dependency on the system", Fig. 2).

In general, if you get some psychotropic drugs like from the "nice" lady where I am; I say I would like this and that but she doesn't give a damn. She does what she wants to because she has an idea; I say ok, this is too much, yes, it will be ok (female, GD: outpatient care after the transition process).

Participants reported that when they felt in need of care, they wanted to be taken seriously and treated as human beings with emotions. This would be in line with their ideal of care provision but often contrasted with their experiences and perceived reality. This caused a dissonance which they tried to solve. Furthermore, participants expressed the experience of intense social pressure to function and to perform. These expectations had gradually changed their conception of illness and treatment to a more mechanistic perception. They used the metaphor of a mentally ill person as a "dysfunctional machine" which has to go to the "garage" where it quickly gets repaired with medication so that it can return to its "normal" tasks. Facing the system (of care/society) made them feel helpless. Young people described an inner conflict in that on the one hand they were attempting to meet social expectations, while on the other realising that a serious mental illness inevitably causes a disruption to one's life. When confronted with older people and their situation in inpatient mental health settings this inner conflict became apparent and caused feelings of distress and despondency ("cognitive dissonance—ideal of care vs. reality").

Great, now I ended up here again. For me, it is a personal failure somehow. Because those who know me know that I am a person trained to achieve... (female, GD: inpatient care after the transition process).

You get sicker in a locked ward than you were beforehand. Because (...) you go there and you are actually doing well, you only had bad thoughts; and then some random people approach you and they are totally messed up and you think to yourself, yes, great, soon I will be like them (male, GD: outpatient care after the transition process).

Participants revealed that they had a clear understanding of a broad conception of mental illness, accepted different aetiological models, and wanted this diversity to be represented in care provision. But in reality, participants described that they felt they often were confronted with one-sided medication treatment, especially in adult psychiatric inpatient care ("concept of mental illness").

To simply have more options, the feeling that one can do something to help oneself. Because I don't know what to do when I want help (male, GD: inpatient care after the transition process).

Research question 2: health care needs

Participants expressed diverse demands regarding care, i.e. care should address many areas based on a broad conception of mental health problems. Care should be authentic, individualised, supportive, and intensive ("expectations of care").

They described the need for personal closeness to the provider, to their friends as well as to daily life. The development of individualised bonds and the experience of personal support and engagement from providers was an element of the care process that participants appreciated with particular emphasis ("need for closeness").

Good psychologists do more for you than they have to. They appreciate you, show empathy but they also disclose their mistakes to you; they are honest with you, normal psychologists listen to you (...) bad psychologists destroy you (female, GD: currently not in treatment before the transition process).

You go there for one hour per week and you get there and say: yes, I'm fine today. They do not notice when someone's not doing well because they simply do not see you in the rest of your life (female, GD: inpatient care before the transition process).

Furthermore, participants emphasised the importance of recognising their autonomy and their right to be informed about treatment decisions and about the transfer and privacy of their personal data. Further topics addressed were the need for more information about patient rights, mental health diagnosis and treatment options ("maturity and the right to have a voice").

Research question 3: factors influencing health behaviour

Study participants indicated three reasons which might negatively influence their health behaviour. First, they reported stigmatising experiences (from their direct social environment, from society and from their own

view about themselves) and expressed uncertainty regarding how to deal with it ("Stigma").

Then I am allowed to go to my family again, to celebrate Christmas; where everybody is like: Oh, it's not that bad and don't make such a fuss about it (male, GD: outpatient care after the transition process).

Well, society does not like something like that; they always want to see and hear "the normal". What people consider normal is not what I regard as normal, yes, normal things are boring (female, GD: currently not in treatment after the transition process).

Secondly, in their role as patients in the care system, study participants described how they are treated more like objects than individuals. In contrast, they expressed their wish to establish good relationships with care providers on an equal footing and in a care setting that treated them with respect ("objectification of patients through care providers").

Thirdly, as a result of being disappointed by the care system, participants described their reactions in dealing with unaddressed needs or barriers and attitudes towards help-seeking as having become predominantly passive. They highlighted episodes in which they made fun of the system, in which they closed themselves up or were not telling the truth about their real inner state, in which they broke off contact with the system or sought help elsewhere, e.g. by believing in God ("strategies for coping with burden").

I'm not someone who doesn't believe in medical treatment... I say that medical care comes from God, and the sciences and the intelligence of many doctors; I think all these things are a gift. But I found that for me psychotherapy is not necessary. I have tried it, but I think it is not beneficial for me now (female, single interview: currently not in treatment after the transition process)

Discussion

The study provides insights into the young user perspective of mental health care during the transition from child and adolescent to adult care, on health care needs and on factors influencing health behaviour.

Perception of health care

A principal finding is that the basic attitude of the participants in our study toward professional mental health care services is that they are pessimistic and disillusioned. This is not directly in line with previous research which had a greater focus on either the practical aspects of transitioning [22, 23] or involvement in a supporting environment

[20, 21]. Young people in our study felt more isolated and focussed on drawbacks and discrepancies between their perception of the care system and reality as perceived by others. Beyond that aspect, young people in our study rather focussed on themselves as independent individuals instead of on being part of a supporting environment (e.g. caregivers).

Participants expressed their wish for an attentive and open contact with professionals on equal terms. They also emphasised the importance of empathy and professional, "parental-like" support which they felt was rarely provided. These experienced shortcomings tended to leave them feeling hopeless and powerless, especially when they perceived the system as 'superior' and lacking any room for them to act. Moreover, the experience of failing to meet expectations of self-optimisation might have caused frustration and anger towards the mental health services system. These results indicate that integrating the mental illness into their personal identities and lives in terms of a recovery process is a permanent challenge for transition-age youth [29].

Health care needs
Participants expressed complex and demanding health care needs for trusting and close therapeutic connections. In line with previous findings [17, 18, 30], participants strongly emphasised relationship issues by referring to numerous examples of positive and negative encounters with mental health care providers. At the same time, participants also stressed their need for interpersonal relationships with family and peers for coping with their mental illness. Previous studies have shown that factors such as feeling connected with significant others and the presence of social support affects health behaviour and protects against mental health risks [31–33]. Social support from any source (family, peers or care providers) can be of great importance to cope with stressors and daily challenges and to promote a sense of hope [32]. Mental health care providers need special therapeutic skills and training to effectively interact with young people and to help them engage with care more. Findings from this study clearly add to existing evidence indicating that professionals in AMHS particularly should be routinely provided with such training [33].

Participants called for a stronger involvement in decisions regarding their own treatment, which seems to contrast with the lack of active coping strategies paralleled by a lack of health literacy, a finding in this study and in previous research [13, 14]. This implies that young patients should be better educated about the health care system, about the transition between care systems in order to strengthen their health competence and self-efficacy [34]. Such programmes should include information

about patient rights and responsibilities when coping with mental health problems, and putting across a clear picture about what AMHS are able to provide in order to avoid frustration [21]. Where needed, AMHS professionals should also provide more "prolonged parenting". This means offering more concrete assistance to young adults, and to initiate discussion about maturation and normative developmental tasks.

Health behaviour
Participants' description of their health behaviour is predominantly characterised by a withdrawal from the system and with mainly passive reactions and coping strategies. One reason for that could be the disappointing experiences which they made in the health care system. The experience of being treated as an impersonal object and the experience of stigmatisation from within the mental health care system as well as from outside (families, relatives, peers, the education system, work, society at large) may account for strategies of avoidance and distancing as emphasised in previous findings [17, 19]. This might lead to young people perceiving professional health care as not beneficial and discontinuing treatment [35].

Self-determination theory is a can be drawn on to provide a better understanding of this [36, 37]. A basic lack of motivation for help-seeking from a professional mental health service in the study seems to be an expression of frustration and lack of satisfaction in terms of the three basic parameters of SDT: autonomy, relatedness and competence. If young patients experience a high system dependency, an indifferent and distant system in which they have no say in their own treatment, then they turn their backs on the system. Previous research has also found that among transition-age youth stigmatising experiences and coping are major issues accompanied by high levels of uncertainty [16, 19]. Social rejection and failing to achieve goals may result in feelings of insufficiency and loneliness. A lack of positive role models for dealing with mental health issues or overcoming crises could lead to young people generalising such experiences, and finally giving up help-seeking due to learned helplessness [7]. Perceiving mental illness as a sign of personal weakness rather than an illness may compromise active help-seeking and reduce positive beliefs about professional sources [38]. One possibility for health care professionals to prevent these negative processes might be putting more emphasis on forming stable relationships in personal encounters. As mentioned above, staff training programmes need to be developed and evaluated in order to address these important issues.

Strengths and limitations

A main strength of the study is its open, narrative approach, which ensured that the group discussions were dynamic through self-monitoring. Implicit knowledge and orientations could thus be accessed. Furthermore, group discussions and interviews with young adults were conducted in different, multi-professional treatment settings (in a university hospital as well as in outreach and community clinics) with varying entry requirements. Hence the spectrum of (user) expert experiences recorded and analysed was wide-ranging. Experiences with care providers in multi-professional teams helped to reflect the reality of current mental health care.

The study's limitations are the following. Because of the unique characteristics of the German health care system, the results from this small qualitative trial must be regarded as country-specific. However, similar themes have been reported in comparable studies from different care systems. We sought to reach theoretical saturation but due to research constraints this could not fully be reached. Group discussion as a qualitative method has some methodological limitations. Due to group dynamic processes, the method implies a risk for dominant personalities to override quiet voices. Some participants might be hesitant about voicing certain opinions when they do not know the other participants. In order to minimise the risk, we offered the possibility of a personal interview in some cases. Since the process of group discussions was supposed to be very self-directed, it supported a process of formulating social consensus and stereotyping which may be shaped by a certain language of authenticity which might sound rigorous and drastic. An extension of the purely qualitative approach would be a mixed-methods approach where a quantitative component would be used to verify the findings. Furthermore, caution must be exercised when drawing conclusions from the results since participants are at different stages of the transition and their individual perceptions reflect a snap-shot of the process. At last, people who did not speak German well enough were excluded but are an interesting group for further research in the field.

Conclusions

Our findings imply that in order to alleviate the disenchantment with professional health care prevalent among transition-age youth, staff training should put more emphasis on how to form and maintain stable connections along with an open style of communication. Such constructive partnerships may constitute the basis for instilling hope and implementing trusting and joint care planning. Our findings also suggest that interventions need to be developed and evaluated to effectively strengthen young people's individual health related competences, behaviour and self-efficacy to enable them to better cope with stigmatising experiences. Such interventions may include the involvement of persons from their more intimate social environment or peer counsellors as partners in treatment. An environment supporting autonomy in treatment with a focus on young people's initiatives, choices and treatment decisions could increase motivation and proactive behaviour. This will help strengthen and encourage transition-age youth with mental illness in their self-reflective capacities and in their right to actively participate in their care process.

Abbreviations

AMHS: adult mental health service; CAMHS: child and adolescent mental health service; COREQ: consolidated criteria for reporting qualitative research; SDT: self-determination theory.

Authors' contributions

SL proposed the project idea. NW and SL conducted the group discussions and analysed the material. SL drafted the manuscript. TB and BP critically revised for important intellectual content. All authors read and approved the final manuscript.

Acknowledgements

We would like to thank all participants who kindly took part in this study. We also would like to thank the following colleagues for their valuable contribution: Silvia Krumm, Isabella Thoma and Julia Zabel.

Competing interests

The authors declare that they have no competing interests.

Funding

The study was funded by a grant from the German Research Foundation (DFG, grant number LO 2164/1-1).

References

1. Lipari RN, Hedden SL. Serious mental health challenges among older adolescents and young adults: the CBHSQ report. Rockville: Substance Abuse and Mental Health Services Administration (US); 2013–2014.

2. Holling H, Schlack R, Petermann F, Ravens-Sieberer U, Mauz E. Psychische Auffalligkeiten und psychosoziale Beeintrachtigungen bei Kindern und Jugendlichen im Alter von 3 bis 17 Jahren in Deutschland—Pravalenz und zeitliche Trends zu 2 Erhebungszeitpunkten (2003–2006 und 2009-2012). Ergebnisse der KiGGS-Studie—Erste Folgebefragung (KiGGS Welle 1). [Psychopathological problems and psychosocial impairment in children and adolescents aged 3–17 years in the German population: prevalence and time trends at two measurement points (2003–2006 and 2009–2012). Results of the KiGGS study: first follow-up (KiGGS Wave 1)]. Bundesgesundheitsblatt Gesundheitsforschung Gesundheitsschutz. 2014;57:807–19. https://doi.org/10.1007/s00103-014-1979-3.

3. Kessler RC, Amminger GP, Aguilar-Gaxiola S, Alonso J, Lee S, Ustun TB. Age of onset of mental disorders: a review of recent literature. Curr Opin Psychiatr. 2007;20:359–64. https://doi.org/10.1097/YCO.0b013e32816ebc8c.

4. McGorry P, Bates T, Birchwood M. Designing youth mental health services for the 21st century: examples from Australia, Ireland and the UK. Br J Psychiatry Suppl. 2013;54:s30–5. https://doi.org/10.1192/bjp.bp.112.119214.

5. Signorini G, Singh SP, Boricevic-Marsanic V, Dieleman G, Dodig-Ćurković K, Franic T, et al. Architecture and functioning of child and adolescent mental health services: a 28-country survey in Europe. Lancet Psychiatry. 2017. https://doi.org/10.1016/S2215-0366(17)30127-X.

6. Zachrisson HD, Rodje K, Mykletun A. Utilization of health services in relation to mental health problems in adolescents: a population based survey. BMC Public Health. 2006;6:34. https://doi.org/10.1186/1471-2458-6-34.

7. Yap MBH, Reavley N, Jorm AF. Where would young people seek help for mental disorders and what stops them? Findings from an Australian national survey. J Affect Disord. 2013;147:255–61. https://doi.org/10.1016/j.jad.2012.11.014.

8. Mulvale GM, Nguyen TD, Miatello AM, Embrett MG, Wakefield PA, Randall GE. Lost in transition or translation? Care philosophies and transitions between child and youth and adult mental health services: a systematic review. J Ment Health. 2016;6:1–10. https://doi.org/10.3109/09638237.2015.1124389.

9. McLaren S, Belling R, Paul M, Ford T, Kramer T, Weaver T, et al. 'Talking a different language': an exploration of the influence of organizational cultures and working practices on transition from child to adult mental health services. BMC Health Serv Res. 2013;13:254. https://doi.org/10.1186/1472-6963-13-254.

10. Paul M, Ford T, Kramer T, Islam Z, Harley K, Singh SP. Transfers and transitions between child and adult mental health services. Br J Psychiatry Suppl. 2013;54:s36–40. https://doi.org/10.1192/bjp.bp.112.119198.

11. Hatfield M, Falkmer M, Falkmer T, Ciccarelli M. Effectiveness of the BOOST-A™ online transition planning program for adolescents on the autism spectrum: a quasi-randomized controlled trial. Child Adolesc Psychiatry Ment Health. 2017;11:54. https://doi.org/10.1186/s13034-017-0191-2.

12. Embrett MG, Randall GE, Longo CJ, Nguyen T, Mulvale G. Effectiveness of health system services and programs for youth to adult transitions in mental health care: a systematic review of academic literature. Adm Policy Ment Health. 2016;43:259–69. https://doi.org/10.1007/s10488-015-0638-9.

13. Biddle L, Donovan J, Sharp D, Gunnell D. Explaining non-help-seeking amongst young adults with mental distress: a dynamic interpretive model of illness behaviour. Sociol Health Illn. 2007;29:983–1002. https://doi.org/10.1111/j.1467-9566.2007.01030.x.

14. Gulliver A, Griffiths KM, Christensen H. Perceived barriers and facilitators to mental health help-seeking in young people: a systematic review. BMC Psychiatr. 2010;10:113. https://doi.org/10.1186/1471-244X-10-113.

15. Lal S, Ungar M, Malla A, Leggo C, Suto M. Impact of mental health services on resilience in youth with first episode psychosis: a qualitative study. Adm Policy Ment Health. 2017;44:92–102. https://doi.org/10.1007/s10488-015-0703-4.

16. Bluhm RL, Covin R, Chow M, Wrath A, Osuch EA. "I just have to stick with it and it'll work": experiences of adolescents and young adults with mental health concerns. Community Ment Health J. 2014;50:778–86. https://doi.org/10.1007/s10597-014-9695-x.

17. Gill F, Butler S, Pistrang N. The experience of adolescent inpatient care and the anticipated transition to the community: young people's perspectives. J Adolesc. 2016;46:57–65. https://doi.org/10.1016/j.adolescence.2015.10.025.

18. Jivanjee P, Kruzich J, Gordon LJ. Community integration of transition-age individuals: views of young with mental health disorders. J Behav Health Serv Res. 2008;35:402–18. https://doi.org/10.1007/s11414-007-9062-6.

19. Leavy JE. Youth experience of living with mental health problems: emergence, loss, adaption and recovery (elar). Can J Community Ment Health. 2005;24:109–26.

20. Lindgren E, Söderberg S, Skär L. Swedish young adults' experiences of psychiatric care during transition to adulthood. Issues Ment Health Nurs. 2015;36:182–9. https://doi.org/10.3109/01612840.2014.961624.

21. Swift KD, Hall CL, Marimuttu V, Redstone L, Sayal K, Hollis C. Transition to adult mental health services for young people with attention deficit/hyperactivity disorder (ADHD): a qualitative analysis of their experiences. BMC Psychiatr. 2013;13:74. https://doi.org/10.1186/1471-244X-13-74.

22. Gilmer TP, Ojeda VD, Leich J, Heller R, Garcia P, Palinkas LA. Assessing needs for mental health and other services among transition-age youths, parents, and providers. Psychiatr Serv. 2012;63:338–42. https://doi.org/10.1176/appi.ps.201000545.

23. Hovish K, Weaver T, Islam Z, Paul M, Singh SP. Transition experiences of mental health service users, parents, and professionals in the United Kingdom: a qualitative study. Psychiatr Rehabil J. 2012;35:251–7. https://doi.org/10.2975/35.3.2012.251.257.

24. Polanyi M. The tacit dimension. Chicago: University of Chicago Press; 2009.

25. Peterson-Sweeney K. The use of focus groups in pediatric and adolescent research. J Pediatr Health Care. 2005;19:104–10.

26. Tong A, Sainsbury P, Craig J. Consolidated criteria for reporting qualitative research (COREQ): a 32-item checklist for interviews and focus groups. Int J Qual Health Care. 2007;19:349–57. https://doi.org/10.1093/intqhc/mzm042.

27. Bohnsack R. Documentary method and group discussions. In: Bohnsack R, Pfaff N, Weller W, editors. Qualitative analysis and documentary method in international educational research. Opladen: B. Budrich; 2010. p. 99–124.

28. van Nes F, Abma T, Jonsson H, Deeg D. Language differences in qualitative research: is meaning lost in translation? Eur J Ageing. 2010;7:313–6. https://doi.org/10.1007/s10433-010-0168-y.

29. McCauley CO, McKenna HP, Keeney S, McLaughlin DF. Concept analysis of recovery in mental illness in young adulthood. J Psychiatr Ment Health Nurs. 2015;22:579–89. https://doi.org/10.1111/jpm.12245.

30. Blum RW, Garell D, Hodgman CH, Jorissen TW, Okinow NA, Orr DP, Slap GB. Transition from child-centered to adult health-care systems for adolescents with chronic conditions. A position paper of the society for adolescent medicine. J Adolesc Health. 1993;14:570–6.

31. Sawyer SM, Afifi RA, Bearinger LH, Blakemore SJ, Dick B, Ezeh AC, Patton GC. Adolescence: a foundation for future health. Lancet. 2012;379:1630–40. https://doi.org/10.1016/S0140-6736(12)60072-5.

32. Cheng Y, Li X, Lou C, Sonenstein F, Kalamar A, Jejeebhoy S, et al. The association between social support and mental health among vulnerable adolescents in five cities: findings from the study of the well-being of adolescents in vulnerable environments. J Adolesc Health. 2014;55:31–8.

33. Patel V, Flisher AJ, Hetrick S, McGorry P. Mental health of young people: a global public-health challenge. Lancet. 2007;369:1302–13. https://doi.org/10.1016/S0140-6736(07)60368-7.

34. Mulfinger N, Müller S, Böge I, Sakar V, Corrigan PW, Evans-Lacko S, et al. Honest, open, proud for adolescents with mental illness: pilot randomized controlled trial. J Child Psychol Psychiatry. 2018;59:684–91. https://doi.org/10.1111/jcpp.12853.

35. O'Connor PJ, Martin B, Weeks CS, Ong L. Factors that influence young people's mental health help-seeking behaviour: a study based on the health belief model. J Adv Nurs. 2014;70:2577–87. https://doi.org/10.1111/jan.12423.

36. Ryan RM, Deci EL. Self-determination theory and the facilitation of intrinsic motivation, social development, and well-being. Am Psychol. 2000;55:68–78.

37. Ng JYY, Ntoumanis N, Thøgersen-Ntoumani C, Deci EL, Ryan RM, Duda JL, Williams GC. Self-determination theory applied to health contexts: a meta-analysis. Perspect Psychol Sci. 2012;7:325–40. https://doi.org/10.1177/1745691612447309.

38. Yap MBH, Reavley NJ, Jorm AF. Associations between stigma and help-seeking intentions and beliefs: findings from an Australian national survey of young people. Psychiatry Res. 2013;210:1154–60. https://doi.org/10.1016/j.psychres.2013.08.029.

19

Feasibility study of a family- and school-based intervention for child behavior problems in Nepal

Ramesh P. Adhikari[1,2]*(ID), Nawaraj Upadhaya[2], Emily N. Satinsky[2], Matthew D. Burkey[3,4], Brandon A. Kohrt[5] and Mark J. D. Jordans[6]

Abstract

Background: This study evaluates the feasibility, acceptability, and outcomes of a combined school- and family-based intervention, delivered by psychosocial counselors, for children with behavior problems in rural Nepal.

Methods: Forty-one children participated at baseline. Two students moved to another district, meaning 39 children, ages 6–15, participated at both baseline and follow-up. Pre-post evaluation was used to assess behavioral changes over a 4-month follow-up period (n = 39). The primary outcome measure was the Disruptive Behavior International Scale—Nepal version (DBIS-N). The secondary outcome scales included the Child Functional Impairment Scale and the Eyberg Child Behavior Inventory (ECBI). Twelve key informant interviews were conducted with community stakeholders, including teachers, parents, and community members, to assess stakeholders' perceptions of the intervention.

Results: The study found that children's behavior problems as assessed on the DBIS-N were significantly lower at follow-up (M = 13.0, SD = 6.4) than at baseline (M = 20.5, SD = 3.8), p < 0.001, CI [5.57, 9.35]. Similarly, children's ECBI Intensity scores were significantly lower at follow-up (M = 9.9, SD = 8.5) than at baseline (M = 14.8, SD = 7.7), p < 0.005, 95% CI [1.76, 8.14]. The intervention also significantly improved children's daily functioning. Parents and teachers involved in the intervention found it acceptable and feasible for delivery to their children and students. Parents and teachers reported improved behaviors among children and the implementation of new behavior management techniques both at home and in the classroom.

Conclusions: Significant change in child outcome measures in this uncontrolled evaluation, alongside qualitative findings suggesting feasibility and acceptability, support moving toward a controlled trial to determine effectiveness.

Keywords: Children, Behavior problems, School and family based intervention, Feasibility study, Psychosocial support, Nepal

Background

In low- and middle-income countries (LMICs), about 20% of children and adolescents suffer from mental illness [1]. Child behavior problems, including oppositional defiant disorder (ODD), conduct disorder (CD), and attention deficit-hyperactivity disorder (ADHD), are important to public health and human development as they are early indicators of later educational, social, emotional, and economic problems [2, 3]. Child behavior problems cause significant burden to families and societies through violence, disrupted relationships, and criminal acts [2]. Difficulties controlling impulses and behaviors often occur early in life [4], and commonly contribute to other mental health problems. These behavior problems comprise the major diagnostic risk factor for suicide [5]. Studies have shown that behavioral problems during childhood predict poorer social, educational, and economic outcomes as adults [6–9]. A meta-analysis of worldwide prevalence

*Correspondence: rameshadhikaria@gmail.com
[2] Research Department, Transcultural Psychosocial Organization (TPO), Baluwatar, Kathmandu, Nepal
Full list of author information is available at the end of the article

of ODD and CD showed similar incidence across geographic regions [10].

Behavior problems result from a complex interplay of biological, environmental, and experiential factors. Poverty, through exacerbating family dysfunction, has been associated with increased risk for CD and delinquency in children and adolescents [11, 12]. Exposure to violence, particularly frequent violent events, can also have adverse effects on children's behavior, leading to school problems and an underdeveloped sense of right and wrong [13].

While Nepal's economy rebounded during 2017, the South Asian country has been affected by a 10-year civil war, political uncertainty, and devastating earthquakes in 2015 [14]. The majority of the country's population lives in rural areas and many of them experience mental health concerns [15]. Behavior problems have not been thoroughly assessed among children less than 18 years in Nepal. Previous research suggests that children with behavior problems in Nepal rarely seek or receive help [16, 17]. A study of physically disabled Nepali children found aggressive behavior (above the 98th percentile on the standard Child Behavior Check List (CBCL) criteria) in 12.5 percent of children [18]. Despite a need for programs to address behavior problems among children and adolescents in rural areas, mental health services in Nepal are concentrated in big cities [19].

Evidence suggests that behavior problems in children can be effectively addressed through parenting interventions. A systematic review of family and parenting interventions in high-income countries (HICs) found that positive effects can last through adolescence and into adulthood, as interventions reduced time spent in juvenile delinquent institutions and minimized re-arrest [20]. Similarly, a randomized controlled trial (RCT) of parent groups targeting child antisocial behavior demonstrated reduced ADHD symptoms in children [21]. While the majority of research on child behavior problems and the impact of treatments derives from HICs, recent interventions and evaluations have been performed in disadvantaged areas of HICs and in LMICs. Trials in LMICs have led to significant reductions in externalizing behaviors and adolescent risk-taking behaviors [22]. By providing parents with education, counselors are able to equip parents with skills to manage defiant behaviors and reduce rates of child non-compliance. Teaching parents pre-emptive strategies to address behavior problems, for example, has been shown to minimize children's non-compliant behavior [23]. Parent Child Interaction Therapy (PCIT) in Puerto Rico boosted parent's confidence in child behavior management and reduced impulsive, aggressive, and defiant behavioral patterns among children [3]. Another study, conducted in disadvantaged

areas of the UK found that children's behavior problems were significantly reduced at both 12 and 18 month follow-up assessments after a parenting intervention [11].

In addition to family-based programs, school-based interventions have been employed in LMICs to address child behavior problems. Studies have demonstrated mixed results. A school-based intervention in inner-city Kingston, Jamaica resulted in significant improvements in attendance and reductions in externalizing behaviors [24]; while a school-based intervention in Santiago, Chile failed to demonstrate a difference in mental health outcomes between the intervention and usual care groups [25]. A classroom-based psychosocial intervention in Nepal demonstrated reduced psychological difficulties and aggression among boys and increased prosocial behavior in girls [26].

Moreover, some literature suggests benefits of a multitiered approach where by intervention modalities are combined: generalized, school- or community-wide interventions with targeted components for high-risk individuals and their families [1, 27]. The present study aimed to evaluate the feasibility, acceptability, and outcomes of a combined school- and family-based intervention for child behavior problems in rural Nepal.

Methods
Identification of priority behavior problems
From 2013 to 2014, 72 free list interviews and 30 key informant interviews (KII) were conducted with community members of Chitwan District, Nepal, to assess parents' and family members' childcare customs and perceptions of child behavior problems [17, 28]. The interviews suggested a number of commonly experienced behavior problems among children in the community. The top five problems reported included; (1) addictive behavior, (2) not paying attention to studies, (3) getting angry easily and fighting over small issues, (4) disobedience, and (5) stealing [28]. Community informants suggested a combined school, family, and individual-based intervention to address the identified child behavior problems [16].

Intervention selection and contextualization
To identify best practice in dealing with child behavior problems in LMICs, a scoping review was conducted using PsychINFO, CENTRAL, and Google Scholar. Altogether, eleven articles were identified. Three were review articles and the remaining eight were randomized control trials (RCTs) (Fig. 1). The findings of the review and results of the formative study guided the selection of the intervention, which was adapted for the Nepalese context through a workshop with Nepalese clinicians.

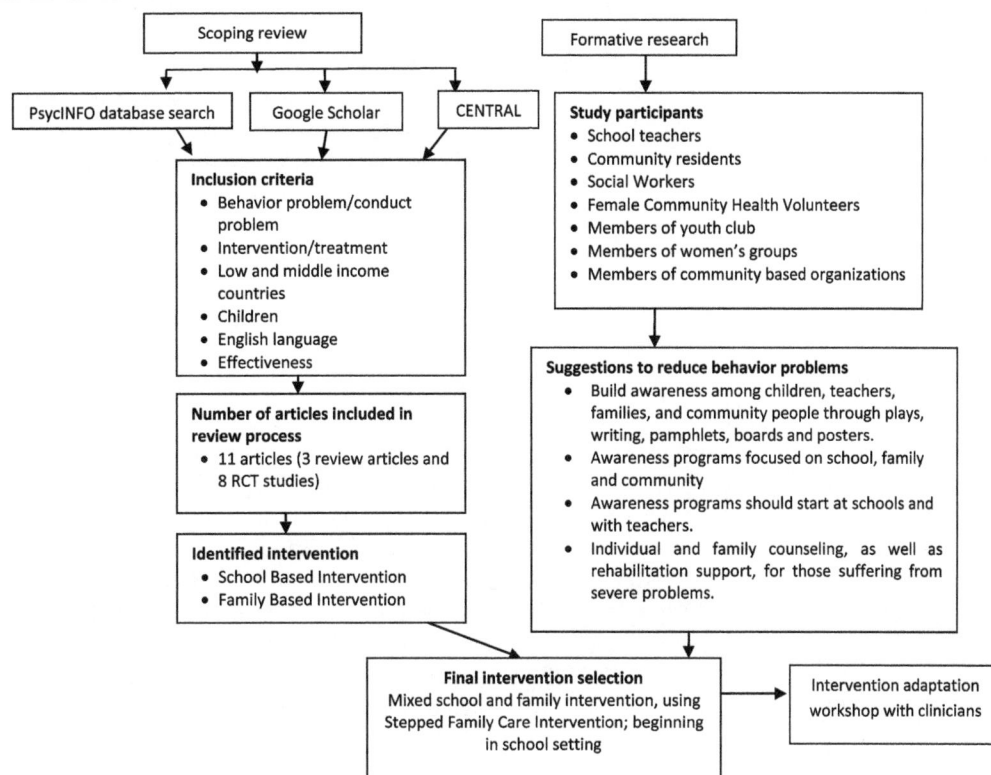

Fig. 1 Selection process of intervention

Intervention adaptation workshop

The Stepped Care Family Intervention (SCFI) developed and implemented by Jordans et al. [29] was used as the basis for the family-based portion of the intervention. This tiered intervention was adapted for the Nepali context during a 1-day workshop at which psychosocial counselors, a teacher, a psychiatrist, and researchers collaborated to culturally adapt the intervention for use in rural Nepal. Altogether nine people with several years of experience in the field participated in the workshop. Based on the different intervention levels (school, family, and individual), three group discussions were established to discuss feasibility and acceptability. Following these discussions, the individual-focused level was removed, as participants agreed that it required substantial resources with only limited evidence for efficacy or potential for population-level impact (Fig. 2). The community-based intervention from the original SCFI was replaced with school based activities (for details see Additional file 1). Below we describe the adapted intervention in more detail.

Step 1: School level prevention

Psycho-education and awareness activities are provided for parents and teachers. The major objectives are to assess the externalizing behaviors and psychosocial problems displayed by children at school and in the household, and to teach parents and teachers how to deal with

such behaviors. A psychosocial counselor conducts initial evaluations of the parent's and teacher's understanding of child behavior problems using emotion cards. During a group discussion, the counselor, teachers, and parents discuss major causes and impacts of these behaviors and current disciplinary practices. After the assessment, the psychosocial counselor provides psycho-education classes to groups based on identified needs. These classes include a brief introduction to child behavior problems, causes, impacts, and skills to effectively deal with specific behaviors (classroom management skills, student–teacher relationships, communication skills, rewards etc.).

Step 2: Family level intake and parent engagement

Family-level treatment is provided for children presenting with moderate-to-severe behavior problems. Trained psychosocial counselors work with parents to provide management strategies, enhance social support, improve family functioning, and reduce child behavior problems. The psychosocial counselors form parent support groups with parents of children with behavior problems. Based on geographic location, four to six parents are included in each support group. Psychosocial counselors facilitate a minimum of three group sessions and one follow-up session with each group. During these sessions, parents build social connectedness and support by sharing their

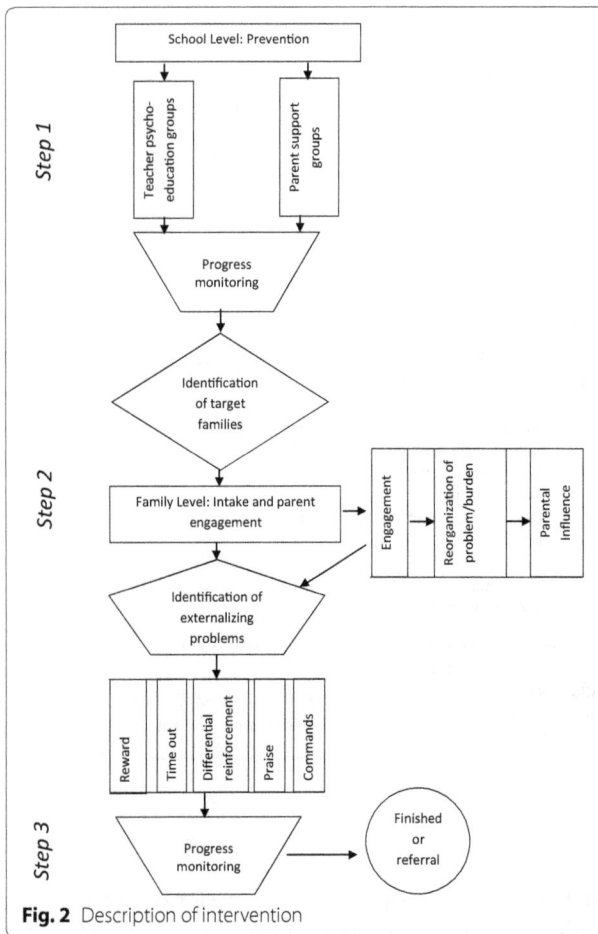

Fig. 2 Description of intervention

stories, exchanging ideas, and exploring alternative ways of addressing family challenges and behavior problems.

Step 3: Progress monitoring

The counselors make home visits to assess the home environment and provide onsite support to both children and parents. Depending on the nature and severity of the child's behavior problems, the counselors complete one to three home visits, during which the counselor works with the parents on behavior modification techniques: (1) training parents in a specific technique, (2) supervising implementation of the technique in the home setting, and (3) evaluating the impact of the technique. Techniques include: (a) selection of desired behaviors, (b) selection of reward system (chocolate or chewing gum, books, clothes, verbal reinforcement, cooking favorite food, physical affection), (c) using reward system *immediately* after desired behavior is shown, (d) explanation of reason for reward (labeling), and (e) consistency. To evaluate the impact of the technique, counselors use personalized outcome indicators based on which behaviors parents most want to see changed. These indicators are measured

before and after the intervention. If low intensity care does not provide the expected gains (i.e. improvement in family functioning and reduction in the child's behavior problems), counselors step-up to the next level of care. Stepping-up requires making decisions on the child's progress based on judgments of 'significant health gain' or 'improvement' (for details see Additional file 1).

Study setting and population

This study was conducted in the Meghauli Village Development Committee (VDC) of Chitwan District, Nepal. The study population consisted of children, parents, and teachers in the Meghauli VDC. After approval from the District Education Office and school principals, all teachers associated with government and private schools in the district were included. Self-referred parents of children ages 5–15 who voluntarily agreed to participate were also included. Although many children live in extended households with multiple adult figures, only parents were included. Children ages 5–15 with disruptive behaviors based on the Disruptive Behavior International Scale—Nepal version (DBIS-N) [30], and their parents were included if both children and parents provided consent.

Initially, psychosocial counselors provided 1 day of psycho-education on child behaviour problems to 201 teachers from 12 schools, and 100 parents, after which psychosocial counselors requested teachers and parents to refer children with behavior problems, based on judgement. Altogether, 104 children were referred. Using the DBIS-N, two researchers conducted screening interviews with parents of all 104 children. After screening, 41 children scored above the cutoff (≥ 17). All were included in the intervention after parents and children gave consent. At follow-up, 39 of the 41 children who participated at baseline were interviewed. The two children who did not participated moved to another district.

Instruments

The baseline interview was conducted using the DBIS-N, the Child Functional Impairment Scale (CFIS), and the Eyberg Child Behavior Inventory (ECBI). After 1 week of the last intervention session, follow-up assessments were conducted using the same instruments.

Disruptive Behavior International Scale—Nepal version (DBIS-N)

The DBIS-N is a 20-item instrument which measures child behavior problems and which has been validated for use in rural Nepal. It includes 4 items assessing pro-social behaviors and 16 items assessing problem behaviors. The items are rated on a 0–3 scale based on frequency of occurrence (0 = "Never" to 3 = "Very Often"). Higher overall scores on the problem scale represent a greater number and/or frequency of behavior problems. The highest possible score for the DBIS problem subscale is 48 [30]. A score of 17 or above was used as the cutoff for inclusion, indicating moderate to severe behavior problems [31].

Child Functional Impairment Scale

Functional impairment was assessed using the CFIS, a tool that has previously been used in Nepal to assess a child's ability to complete 11 routine daily functions expected of children in the study age range [32]. Each item is rated on a 0–3 scale with 0 representing no difficulty and 3 representing difficulty completing the task "most of the time". Therefore, the range of potential scores on the CFIS is 0–33, with 33 representing the highest level of functional impairment across tasks.

Eyberg Child Behavior Inventory

The ECBI is a 36-item parent-report questionnaire that assesses child behavior problems using a 7-point scale to assess frequency and "yes/no" responses to assess the current presence of specific problems. The ECBI is scored according to "intensity" and "problem" domains, with "intensity" representing the summed numerical scores (range 36–252, where higher numbers indicates greater "intensity" of behavior problems) and "problem" representing the total number of items that are reported as being a "problem" for the informant (range 0–36, where higher numbers indicate a greater number of "problem" items) [33]. The ECBI was translated into Nepali by the authors of this study and approved by the authors of the ECBI.

Implementation and supervision

Two counselors were mobilized for the three steps of intervention-delivery under the direct supervision of a clinical supervisor and the principal investigator (RPA). A clinical psychologist with knowledge of the intervention provided a 1-week training to both counselors. To further strengthen the quality of services and the uniformity of intervention delivery, the clinical supervisor visited the study community each week to provide supervision and feedback, with additional supervision via phone contact when necessary. Behavior changes were assessed at 4-month follow-up period.

Qualitative methods

To assess stakeholders' perceptions of the acceptability and feasibility of the intervention, a qualitative process evaluation was conducted. Using purposive sampling, a total of 12 people 4 teachers, 4 parents, and 4 community members participated in key informant interviews (KIIs) by the researcher. Semi-structured interviews explored stakeholder perceptions of the program, changes in children's behavior, changes in behavior management, logistical concerns with the intervention, and recommendations for future delivery/scale-up of the intervention.

Data collection

Two trained researchers with 2 years of experience in mental health research conducted the screening, baseline, and follow-up interviews. Both researchers received a 1-week training on the study objectives, design, overview of the intervention, ethics, and study instruments and semi-structured interview guide. At first, they conducted the screening interviews using the DBIS-N. If the screening instrument suggested that the children had behavior problems, they then conducted baseline interviews to collect household socio-economic information, the CFIS, and the ECBI. After the intervention, the same researchers conducted follow-up interviews.

Data analysis

The quantitative data was entered into SPSS software and paired t-tests were conducted to assess differences in mean scores between pre- and post-intervention. Regression analyses were performed to explore predictors of child behavior problems. Thematic analyses were conducted with the qualitative data to establish themes on related topics. The collected qualitative data was first transcribed in the original language (Nepali) and then translated into English. After translation, the data was analyzed through creation of themes and subthemes.

Results
Background information

Of the total 41 children who participated at baseline, 31 (75.6%) were boys and 10 (24.4%) were girls. Participating children's ages ranged from 6 to 15 years (mean = 10.7, SD = 2.8). Most children lived in nuclear families (65.9%) and a large proportion were from the Brahman/Chhetri caste (46.3%). Almost half of the children (41.7%) had fathers working in foreign employment. About two-thirds of the children (65.9%) had low food sufficiency status based on household production (Table 1).

Intervention outcomes

The paired sample t-test among the 39 children showed statistically significant reductions in mean DBIS-N problem scores, CFIS, and the ECBI. The change in the mean scores assessing impairment in daily functioning suggested that the intervention significantly improved children's daily functioning. On average, the intervention reduced the DBIS-N score by 7.5, the CFIS score by 3.2, the ECBI problem score by 16.1, and the ECBI intensity score by 4.9 (Table 2).

Table 1 Socio-economic characteristics of study participants

	N	%
Age		
Less than 10	13	31.7
10–12	16	39.0
13–16	12	29.3
Total	41	100.0
Range and standard deviation	5–15 (2.8)	
Gender		
Girls	10	24.4
Boys	31	75.6
Total	41	100.0
Types of family		
Single parent	5	12.2
Nuclear	27	65.9
Extended	9	22.0
Total	41	100.0
Caste/ethnicity		
Brahman/Chhetri	19	46.3
Janajati	18	43.9
Dalit	4	9.8
Total	41	100.0
Father occupation		
Foreign employment	15	41.7
Daily wage labor	9	25.0
Service	7	19.4
Others (agriculture, business, self-employed)	5	13.9
Total	36	100.0
Sources of family income		
Own agriculture	4	9.8
Fieldwork for other landowner	4	9.8
Daily wage labor non-farming	6	14.6
Service	8	19.5
Foreign employment	16	39.0
Others	3	7.3
Total	41	100.0
Food sufficiency for the whole year		
Yes	14	34.1
No	27	65.9
Total	41	100.0

The intervention resulted in better outcomes in reducing DBIS-N scores among children from extended families compared to single parents, and among children from the Brahman/Chhetri caste compared to the Dalit caste. Likewise, the intervention resulted in a significantly larger reduction of the Eyberg problem score and intensity score in older children than in younger children, and in children from the Brahman/Chhetri caste than the Dalit caste. The intervention resulted in significantly larger improvements in daily functioning among children belonging to the Brahman/Chhetri caste compared with children from the Dalit caste (Table 3).

Perspective on parent management training

A mother of three children learned to replace her typical scolding and beating with loving and sweet words. Her youngest child, stubborn and disobedient before the intervention, showed behavioral improvements when the mother started asking him to do things from a closer distance (rather than yelling across a room), and by taking him gently by the hand. Instead of getting annoyed and impatient, she learned to show her child love and be more attentive in helping him study and read. She explained, "*If we bring changes in our behavior, we could also bring changes in their behavior.*" As the psychosocial counselors taught parents and teachers to demonstrate love and patience to the children, instead of instilling fear through beating and scolding, intervention participants saw tangible changes in children's behaviors.

Restructuring routines

In addition to changes in disciplinary practices, parents were also instructed in creating daily schedules so that their children could follow structured day-to-day routines. Many parents stressed behavior changes seen as a result of instilling routine into their child's lives. Post-intervention, children more consistently washed, did homework, attended school, and ate meals in a scheduled manner. By allowing children to play after eating, instead of forcing them to immediately start work, parents noticed that their children demonstrated increased focus when it came time to study.

Table 2 Comparisons of mean changes between baseline and follow-up (N = 39)

	Baseline Mean (SD)	Follow-up Mean (SD)	T (df); p	CI	% change
DBIS	20.5 (3.8)	13.0 (6.4)	8.0 (38); 0.000	5.57–9.35	−36.6
CFIS	12.3 (6.1)	9.1 (5.6)	3.1 (38); 0.003	1.13–5.23	−26.0
ECBI problem score	107.9 (32.7)	91.7 (36.1)	3.2 (38); 0.003	5.84–26.41	−15.0
Eyberg Intensity Scale	14.8 (7.7)	9.9 (8.5)	3.1 (38); 0.003	1.76–8.14	−33.1

df, degrees of freedom; SD, standard deviation; CI, confidence interval

Table 3 Impact of the intervention by background characteristics (N = 39)

	DBIS		CFIS		ECBI problem score		Eyberg intensity scale	
	Beta (CI)	T (p)	Beta (CI)	T (p)	Beta (CI)	T (p)	Beta (CI)	T (p)
Time effects [baseline (ref.); end line]	−8.0* (−10.4 to −5.6)	−6.6 (0.000)	−3.0* (5.6 to 0.4)	−2.3 (0.02)	−14.0* (−28.1 to 0.1)	−2.0 (0.05)	−3.9* (−7.3 to −0.4)	−2.2 (0.03)
Age	−0.11 (−0.6 to 0.4)	−0.4 (0.67)	0.2 (−0.3 to 0.7)	0.8 (0.44)	−3.3* (−6.2 to 0.3)	−2.2 (0.03)	−0.7* (−1.4 to 0.1)	−2.0 (0.05)
Gender [girl (ref.); boys]	2.3 (−0.7 to 5.2)	1.5 (0.13)	2.3 (0.8 to 5.4)	1.5 (0.14)	2.2 (−14.9 to 19.2)	0.3 (0.80)	−0.8 (−5.0 to 3.3)	−0.4 (0.69)
Types of home [single parent (ref.); Nuclear; Joint]	−2.8* (−5.9 to 0.3)	−1.8 (0.07)	−1.5 (−4.8 to 1.7)	−0.9 (0.36)	−32.7* (−50.8 to −14.7)	−3.6 (0.001)	−2.4 (−6.9 to 2.0)	−1.1 (0.27)
Mother caste [Dalit (ref.); Janajati; Brahman/Chhetri]	−3.3* (−5.3 to −1.3)	−3.3 (0.002)	−2.4* (−4.5 to −0.3)	−2.3 (0.03)	−23.2* (−34.9 to −11.5)	−4.0 (0.000)	−5.8* (−8.7 to −3.0)	−4.1 (0.000)
Mother education [illiterate (ref.); primary; secondary; SLC and above]	−0.4 (−2.1 to 1.4)	−0.4 (0.66)	−1.2 (−3.1 to 0.6)	−1.3 (0.20)	2.9 (−7.2 to 13.1)	0.6 (0.56)	0.5 (−2.0 to 3.0)	0.4 (0.67)
Father occupation [foreign labor migration (ref.); labor; service; other]	1.0 (−0.2 to 2.3)	1.6 (0.11)	0.1 (−1.2 to 1.5)	0.2 (0.83)	4.6 (−2.6 to 11.8)	1.3 (0.21)	−0.1 (−1.8 to 1.7)	−0.1 (0.94)

CI, confidence interval

* Statistically significant at p < 0.05

Classroom changes

A teacher commented that instead of carrying a stick into the classroom, she started using inspirational methods to encourage students to work hard. She told her students: *"Whether you are here to play or to study, tomorrow you will need to be a doctor or an engineer".* By giving examples of people in society who were on the wrong track because of poor habits developed early in life, she motivated her students to study and work hard. Another teacher explained that through a developed understanding of child psychology, teachers learned to create more favorable learning environments. They worked more closely with parents, let guardians know if there was a problem, and treated each child as an individual. Rather than using harsh techniques on the entire classroom, they made specific action plans to help struggling students. A high school teacher enacted a "No Punishment Zone" at his school, noting that the *"behavior of one teacher determines the future of the child".* Following the intervention, if teachers beat their students they were liable to be punished, suggesting that the intervention led to sustained attitudinal and behavior change amongst teachers in the district. Teachers introduced new teaching methods and exercises to their classrooms based on psycho-education training. Before the intervention, some teachers had students copy answers even if children did not understand the questions—these teachers stopped this practice. One of the school principals started holding regular staff meetings to reiterate behavioral management techniques and to discuss challenges. During these meetings, teachers were encouraged to leave their stress at home and work toward a better understanding of child psychology.

Child behavior problems

As a result of changes both at home and in the classroom, teachers, parents, the principal, and the counselor, saw reductions in child externalizing behaviors. A teacher noted that the children in his classroom *"used to have a 90% habit of getting angry, and now it [had] fallen to 60%".* Other parents explained that their children started washing-up and studying without prompting. However, one mother noted that her child had reverted to his previous, disobedient state. She mentioned that children whose parents were not involved in the intervention were a bad influence on her son. While some children continued to lie and curse, all but one was significantly better behaved than before the intervention.

Feasibility and community perceptions of intervention

Community informants were asked how community members perceived the intervention. The participants reported that community members generally appreciated the intervention. For example, one teacher said, *"when*

I talked with my students' parents about the program, many laughed with joy as they were very pleased with the intervention". When asked whether the participants experienced any difficulties during the intervention, a few commented that they had difficulty attending meetings because of hectic work schedules. However, almost all informants mentioned that the counselors were flexible with their time and were willing to meet parents and teachers wherever and whenever was most convenient.

Recommendations

Participants recommended that counselors work with more parents in the community. While the intervention primarily targeted parents of children presenting with behavior problems, participants reported that other parents may have similarly benefitted from psycho-education. Additionally, some informants suggested ongoing follow-up. For instance, one of the school principals explained that teachers would benefit from continued education and psychosocial support on child psychology and behavior. One of the intervention counselors mentioned that she and her team had to make adjustments to classroom management skills, teacher–student relationships, communication skills, and reward and reinforcement systems. This counselor suggested that future programs add more information on self-care. Extremely happy with the intervention, a school teacher advocated for more training sessions in order to include the entire village—parents, teachers, and students alike. While the Nepali conflict caused a huge economic and societal burden, he explained that *"this kind of program,"* can make society *"more effective, trustworthy, and fruitful".*

Discussion

This study examined the feasibility, acceptability, and outcomes of a stepped school- and family-based intervention for child behavior problems in rural Nepal. In both quantitative measures and qualitative reports, parents and teachers of children with behavior problems reported substantial improvements in children's behaviors and functioning from baseline to follow-up. Parents and teachers both found the intervention feasible and acceptable to be implemented within a rural setting. Stakeholders in the community reported that the intervention brought important improvements in disciplinary practices both at home and at school. Improvements in behaviors at home were not isolated to participating families; rather, parents spread psycho-education to other community members, creating an environment supportive of positive behaviors among children and positive discipline and management among parents. Effectiveness studies assessing stepped family care models in India have shown similar findings; family-based interventions are appropriate even in poor and rural communities [34, 35]. This is consistent with the literature, including systematic reviews, observational studies, and randomized controlled trials, which suggests that positive parenting is a key factor in reducing child externalizing behaviors [11, 20, 36–39].

The mean score reductions on both the DBIS-N and the ECBI suggest significant improvements in children's behavior problems. However, demonstration of effectiveness will require demonstration of statistical significance when compared with a control group. It is important to note that regression analysis suggested that the intervention was most effective among children belonging to extended families, among children from the Brahman/Chhetri caste, and among younger children.

Through the intervention, family members learned to deal with their children's behavior problems through positive parenting and family adjustment. Family members were taught social learning techniques to improve children's negative behaviors. The presence of multiple adults caring for children in extended families could potentially explain the greater reductions in negative behaviors seen among children in these groups, when compared to single-parent homes. In extended, or joint family systems in Nepal, several family members are responsible for caring for children and adolescents. Thus, having several adults engaged in positive parenting and family adjustment likely benefited children in extended families.

While school- and family-based interventions are often effective for low-income students with externalizing behaviors [40], class differences can impact effectiveness [41]. Children from the Brahman/Chhetri caste may have experienced increased reductions in externalizing behaviors compared to children from the Janajati and Dalit castes due to ingrained community- and self-stigma and caste-based discrimination against these groups [42]. Additionally, families from high castes, particularly those with intact family structures, are exposed to fewer effects of social determinants of mental health [43]. Children from lower castes are more likely to be marginalized, live in unstable family situations, and be exposed to poverty. In order to see similar reductions in behavior problems among the Janajati and Dalit castes, these groups may require additional social services.

Younger children may have seen more significant improvements in ECBI because of age differences in environment, brain development, and impulsivity. Older students likely spend more time away from the classroom and home environments. Thus, these students were less frequently exposed to teachers' and parents' new disciplinary practices and behavior management techniques. Furthermore, impulsivity increases dramatically during adolescence [44]. Due to limitations in brain development, adolescents are often unable to control this impulsivity [45]. This pattern may be stronger in emotionally reactive adolescents [45]. As the students involved in the present study demonstrated emotional reactivity, it is likely that older individuals demonstrated worse outcomes than their younger counterparts due to age discrepancies in brain development and impulsivity.

The pilot intervention had a number of strengths. The intervention was delivered by community psychosocial counselors who received an extensive, week-long training. Quality assurance was continually ensured through regular supervision by a clinical psychologist with knowledge of the intervention. The intervention was successful in mobilizing qualified psychosocial counselors. In future stepped-care implementation in Nepal, programs can maximize intervention reach (contact coverage) by employing community psychosocial workers. If strong support and supervision mechanisms are established, community psychosocial workers can more efficiently reach parents and teachers.

In addition to the strengths noted above, the intervention also had limitations. Due to a lack of control group, this study was unable to infer causality, and therefore determine effectiveness. Thus, this study was only able to assess feasibility and acceptability. Another limitation stemmed from the short follow-up period, as behaviors were only measured after 4 months. Future research should employ a longer follow-up period, whereby children's behaviors are assessed on the three instruments at 6- and 12-month follow-up. Lastly, KII assessing stakeholders' perceptions of the acceptability and feasibility of the intervention were overwhelmingly positive. These results could potentially be skewed due to social desirability bias.

As this study served as an initial feasibility test of the intervention, follow-up research employing an adequately powered sample size and a control group should be implemented to determine intervention effectiveness. If the intervention is deemed effective, future scaling-up of the intervention in surrounding VDCs should monitor and evaluate progress using larger sample sizes and assessing socioeconomic differences and other potential moderating factors more rigorously.

In future studies, parents of children without moderate-to-severe behavioral problems could be reached through further peer support, for example by training and supervising parents to lead parent peer-groups on Parent Management Training. By relieving the resources required by having psychosocial counselors or community psychosocial workers lead sessions, parent-led groups could give parents agency and provide more parents with necessary strategies in dealing with child behavioral problems.

Conclusion

This study evaluated a stepped school- and family-based intervention for reducing child behavior problems in rural Nepal. The quantitative results demonstrated reductions in child externalizing behaviors, and parents and teachers involved in the intervention found the intervention acceptable and feasible for use with their children and students. Based upon the findings from this pilot testing, an RCT should be designed and implemented to determine the effectiveness of the intervention. If the intervention is shown to be effective for the Nepali setting, it should be further scale-up in surrounding VDCs and beyond to further reduce child externalizing behaviors, and subsequently, negative impacts at the family and community levels.

Authors' contributions

RPA and MJ designed the study. RPA supervised the data collection, conducted the analysis. The first draft was prepared by RPA, NU and ENS. NU, MDB and BK contributed in the design. All authors reviewed the manuscript. All authors read and approved the final manuscript.

Author details

[1] Padma Kanya Multiple Campus, Tribhuvan University Kathmandu, Bagbazar, Kathmandu, Nepal. [2] Research Department, Transcultural Psychosocial Organization (TPO), Baluwatar, Kathmandu, Nepal. [3] Global Mental Health and Addiction Program, University of Maryland College Park, College Park, USA. [4] Johns Hopkins University, Baltimore, MD, USA. [5] Department of Psychiatry and Behavioral Sciences, George Washington University, Washington, DC, USA. [6] Centre for Global Mental Health, Institute of Psychiatry, Psychology & Neuroscience, King's College London, London, UK.

Acknowledgements

We are thankful to Pragya Shrestha, Bina Chaudhary and Ambikalasalami Magar from Transcultural Psychosocial Organization (TPO) Nepal for their support in implementing the intervention. We are also grateful to Nagendra P. Luitel for technical guidance, Anup Adhikari for coordination support and researchers from TPO Nepal Chitwan District office for their support in data collection. We would like to thank Anna Louise Chiumento, University of Liverpool, UK, for reviewing the final manuscript and helping with the English editing.

Competing interests

The authors declare that they have no competing interests.

Funding

This research was supported by a fellowship to the first author under the South Asian Hub for Advocacy, Research and Education on Mental Health (SHARE), the U.S. National Institute of Mental Health (NIMH) Grant No. U19MH095687. BAK was supported by the US NIMH, Grant No. K01MH104310. The funder played no role in the design, data collection, analysis, or writing of the manuscript. The content is solely the responsibility of the authors and does not necessarily represent the official views of the National Institutes of Mental Health.

References

1. Klasen H, Crombag A. What works where? A systematic review of child and adolescent mental health interventions for low and middle income countries. Soc Psychiatry Psychiatr Epidemiol. 2013;48:595–611.
2. Fergusson DM, Horwood LJ, Ridder EM. Show me the child at seven: the consequences of conduct problems in childhood for psychosocial functioning in adulthood. J Child Psychol Psychiatry. 2005;46(8):837–49.
3. Matos M, Bauermeister JJ, Bernal G. Parent-Child Interaction Therapy for Puerto Rican preschool children with ADHD and behaviour problems: a pilot efficacy study. Parent Process. 2009;48(2):232–52.
4. Kessler RC, Amminger GP, Aguilar-Gaxiola S, Alonso J, Lee S, Ustün TB. Age of onset of mental disorders: a review of recent literature. Curr Opin Psychiatry. 2007;20(4):359–64.
5. Nock MK, Borges G, Bromet EJ, Cha CB, Kessler RC, Lee S. Suicide and suicidal behaviour. Epidemiol Rev. 2008;30(1):133–54.
6. Loeber R, Dishion T. Early predictors of male delinquency: a review. Psychol Bull. 1983;94(1):68–99.
7. Kessler RC, Berglund P, Demler O, Jin R, Walters EE. Lifetime prevalence and age-of-onset distributions of DSM-IV disorders in the National Comorbidity Survey Replication. Arch Gen Psychiatry. 2005;62(5):593–602.
8. Barkley RA, Fischer M, Smallish L, Fletcher K. Young adult outcome of hyperactive children: adaptive functioning in major life activities. J Am Acad Child Adolesc Psychiatry. 2006;45(2):192–202.
9. Rey JM, Morris-Yates A, Singh M, Andrews G, Gavin W. Continuities between psychiatric disorders in adolescents and personality disorders in young adults. Am J Psychiatry. 1995;152(6):895–900.
10. Canino G, Polanczyk G, Bauermeister JJ, Rohde LA, Frick PJ. Does the prevalence of CD and ODD vary across cultures? Soc Psychiatry Psychiatr Epidemiol. 2010;45(7):695–704.
11. Bywater T, Hutchings J, Daley D, Whitaker C, Yeo ST, Jones K, et al. Long-term effectiveness of a parenting intervention for children at risk of developing conduct disorder. Br J Psychiatry. 2009;195:318–24.
12. Sheldrick CE. Delinquency: risk factors and treatment interventions. Curr Opin Psychiatry. 1995;8(6):362–5.
13. Wallen J, Rubin RH. The role of the family in mediating the effects of community violence on children. Aggress Violent Behav. 1997;2(1):33–41.
14. IFRC. World disasters report. Geneva: International Federation of Red Cross and Red Crescent Societies; 2016. p. 2016.
15. Luitel NP, Jordans MJD, Sapkota RP, Tol WA, Kohrt BA, Thapa SB, et al. Conflict and mental health: a cross-sectional epidemiological study in Nepal. Soc Psychiatry Psychiatr Epidemiol. 2013;48(2):183–93.
16. Adhikari RP, Upadhaya N, Gurung D, Luitel NP, Burkey MD, Kohrt BA, et al. Perceived behavioural problems of school aged children in rural Nepal: a qualitative study. Child Adolesc Psychiatry Ment Health. 2015;9(25):1–9.
17. Burkey MD, Ghimire L, Adhikari RP, Wissow LS, Jordans MJ, Kohrt BA. The ecocultural context and child behavior problems: a qualitative analysis in rural Nepal. Soc Sci Med. 2016;159:73–82.
18. Ojha SP, Khalid A, Nepal MK, Koirala NR, Regmi SK, Gurung CK. An exploratory study of emotional and behavioural problems in physically disabled children and adolescents. J Inst Med. 2000;22(3&4):212–20.
19. Luitel NP, Jordans MJ, Adhikari A, Upadhaya N, Hanlon C, Lund C, et al. Mental health care in Nepal: current situation and challenges for development of a district mental health care plan. Confl Health. 2015;9:3.
20. Woolfenden S, Williams KJ, Peat J. Family and parenting interventions in children and adolescents with conduct disorder and delinquency aged 10–17. Cochrane Database Syst Rev. 2001;2:1–37.
21. Scott S, Sylva K, Doolan M, Price J, Jacobs B, Crook C, et al. Randomised controlled trial of parent groups for child antisocial behaviour targeting multiple risk factors: the SPOKES project. J Child Psychol Psychiatry. 2010;51:48–57.
22. Klasen H, Crombag AC. What works where? A systematic review of child and adolescent mental health interventions for low and middle income countries. Soc Psychiatry Psychiatr Epidemiol. 2013;48(4):595–611.
23. Gardner FEM. Parents anticipating misbehaviour: observational study of strategies parents use to prevent conflict with behaviour problem children. J Child Psychol Psychiatry. 1999;40(8):1185–96.
24. Baker-Henningham H, Scott S, Jones K, Walker S. Reducing child conduct problems and promoting social skills in a middle-income country: cluster randomised controlled trial. Br J Psychiatry. 2012;201:101–8.
25. Araya R, Fritsch R, Spears M, et al. School intervention to improve mental

health of students in Santiago, Chile: a randomized clinical trial. JAMA Pediatr. 2013;167(11):1004–10.

26. Jordans MJD, Kamproe I, Tol W, Kohrt B, Luitel N, Macy R, et al. Evaluation of a classroom-based psychosocial intervention in conflict-affected Nepal: a cluster randomized controlled trial. J Child Psychol Psychiatry. 2010;51(7):818–26.

27. Jordans MJD, Tol WA, Komproe IH, Susanty D, Vallipuram A, Ntamatumba P, et al. Development of a multi-layered psychosocial care system for children in areas of political violence. Int J Ment Health Syst. 2010;4(15):1–12.

28. Adhikari RP, Upadhaya N, Gurung D, Luitel NP, Burkey MD, Kohrt BA, et al. Perceived behavioral problems of school aged children in rural Nepal: a qualitative study. Child Adolesc Psychiatry Ment Health. 2015;9:25.

29. Jordans MJD, Tol WA, Komproe IH. Mental health interventions for children in adversity: pilot-testing a research strategy for treatment selection in low-income settings. Soc Sci Med. 2011;73(3):456–66.

30. Burkey MD, Ghimire L, Adhikari RP, Kohrt BA, Jordans MJD, Haroz EE, et al. Development process of an assessment tool for disruptive behavior problems in cross-cultural settings: the Disruptive Behavior International Scale—Nepal version (DBIS-N). Int J Cult Ment Health. 2016;9(4):387–98.

31. Burkey MD, Adhikari RP, Ghimire L, Kohrt BA, Wissow LS, Luitel N, et al. Validity and psychometric properties of the Disruptive Behavior International Scale—Nepal Version: a scale developed using local stakeholder participation **(Draft submitted)**.

32. Tol WA, Barbui C, Galappatti A, Silove D, Betancourt TS, Souza R, et al. Mental health and psychosocial support in humanitarian settings: linking practice and research. Lancet. 2011;378(9802):1581–91.

33. Eyberg SM, Ross AW. Assessment of child behavior problems: the validation of a new inventory. J Clin Child Psychol. 1978;7(2):113–6.

34. Van Ginneken N, Maheedharia MS, Ghani S, Ramakrishna J, Raja A, Patel V. Human resources and models of mental healthcare integration into primary and community care in India: case studies of 72 programmes. PLoS ONE. 2017;12(6):e0178954.

35. Patel VH, Kirkwood BR, Pednekar S, Araya R, King M, Chisholm D, et al. Improving the outcomes of primary care attenders with common mental disorders in developing countries: a cluster randomized controlled trial of a collaborative stepped care intervention in Goa, India. Trials. 2008;9:4.

36. Gardner F, Hutchings J, Bywater T, Whitaker C. Who benefits and how does it work? Moderators and mediators of outcomes in an effectiveness trial of a parenting intervention. J Clin Child Adolesc Psychol. 2010;39:568–80.

37. Haggerty KP, McGlynn-Wright A, Klima T. Promising parenting programmes for reducing adolescent problem behaviours. J Child Serv. 2013;8(4):229–43.

38. Furlong M, McGilloway S, Bywater T, Hutchings J, Smith SM, Donnelly M. Behavioural and cognitive-behavioural group based parenting programmes for early-onset conduct problems in children aged 3 to 12 years. Cochrane Database Syst Rev. 2012;2:CD008225.

39. Scott S, Knapp M, Henderson J, Maughan B. Financial cost of social exclusion: follow up study of antisocial children into adulthood. BMJ. 2001;323(7306):191.

40. O'Donnell J, Hawkins JD, Catalano RF, Abbott RD, Day LE. Preventing school failure, drug use, and delinquency among low-income children: long-term intervention in elementary schools. Am J Orthopsychiatry. 1995;65(1):87–100.

41. Cutler D. Behavioral health interventions: what works and why? In: Bulatao R, Anderson N, editors. Understanding racial and ethnic differences in health in late life: a research agenda. Washington, DC: National Academies Press; 2004.

42. OHCHR. Shadow of caste and its stigma continue to violate all aspects of human rights. 2016. http://www.ohchr.org/EN/NewsEvents/Pages/Shadowofcaste.aspx. Accessed 15 Sept 2017.

43. WHO. Social determinants of mental health. Geneva: World Health Organization and Calouste Gulbenkian Foundation; 2014.

44. Romer D. Adolescent risk taking, impulsivity, and brain development: implications for prevention. Dev Psychobiol. 2010;52(3):263–76.

45. Casey BJ, Jones RM, Hare TA. The adolescent brain. Ann NY Acad Sci. 2008;1124:111–26.

Cost-effectiveness of dialectical behaviour therapy vs. enhanced usual care in the treatment of adolescents with self-harm

Egil Haga[1]* ⓘ, Eline Aas[2], Berit Grøholt[1], Anita J. Tørmoen[1] and Lars Mehlum[1]

Abstract

Background: Studies have shown that dialectical behaviour therapy (DBT) is effective in reducing self-harm in adults and adolescents.

Aims: To evaluate the cost-effectiveness of DBT for adolescents (DBT-A) compared to enhanced usual care (EUC).

Methods: In a randomised study, 77 adolescents with repeated self-harm were allocated to 19 weeks of outpatient treatment, either DBT-A ($n = 39$) or EUC ($n = 38$). Cost-effective analyses, including estimation of incremental cost-effectiveness ratios, were conducted with self-harm and global functioning (CGAS) as health outcomes.

Results: Using self-harm as effect outcome measure, the probability of DBT being cost-effective compared to EUC increased with increasing willingness to pay up to a ceiling of 99.5% (threshold of € 1400), while with CGAS as effect outcome measure, this ceiling was 94.9% (threshold of € 1600).

Conclusions: Given the data, DBT-A had a high probability of being a cost-effective treatment.

Keywords: Cost-effectiveness, Self-harm, Psychotherapy, Longitudinal, Randomised trial

Background

Repeated self-harm is strongly associated with mental health problems [1, 2], and a large proportion of self-harming adolescents report having been in contact with mental health services, if not necessarily in relation to their self-harm episodes [3–5]. Psychosocial treatments that effectively reduce self-harm in adolescents have only recently emerged. Such treatments seem to be characterised by a sufficient dose of treatment and family involvement [6]. Repeated self-harm is resource-demanding, as it involves a broad range of health services for shorter or longer periods of time. Resources are, however, always limited, and there is a strong consensus that our clinical priorities should be made on the basis of the severity of the disorder, expected benefits of the treatments, and assessment of the relationship between costs and effects.

Studies of cost-effectiveness involve the systematic measurement of the inputs (treatment costs) and outcomes (health) of two alternative treatments, commonly the new experimental treatment and standard treatment. The subsequent comparative analysis provides decision-makers with information on between-treatments differences with respect to costs and health effects. The results thus form the basis for evaluating whether the new treatment produces a better health effect to a lower or similar cost compared to standard treatment, alternatively that a higher cost is acceptable for added health effect. In the present study the cost-effectiveness of DBT-A is analyzed based on the incremental cost-effectiveness ratio (ICER), given by the ratio of between-group differences in costs and effects.

Several trials have shown that dialectical behaviour therapy (DBT) is effective in reducing self-harm [7–11] compared to treatment as usual (TAU). Two previous RCT studies, both comparing DBT with treatment as usual (TAU) over a period of 12 months, have included an economic evaluation. A study with female adult

---

*Correspondence: egil.haga@medisin.uio.no
[1] National Centre for Suicide Research and Prevention, University of Oslo, Sognsvannsveien 21, Bygg 12, 0372 Oslo, Norway
Full list of author information is available at the end of the article

patients (N = 44) showed that DBT treatment incurred significantly higher psychotherapy costs, but lower inpatient care and emergency room costs than TAU over a period of 12 months. However, the results indicated no statistically significant differences in total treatment costs [12]. Another economic evaluation of DBT (age > 16 years, N = 40), yielded a similar result as it showed no significant differences in total treatment costs [13]. In a review of the cost-effectiveness of treatments for people with borderline personality disorder (BPD), treatment studies were included by estimating cost data on the basis of available resource use data thus enabling analyses of cost-effectiveness. The authors conclude that none of the reviewed treatments, including DBT, were cost-effective, but that DBT has a potential for being cost-effective [14]. A shortened version of DBT, delivered in the outpatient setting, has been adapted for adolescents (DBT-A). With a strong focus on teaching distress tolerance skills and enhancing family functioning, the treatment is expected to use more resources in the outpatient setting than usual care, one of the aims being to reduce the need for hospitalizations. Recently, we have shown that DBT-A is more effective than enhanced usual care (EUC) in reducing frequency of self-harm episodes [15, 16]. To our knowledge, no study has conducted an economic evaluation of DBT-A. It is important to establish whether such a relatively brief intervention with intensified use of resources would lead to reduced needs for resources in the longer term, and particularly whether DBT-A is associated with a reduced need for hospitalizations, thus, reducing treatment costs substantially. The aims of the present study were: to assess the total treatment costs of DBT-A compared to EUC, both over the treatment trial period of 19 weeks and over a subsequent follow-up year of 52 weeks, and to evaluate in a health care perspective the cost-effectiveness of DBT-A compared to EUC, with number of self-harm episodes and global functioning as health outcomes. To examine the economic impact of the intervention after the relatively short trial period the cost-effectiveness analysis will be conducted on the entire observational period from treatment start to follow-up assessment, altogether 71 weeks.

Methods

Methods have been described in separate papers [15, 16]. The core issues relevant to this cost-effectiveness study are presented below. The study is registered at Clinical-Trials.gov (Identifier NTC00675129).

Design

Participants were randomised to receive either DBT-A or EUC, stratified according to the presence of major depression, suicide intent at the most severe self-harm episode in the 4 months prior to enrollment, and gender.

Participants

A total of 77 adolescents (39 to DBT-A and 38 to EUC) were enrolled, from June 2008 to March 2012, mainly from child and adolescent psychiatric outpatient clinics in the Oslo area. Inclusion criteria were repeated self-harm (two or more episodes, the last episode within the past 4 months), age 12–18 years, and meeting at least three criteria of borderline personality disorder (assessed by SCID-II). The study was approved by the Regional Committee for Medical Research Ethics, South-East Norway. All patients and parents provided written informed consent prior to inclusion in the study.

Treatments

All participants received 19 weeks of treatment (trial period) in one of the publicly funded child and adolescent outpatient psychiatric clinics in the Oslo region/Norway. As is all publicly funded health care in Norway, treatments were free of charge for the participants in both treatment conditions.

The patients allocated to DBT-A received treatment according to the adolescent version of DBT [17]. The programme consisted of 19 weeks of weekly sessions (60 min) of individual therapy and weekly sessions (120 min) of skills training in a multifamily format. Family therapy sessions and telephone coaching were provided as needed according to the DBT-A protocol [18]. After 19 weeks, DBT-A treatment was ended and in cases where further treatment was needed, patients were referred to standard outpatient treatment (non-DBT) in one of the participating clinics. EUC was non-manualized, but was mainly psychodynamical or cognitive behaviour-oriented therapy, enhanced for the purpose of the trial through providing all therapists with training in suicide risk assessment and management and implementing a patient safety protocol [15]. Furthermore, EUC therapists were required to provide weekly treatment over a period of a minimum of 19 weeks. The termination of EUC-patients' treatment was decided by each therapist, so that outpatient treatment was continued beyond 19 weeks when needed. In the follow-up period (week 20–71) the participants in both groups received standard outpatient treatment as needed, which would be of different length and frequency. Some of the patients did not receive any outpatient treatment (23% of the DBT-A patients and 14% of the EUC patients).

Health outcomes

The participants were clinically assessed before treatment-start, at the end of the trial (19 weeks), and at a follow-up assessment 52 weeks after end of the trial, so that the entire observational period was 71 weeks. The clinical outcomes were evaluated by using the Lifetime Parasuicide Count (LPC) interview [19] for number of self-harm episodes (from treatment start to follow-up assessment), and the researcher rated Children's Global Assessment Scale (CGAS) [20] for global functioning.

Costs

Data on outpatient treatment resources (number of individual therapy sessions, family therapy sessions, group sessions, telephone consultations and the amount of medication) were collected from clinical records for the intervention period (week 0–19). Additionally, we monitored use of other health services due to self-harm or risk of self-harm (in the results section referred to as emergency treatment), which included inpatient treatment, emergency room visits, and general practitioner (GP) consultations. These data were collected from the adolescents on the basis of both interview and self-report, as well as from registry data obtained from the National Patient Registry (NPR). In the follow-up period (week 20–71) data on outpatient treatment and inpatient treatment were obtained from the NPR and from self-report questionnaires and interview. Data on GP consultations and emergency room visits were based on self-report and interview for this period.

The National Patient Registry (NPR) contains information on specialized treatment in psychiatric outpatient clinics and inpatient hospitalizations (psychiatric and somatic). The registry provides reliable records of resource use per patient, since the accurate registering of treatment contacts is mandatory and is the basis for funding of the clinics.

The data on the use of health service resources were collected over a 4-year period. The costs per resource unit were estimated on the basis of cost information from the financial year 2012. Costs are presented in EUR, converted from NOK by the average exchange rate of 2012. The mean total cost per patient in each group was estimated for the trial period (week 0–19) and for the follow-up period from end of trial period to follow-up assessment (week 20–71). Total treatment costs for the entire observational period from baseline to follow-up assessment (71 weeks) were calculated on the basis of these estimates. The estimation of cost for one specific resource unit, e.g. one individual therapy session in an outpatient clinic, was based on an approach that includes all actual costs that were required to produce the total number of individual therapy sessions within a given time period, divided by the number of sessions that were produced during that period. Thus, the cost for a resource unit includes wages for staff (clinical/administrative),

equipment, IT, house rent, etc. Data on these costs were obtained from annual accounts from the participating clinics.

The specific costs related to DBT-A include the cost of telephone coaching (implying availability after regular working hours) and weekly therapist team consultations. The average cost per patient for telephone coaching was estimated on the basis of an annual extra fee which each therapist in the participating DBT-A teams received, and was added to the total outpatient cost (week 0–19) for each DBT-A patient. Similarly, the average cost per patient for DBT-A therapist team consultation was estimated and added to the outpatient cost (week 0–19) per DBT-A patient. Since there was no available data on supervision received by the EUC therapists, we have assumed that supervision received by EUC therapists was less resource-intensive compared to DBT-A by a factor of 0.5 (based on a previous economic evaluation of DBT [14]), and added this average cost to all EUC patients.

The average unit cost of one general practitioner (GP) visit (due to self-harm or risk of self-harm) was estimated based on information from the Norwegian Health Economics Administration (HELFO), and is the sum of what each patient pays the GP for the consultation, the amount of health insurance reimbursement the GP on average receives per consultation, and the average annual reimbursement the GP receives from the municipality per consultation. Data on the use of medication was collected for the trial period, and costs per patient were estimated on the basis of price per tablet for a specific psychotropic drug used by the patient (cf. records of Norwegian Medicines Agency [21]) and assumed number of tablets used, i.e. the patient's days of receiving medication treatment and recommended daily dosage, as per The Norwegian Pharmaceutical Product Compendium [22].

Statistical analyses

Analyses were carried out on an intention-to-treat basis. Means and standard deviations or median and interquartile ranges were computed for normally and non-normally distributed clinical/sociodemographic variables. Between-group differences were tested by independent samples t tests or Mann–Whitney U tests. Differences between group proportions were tested by Pearson's Chi squared or Fisher's exact tests.

Costs of treatment are presented as mean total treatment costs per patient. Long inpatient hospitalizations incur high costs by relatively few patients, so that the costs for a single patient may affect the mean of the treatment group substantially. Such hospitalizations have been treated as rare but plausible events, and we have presented results regarding emergency treatment costs both with and without costs incurred by hospitalizations.

For analysis of cost-effectiveness we estimated incremental cost-effect ratios (ICER). The ICER is given as the difference in mean costs $(\overline{C}_{DBT} - \overline{C}_{EUC})$ divided by the difference in mean effect $(\overline{E}_{DBT} - \overline{E}_{EUC}$ on a given health outcome), i.e. $ICER = \overline{C}_{DBT} - \overline{C}_{EUC}/\overline{E}_{DBT} - \overline{E}_{EUC}$. A treatment is considered cost-effective if the treatment is more effective at a lower or similar cost than the comparator. The more effective treatment may also be considered cost-effective despite a higher cost, depending on the willingness-to-pay for health gains [23].

Because of the difficulties related to estimation of confidence intervals for the ICER [24], we have used bootstrapping to simulate a distribution of mean incremental costs and mean incremental effects, thus illustrating the uncertainty of the point estimate of the ICER. This was done by bootstrapping the costs and effect for each group separately (1000 replications). Incremental cost $(\Delta\overline{C} = \overline{C}_{DBT} - \overline{C}_{EUC})$ and incremental effect $(\Delta\overline{E} = \overline{E}_{DBT} - \overline{E}_{EUC})$ were calculated for each bootstrap sample and were plotted on the incremental cost-effectiveness plane (see Fig. 1), where each data-point represents one simulated $\Delta\overline{C}$ (y-axis) on $\Delta\overline{E}$ (x-axis). Finally, cost-effectiveness acceptability curves (CEAC) were constructed to summarize the uncertainty in cost-effectiveness estimates [25]. The CEAC represents the probability that DBT-A is cost-effective compared to EUC with increasing threshold values of willingness to pay for one unit incremental effect.

In the efficacy study group-differences in self-harm episodes were analysed separately for the intervention period and the follow-up period. Mixed-effect Poisson regression with robust variance was used to test for differences [16]. For estimation of incremental effectiveness in terms of self-harm, to be included in the cost-effectiveness analysis, we assumed that the groups had the same mean number of self-harm episodes at baseline, so that the effect difference was given by the difference in the mean total number of self-harm episodes per group from treatment start to the 71 weeks' assessment.

We have missing data for some participants on specific sub-categories of outpatient treatment costs (e.g. for five patients on phone calls to patients). We also had missing data for the main cost categories: one patient in the intervention period and three patients in the follow-up period for outpatient treatment costs, and two patients in the follow-up for emergency treatment costs. We have used the mean cost for the patient's treatment group to impute missing data. Missing data on self-harm episodes (two DBT-A patients and six EUC patients) have been imputed by using the expectation–maximization (EM) method. All analyses were performed with STATA 13 [26] and IBM SPSS Statistics 22 for Windows [27].

Results

Baseline characteristics

Mean age of the 77 patients was 15.6 years $(SD = 1.5)$ and 88.3% were girls. There were no differences between the 39 allocated to DBT-A and the 38 participants allocated to EUC on any of the reported sociodemographic and clinical variables before treatment start (Table 1). There were also no between-group differences with respect to proportion of patients having received any psychiatric treatment (68.0% of the total sample) and having been admitted to inpatient psychiatric treatment (7.8% of the total sample) prior to participation in the study.

Main results of the efficacy study

In the first 19 weeks, DBT-A was superior to EUC in reducing the number of self-harm episodes and the level of suicidal ideation and depressive symptoms [15]. At 71 weeks, participants who had received DBT-A still had a statistically significantly larger reduction in self-harm episodes than participants in the EUC-group, however for the other outcomes there were no longer significant differences; this was caused by EUC participants having reached an equal level of improvement over the 1 year follow-up interval [16].

Incremental costs

DBT-A had significantly higher outpatient treatment costs at 19 weeks (Table 2), mainly due to the costs incurred by the DBT-A multifamily skills training (group sessions). The costs of emergency treatment due to self-harm or risk of self-harm were higher in the EUC group due to one long hospitalization. Because of the low number of patients and incidents, the difference was not tested statistically. The average cost per patient for medication in the trial period was included in the outpatient treatment costs and was 7 € in both groups $(SD = 42$ for the DBT-A group and $SD = 19$ for the EUC group). DBT-A incurred higher total treatment costs. The mean difference € 2981 (95% CI = − 4666 to 10,629) was statistically significant $(p < 0.000)$.

The EUC patients incurred significantly higher outpatient costs than the DBT-A patients in the follow-up period (week 20–71). The EUC emergency treatment costs were higher because of one long inpatient hospitalization (difference not tested statistically). The total treatment costs were higher in the EUC group in this period, and the mean difference € − 10787 (95% CI = − 20023 to − 1550) was statistically significant $(p = 0.007)$.

For the entire observation period from treatment start to follow-up assessment (week 0–71), the difference in outpatient treatment costs between the DBT-A patients and the EUC patients was not statistically significant $(p = 0.555)$. Although the EUC group incurred on average

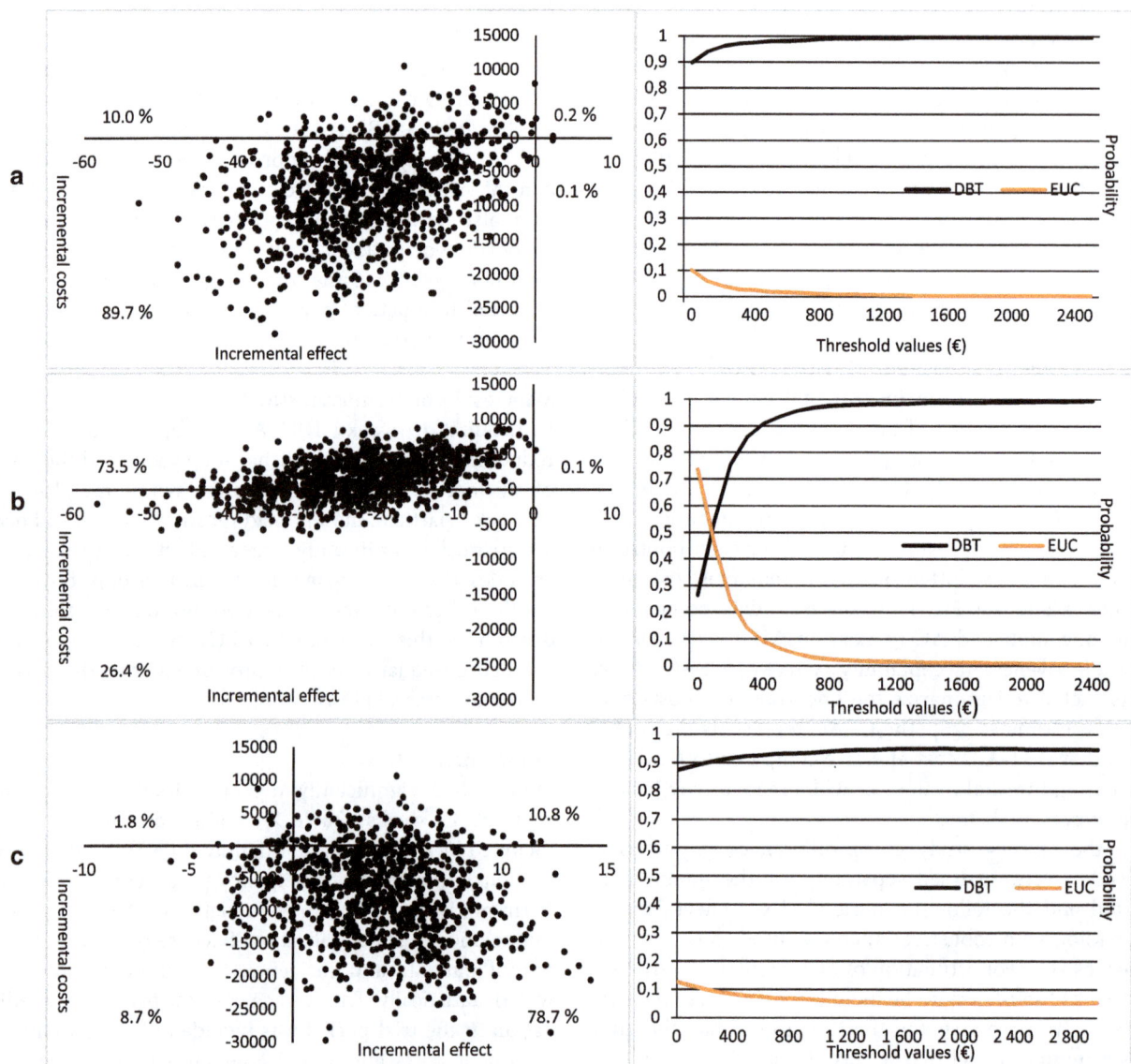

Fig. 1 The figure shows plots of simulated ICERs, mean incremental costs on the y-axis, and mean incremental effect on the x-axis (per bootstrap sample, 1000 replications), on the left hand side. On the right hand side, the corresponding CEACs show changes in probability of DBT-A being cost-effective compared to EUC (y-axis) as a function of increasing threshold values (x-axis). **a** Plot of simulated ICERs and CEAC with incremental total treatment costs and mean incremental effect in terms of mean number of self-harm episodes. Note that increased effect is indicated by negative values on the x-axis. **b** Plot of simulated ICERs and CEAC with incremental outpatient costs (emergency treatment costs excluded) and mean incremental effect in terms of mean number of self-harm episodes. Note that increased effect is indicated by negative values on the x-axis. **c** Plot of simulated ICERs and CEAC with incremental total treatment costs and mean incremental effect in terms of change in global functioning (CGAS)

higher emergency treatment costs, the difference was not statistically significant ($p=0.261$). EUC incurred higher total treatment costs, but the mean difference € -7805 (95% CI = -21622 to 6012) was not statistically significant ($p=0.508$).

Incremental effectiveness
The EUC patients reported a mean of 22.5 (95% CI = 11.4–33.5) episodes in the 19 weeks trial period and

14.8 (95% CI = 7.3–22.3) episodes during the subsequent follow-up period, whereas the DBT-A patients reported a mean of 9.0 (95% CI = 4.7–13.2) and 5.5 (95% CI = 1.7–9.1) in the corresponding time intervals. The between-group difference was statistically significant at both time intervals ($p<0.05$) [16]. For estimation of incremental effectiveness in terms of self-harm, we analysed the frequency of self-harm episodes for the entire observation period of 71 weeks. Since we did not have comparable

Table 1 Sample characteristics before treatment start

	DBT-A (N = 39)		EUC (N = 38)		Total sample (N = 77)	
	N	%[a]	N	%[a]	N	%[a]
Female sex	34	87.2	34	89.5	68	88.3
Child protection (current)	6	15.4	7	18.4	13	16.9
Child protection (past)	10	26.3	11	28.9	21	27.6
Past psychiatric treatment	28	73.7	23	62.2	51	68.0
Past inpatient psychiatric treatment	3	8.6	3	7.9	6	7.8
Current DSM-IV Axis I and II diagnoses						
Major depression	9	23.1	8	21.1	17	22.1
Other depressive disorder	16	41.0	13	34.2	29	37.7
Panic disorder	2	5.1	5	13.2	7	9.1
Posttraumatic stress disorder	7	17.9	6	15.8	13	16.9
Any anxiety disorder	18	46.2	15	39.5	33	42.9
Any substance use disorder	1	2.6	1	2.6	2	2.6
Any eating disorder	3	7.7	3	7.9	6	7.8
Borderline personality disorder	10	26.3	5	14.3	15	20.5
Suicide attempts, last 4 months (n)	11	28.2	9	23.7	20	26.0
	Mean	SD	Mean	SD	Mean	SD
Age (years)	15.9	1.4	15.3	1.6	15.6	1.5
C-GAS score	55.3	8.0	57.9	10.1	56.1	8.3
CBCL total, by parent (n)	69.6	11.0	68.4	8.9	69.0	9.8
Suicide attempts, lifetime (n)[c]	2.1	5.2	1.3	2.8	1.7	4.2
Non-suicidal self-harm, lifetime (n)[b]	49.5	159.5	25.0	45.5	34.0	88.0

[a] Due to missing data in some cells there were slight variations in the percentage basis

[b] Median and interquartile range

[c] The median was zero for both groups. The interquartile ranges were 1.0 and 1.3 in the DBT and EUC group, respectively

data on number of self-harm episodes at baseline, the effect difference was given by the between-group difference at 71 weeks based on the assumption that baseline levels of self-harm were similar in both groups. The mean number of self-harm episodes was 15.0 ($SD = 17.5$) for the DBT-A patients and 37.5 ($SD = 52.9$) for the EUC patients. The mean effect difference was -22.5 (95% CI $= -40.6$ to -4.3) (Table 3).

Global functioning was measured by CGAS, and effect was calculated as change in CGAS from baseline to follow-up assessment (week 0–71). Mean improvement in CGAS was 10.4 ($SD = 13.4$) for the DBT group and 6.3 ($SD = 14.9$); the mean effect difference 4.1 (95% CI $= -2.3$ to 10.6) was not statistically significant ($p = 0.204$).

Incremental cost-effectiveness with number of self-harm episodes as effect outcome measure

The incremental cost-effectiveness ratio (ICER) was estimated to € $-7805/-22.5 = €\,346$; i.e. the cost reduction for DBT-A compared to EUC was € 346 per reduction of 1 self-harm episode (Table 3). Bootstrapping (1000 replications) was performed, and the incremental mean

cost and effect of each bootstrap sample were plotted on the incremental cost-effectiveness plane (Fig. 1a). A proportion of 89.7% of the simulated ICERs falls into the quadrant where a reduction in self-harm is achieved by DBT-A for less cost compared to EUC. Additionally, 10.0% of the simulated ICERs fall into the quadrant with better effect to a higher cost.

The cost effectiveness acceptability curve (CEAC, Fig. 1a) shows the probability of DBT-A being cost-effective in reducing the number of self-harm episodes, compared to EUC, as a function of increasing threshold values of willingness to pay for reduction of one self-harm episode. With a zero threshold, i.e. no willingness to pay, the probability of DBT-A being cost-effective is 89.8% (the proportion of the simulations below the x-axis). With increasing threshold values, the probability of DBT being cost-effective increases, since a proportion of the simulated ICERs in the quadrant above the x-axis is added to the proportion considered cost-effective. The probability of DBT-A being cost-effective increases to 97.5% with a threshold value of € 400, and up to a ceiling probability at approx. 99.5%, at a threshold of € 1400.

Table 2 Outpatient, emergency and total treatment costs (EUR) per patient, week 0–19 (trial), week 20–71 (follow-up) and week 0–71 (entire period)

	Week 0–19				Week 20–71				Week 0–71			
	DBT-A	EUC	Mean diff (SE)	p	DBT-A	EUC	Mean diff (SE)	p	DBT-A	EUC	Mean diff (SE)	p
	Mean (SD)	Mean (SD)			Mean (SD)	Mean (SD)			Mean (SD)	Mean (SD)		
Outpatient costs	15,850 (5758)	9566 (5782)	6284 (1333)	0.000[a]	5367 (7079)	9938 (9894)	−4571 (1969)	0.010	21,217 (10,906)	19,504 (14,291)	1713 (2892)	0.555[b]
Emergency treatment costs[a]	349 (1726)	3651 (21,644)	−3303 (3476)		541 (2996)	6757 (22,503)	−6215 (3682)		890 (4701)	10,408 (30,440)	−9518 (4803)	0.261
Emergency treatment costs, hospitalizations excluded	24 (73)	90 (187)	−66 (33)		63 (171)	20 (74)	43 (30)		87 (206)	110 (217)	−23 (46)	0.659
Emergency treatment: number of patients and incidents	6 patients (2 inpatients) 10 incidents	10 patients (2 inpatients) 23 incidents			8 patients (1 inpatient) 11 incidents	8 patients (6 inpatients) 10 incidents			11 patients (3 inpatients) 21 incidents	13 patients (8 inpatients) 33 incidents		
Total treatment costs	16,199 (6669)	13,217 (23,006)	2981 (3839)	0.000	5909 (8266)	16,695 (27,042)	−10,787 (4582)	0.007	22,107 (13,358)	29,912 (40,179)	−7805 (6860)	0.508

a Costs of emergency treatment due to self-harm or risk of self-harm, including GP consultations, emergency department visits and hospitalizations

b t test. Other tests of p values of mean difference are tested by Mann–Whitney U

Table 3 Summary of costs (EURO) and effects at follow-up assessment (71 weeks)

	Total costs	Outpatient costs	Number of self-harm episodes	Change in CGAS score
	Mean (SD)	Mean (SD)	Mean (SD)	Mean (SD)
DBT-A	22,107 (13,358)	21,217 (10,906)	15.0 (17.5)	10.4 (13.4)
EUC	29,912 (40,179)	19,504 (14,291)	37.5 (52.9)	6.3 (14.9)
	Mean (CI 95%)	Mean (CI 95%)	Mean (CI 95%)	Mean (CI 95%)
Group differences	−7805 (−21,622 to 6012)	1713 (−4049 to 7475)	−22.5 (−40.6 to −4.3)	4.1 (−2.3 to 10.6)
ICER, total costs/self-harm	346[a]			
ICER, outpatient costs/self-harm	−76[a]			
ICER, total costs/CGAS	−1904[b]			

[a] Cost difference in EURO per reduction of one self-harm episode

[b] Cost difference in EURO per one point improvement in CGAS score (global functioning)

As noted above two long inpatient admissions in the EUC group substantially affected the total mean costs of the EUC patients. In order to study the impact of such costs on the ICER we excluded the inpatient and other emergency treatment costs for both groups, thus including only outpatient costs. The ICER was estimated to €1713/−22.5 = € −76, i.e. the extra cost for a reduction of one self-harm episode was € 76. The CEAC (Fig. 1b) showed that, with costs associated with inpatient and other emergency treatments excluded from the analysis, EUC had a higher probability of being cost-effective with no willingness to pay for extra effect. With willingness to pay approximately € 100 per reduction of one self-harm episode, the probability of being cost-effective was equal for the treatment groups; with willingness to pay more than € 100, DBT-A had a higher probability of being cost-effective, i.e. a probability up to a ceiling ratio of 99.9%.

Incremental cost-effectiveness with global functioning (CGAS) as effect outcome measure

With CGAS as effect outcome measure, the ICER was estimated to € −7805/4.1 = € −1904, i.e. the cost reduction for DBT-A vs. EUC was € 1904 per one point improvement in CGAS. The plot of mean costs and effects showed that a majority of the simulated ICERs falls into the quadrant with more effect at a lower cost (78.7%). The CEAC showed that the probability of DBT-A being cost-effective increases up to a ceiling of 94.9% at a threshold of € 1600.

Discussion

This study showed that there were no statistically significant differences between DBT-A and EUC with respect to total treatment costs when taking both the treatment trial period of 19 weeks and the 1-year follow-up interval under consideration. When cost data were analysed

together with our previously published outcome data showing that DBT-A was superior to EUC in reducing self-harm over the relevant time interval [16], we found that DBT-A had a probability of being cost-effective increasing from 89.8% with no willingness to pay extra for extra health gains, up to a ceiling probability at approximately 99.5% with increasing willingness to pay up to a threshold of € 1400. Thus, given the data, DBT-A had a high probability of being cost-effective compared to EUC.

DBT-A had higher outpatient treatment costs during the 19 weeks trial period, whereas EUC had higher outpatient costs during the follow-up period. It is an important finding that the intensified use of resources during the intervention period was followed by a subsequent reduced need for treatment in the follow-up period for the DBT-A group. Our efficacy study showed that DBT-A resulted in a more rapid improvement during the intervention period [15]. The finding that DBT-A improved health at 19 weeks and that there were no statistically significant between-group differences in outpatient treatment costs at 71 weeks, suggests that the initial extra use of resources in the DBT-A group gave good value for money.

Two previous studies have shown higher outpatient psychotherapy costs for DBT compared to the control group [12, 13]. In these studies, the original DBT program for adults was used, so that the intervention had longer duration. The patients in these studies were mainly adults, and although comparison between adult and adolescent samples should be done with caution, our findings suggest that a shorter DBT intervention period may be favourable both from an effect- and a cost-perspective.

There were no between-group differences with respect to emergency intervention costs other than hospitalization. The EUC group incurred considerably higher costs for hospitalizations due to two long inpatient stays. When including the costs of hospitalization, the total treatment costs were higher for EUC for the entire period, but the difference did not reach statistical significance, partly because the impact of long hospitalization costs are ruled out in the rank-order test (Mann–Whitney U). DBT-A has a specific focus on reducing hospitalization, and some previous studies have pointed in the direction that DBT may reduce the need for such hospitalization compared to the control treatment, [7, 8, 28] although this finding has not been replicated by other studies [9, 29–31]. The observed differences in our study are difficult to interpret with respect to between-group differences due to the limited number of hospitalizations. It would not be possible to conclude whether the higher incurred costs in the EUC group were due to treatment differences or a result of mere chance.

The relatively small proportion of patients receiving inpatient treatment in the present study contrasts what has been observed in studies with adult patients [7, 8, 29, 31]. It is, however, important to note that psychiatric hospitalisation of adolescents has in general a much higher threshold in most countries, since such measures are regarded as very drastic in this age group, since most adolescents have a base for care in their own family, and clinicians will normally seek to deliver crisis interventions in an outpatient fashion. To be able to observe analysable differences, a study with more patients and/or longer duration of follow-up would be required.

In this study treatment was free of charge for the participants. Provided that the way treatment is funded in other health care systems does not lead to substantial between-group differences in total treatment costs, we suggest that the findings of the study would generalize to systems where treatment is not publicly funded. However, we may assume that certain factors could affect the costs of DBT-A compared to standard treatment, e.g. the extent to which frequency of inpatient admissions differ across systems, whether one of the treatment methods is more or less available dependent of the healthcare setting, and/or the possibility that the ratio of cost per resource unit for outpatient treatment and inpatient treatment differ across systems. It is beyond the scope of this article to fully examine this complex issue of generalizability.

Limitations

Our sample was of limited size for a cost-effectiveness study. A larger sample combined with a longer observation period would have provided a stronger basis for detecting possible group differences, on both clinical and cost variables. Most importantly it would facilitate

analysis of the use of crisis services, as mentioned above, which is a highly relevant issue for this patient group. Furthermore, we have limited the cost analyses to direct treatment costs and not included societal costs. It would be expected that productivity losses due to, e.g. parents' extra care for their adolescents, would result in indirect costs for this patient group. The adolescents' absenteeism from school would also be a relevant indirect cost unit to study. Although difficult to value within a limited time perspective, this would be relevant to follow-up into adulthood since non-completed education may have an impact on the ability to maintain employment, with substantial indirect costs to society. Finally, quality adjusted life years (QALYs) are commonly included in cost-effectiveness studies as a generic measure of health outcome; but this was not used in the present study, since it was not initially planned as a cost-effectiveness study. Instead we chose CGAS as a measure of global health effect.

Strengths

The liberal inclusion criteria and the delivering of treatments in a community mental health setting with patients recruited from a defined catchment area strengthen the external validity of the findings.

The validity of the findings is increased by the randomised trial design and the rigorous procedures for data collection, providing high-quality data for health outcome measures. A further strength is the high participation rate with only two participants (one in each treatment condition) lost to follow-up at 71 weeks. Finally, the calculation of costs is based on detailed and reliable data for the most resource-intensive treatment categories (outpatient treatment and inpatient hospitalizations), directly derived from records of the clinics where the patients received treatment, as well as from the Norwegian Patient Registry. The data regarding costs for GP consultations and emergency room visits due to self-harm or risk of self-harm were based on self-report and interview, and may be less accurate because of recall bias. However, collecting the data from different sources made it possible to cross-check information, thus minimizing the effect on data quality.

Conclusions

The findings that DBT-A had a higher probability of being cost-effective compared to EUC, and that DBT-A was superior in reducing self-harm at a similar cost, support the choice of DBT-A as a treatment for adolescents with repeated self-harm. The limited sample size and low number of inpatient admissions in our study sample call for further studies to evaluate the cost-effectiveness of DBT-A.

Abbreviations

BPD: borderline personality disorder; CEAC: cost-effectiveness acceptability curve; CI: confidence interval; CGAS: Children's Global Assessment Scale; DBT-A: dialectical behaviour therapy for adolescents; EM: expectation–maximization method; EUC: enhanced usual care; GP: general practitioner; ICER: incremental cost-effectiveness ratio; LPC: Lifetime Parasuicide Count; SCID-II: Structural Clinical Interview for DSM Disorders; TAU: treatment as usual.

Authors' contributions

EH coordinated data-collection, drafted the manuscript and analysed and interpreted the data. LM designed and obtained funding for the study, and reviewed the manuscript and the interpretation of the data-analyses. EA gave advice on how to perform and interpret the cost-effectiveness analysis, and reviewed the manuscript. BG and AJT reviewed the manuscript. All authors read and approved the final manuscript.

Author details

[1] National Centre for Suicide Research and Prevention, University of Oslo, Sognsvannsveien 21, Bygg 12, 0372 Oslo, Norway. [2] Department of Health and Health Economics, University of Oslo, Oslo, Norway.

Acknowledgements

We thank all patients who have participated in the project, as well as the participating clinics for providing resource use data for the economic evaluation. We would also like to thank Lien My Diep for advice on the statistical analyses.

Competing interests

The authors declare that they have no competing interests.

Disclaimer

Data from the Norwegian Patient Registry has been used in this publication. The interpretation and reporting of these data are the sole responsibility of the authors, and no endorsement by the Norwegian Patient Registry is intended nor should be inferred.

Funding

The trial was funded by grants from the Norwegian Directorate of Health, the South Eastern Regional Health Authority, the Extra-Foundation for Health and Rehabilitation, and the University of Oslo.

References

1. Nock M. Self-injury. Annu Rev Clin Psychol. 2010;6:339–63.
2. Jacobson C, Muehlenkamp J, Miller A, Blake Turner J. Psychiatric impairment among adolescents engaging in different types of deliberate self-harm. J Clin Child Adolesc Psychol. 2008;37(2):363–75.
3. Nock M, Green J, Hwang I, McLaughlin K, Sampson N, Zaslavsky A, Kessler R. Prevalence, correlates, and treatment of lifetime suicidal behavior among adolescents. JAMA Psychiatry. 2013;70(3):300–10.
4. Nixon M, Cloutier P, Jansson S. Nonsuicidal self-harm in youth: a population-based survey. CMAJ. 2008;178(3):306–12.
5. Tørmoen A, Rossow I, Mork E, Mehlum L. Contact with child and adolescent psychiatric services among self-harming and suicidal adolescents in the general population: a cross sectional study. Child Adolesc Psychiatry Ment Health. 2014;8:13.
6. Brent D, McMakin D, Kennard B, Goldstein T, Mayes T, Douaihy A. Protecting adolescents from self-harm: a critical review of intervention studies. J Am Acad Child Adolesc Psychiatry. 2013;52(12):1260–71.
7. Linehan M, Armstrong H, Suarez A, Allmon D, Heard H. Cognitive-behavioral treatment of chronically parasuicidal borderline patients. Arch Gen Psychiatry. 1991;48:1060–4.
8. Linehan M, Comtois K, Murray A, Brown M, Gallop R, Heard H, Korslund K, Tutek D, Reynolds S, Lindenboim N. Two-year randomized controlled trial and follow-up of dialectical behavior therapy vs therapy by experts for suicidal behaviors and borderline personality disorder. Arch Gen Psychiatry. 2006;63:757–66.
9. Koons CR, Robins CJ, Tweed JL, Lynch TR, Gonzalez AM, Morse HQ, Bishop GK, Butterfield MI, Bastian LA. Efficacy of dialectical behavior therapy in women veterans with borderline personality disorder. Behav Ther. 2001;32(2):371–90.
10. Verheul R, van den Bosch LMC, Koeter MWJ, de Ridder MAJ, van den Brink W. Dialectical behaviour therapy for women with borderline personality disorder—12-month, randomised clinical trial in The Netherlands. Br J Psychiatry. 2003;182:135–40.
11. Turner RM. Naturalistic evaluation of dialectical behavior therapy-oriented treatment for borderline personality disorder. Cogn Behav Pract. 2000;7:413–9.
12. Heard HL. Cost-effectiveness of dialectical behavior therapy in the treatment of borderline personality disorder. Seattle: Department of Psychology, University of Washington; 2000.
13. Priebe S, Bhatti N, Barnicot K, Bremner S, Gagli A, Katsakou C, Molosankwe I, McCrone P, Zinkler M. Effectiveness and cost-effectiveness of dialectical behaviour therapy for self-harming patients with personality disorder: a pragmatic randomised controlled trial. Psychother Psychosom. 2012;81:356–65.
14. Brazier J, Tumur I, Holmes M, Ferriter M, Parry G, Dent-Brown K, Paisley S. Psychological therapies including dialectical behaviour therapy for borderline personality disorder: a systematic review and preliminary economic evaluation. Health Technol Assess. 2006;10(35).
15. Mehlum L, Tørmoen A, Ramberg M, Haga E, Diep L, Laberg S, Larsson B, Stanley B, Miller A, Sund A, Grøholt B. Dialectical behavior therapy for adolescents with recent and repeated suicidal and self-harming behavior and borderline traits—a randomized trial. J Am Acad Child Adolesc Psychiatry. 2014;53(10):1082–91.
16. Mehlum L, Ramberg M, Tormoen AJ, Haga E, Diep LM, Stanley BH, Miller AL, Sund AM, Groholt B. Dialectical behavior therapy compared with enhanced usual care for adolescents with repeated suicidal and self-harming behavior: outcomes over a one-year follow-up. J Am Acad Child Adolesc Psychiatry. 2016;55(4):295–300.
17. Rathus J, Miller A. Dialectical behavior therapy adapted for suicidal adolescents. Suicide Life Threat Behav. 2002;32(2):146–57.
18. Miller AL, Rathus JH, Linehan MM. Dialectical behavior therapy with suicidal adolescents. New York: The Guilford Press; 2007.
19. Linehan M, Comtois K. Lifetime parasuicide count. Seattle: University of Washington; 1996.
20. Shaffer D, Gould M, Brasic J, Anmbrosini P, Fisher P, Bird H. A children's global assessment scale (CGAS). Arch Gen Psychiatry. 1983;40:1228–31.
21. Statens legemiddelverk: Price- and reimbursement list. 2013. https://legemiddelverket.no/english/price-and-reimbursement/maximum-price#list-of-products-with-maximum-prices. Accessed 1 Sept 2013.
22. Felleskatalogen. Felleskatalogen farmasøytiske preparater markedsført i Norge. 2015. http://www.felleskatalogen.no. Accessed 1 June 2015.
23. O'Brien BJ, Drummond MF, Labelle RJ, Willan A. In search of power and significance: issues in the design and analysis of stochastic cost-effectiveness studies in health care. Med Care. 1994;32(2):150–63.
24. Van Hout BA, Al MJ, Gordon GS, Rutten FFH. Costs, effects and c/e ratios alongside a clinical trial. Health Econ. 1994;3(5):309–19.
25. Fenwick E, Marshall D, Levy A, Nichol G. Using and interpreting cost-effectiveness acceptability curves: an example using data from a trial of management strategies for atrial fibrillation. BMC Health Serv Res. 2006;6(52):106–8.

26. Stata Corporation. STATA Statistical Software. College Station: Stata Corporation LP; 2013.

27. IBM Corporation. IBM SPSS Statistics for Windows. Armonk: IBM Corporation; 2013.

28. Linehan M. Cognitive-behavioral treatment of borderline personality disorder. New York: The Guilford Press; 1993.

29. Carter GL, Wilcox CH, Lewin TJ, Conrad AM, Bendit N. Hunter DBT project: randomized controlled trial of dialectical behaviour therapy in women with borderline personality disorder. Aust N Z J Psychiatry. 2010;44(2):162–73.

30. McMain SF, Guimond T, Streiner DL, Cardish RJ, Links PS. Dialectical behavior therapy compared with general psychiatric management for borderline personality disorder: clinical outcomes and functioning over a 2-year follow-up. Am J Psychiatry. 2012;169(6):650–61.

31. McMain SF, Links PS, Gnam WH, Guimond T, Cardish RJ, Korman L, Streiner DL. A randomized trial of dialectical behavior therapy versus general psychiatric management for borderline personality disorder. Am J Psychiatry. 2009;166(12):1365–74.

21

Children's Perceived Competence Scale: reevaluation in a population of Japanese elementary and junior high school students

Yukiyo Nagai[1*], Kayo Nomura[1], Masako Nagata[2], Tetsuji Kaneko[3] and Osamu Uemura[4,5]

Abstract

Background: It is important for children to maintain high self-perceived competence and self-esteem, and there are few measures to evaluate them through elementary to junior high school days in Japan. To evaluate psychometric properties of the Children's Perceived Competence Scale (CPCS).

Methods: Data were collected from 697 elementary school and 956 junior high school students. Some of these students completed measures for construct validity, whereas others repeated the CPCS.

Results: The results demonstrated the three-factor structure of the CPCS: cognitive (nine items), social (eight items) and physical (nine items). Factorial invariance was confirmed between elementary and junior high school students, as well as between boys and girls. Construct validity was excellent. Scores on the cognitive, physical and general self-worth domains declined with increasing age. Boys scored significantly higher than girls on physical and general self-worth domains.

Conclusions: The CPCS is a valid and reliable measure of perceived competence in Japanese children aged 6–15 years. The CPCS may be applied to students from elementary through junior high school days as a measure of self-perceived and psychological state in Japan.

Keywords: Children's Perceived Competence Scale, Reliability, Validity, Elementary school, Junior high school, Children, Adolescents

Background

Positive self-esteem has been found to protect children and adolescents from distress and despondency, enabling them to cope with difficult and stressful life situations [1]. A positive sense of self is regarded as central to the adaptive function of individuals [2], with self-perceived competence being an indispensable emotion and the central issue for children and adolescents in the educational, psychological and medical fields. At least one study has revealed the positive role of self-esteem in emotional states (depression and anxiety) in adolescents aged 13–18 [3]. Maintaining positive or high self-esteem is a very important aspect in pediatric medicine, especially for children with chronic diseases [4]. Self-perception or quality of life varies with chronic diseases, as scores in adolescents with autism spectrum disorders were significantly lower than those in controls and diabetic adolescents, especially in the factors friendships, leisure time, and affective and sexual relationships [5]. Although the most appropriate method to determine a child's viewpoint by psychological assessment is currently regarded to be a semi-structured interview [6], clinicians and medical workers in the pediatric field have long sought a useful measure of self-esteem as an objective and supplementary yardstick.

Self or self-esteem has been described using different terms, including self-worth, self-perception, self-representation, self-evaluation, and self-perceived competence. The term "perceived competence" was

*Correspondence: ynagai390503@gmail.com
[1] Department of Pediatrics, Japanese Red Cross Nagoya Daini Hospital, 2-9 Myoken-cho Showa-ku, Nagoya, Aichi 466-8650, Japan
Full list of author information is available at the end of the article

selected based on theories of competence and intrinsic motivation [7–9]. Until the 1970s, a single score approach was utilized to evaluate children's general sense of self or self-esteem [10–12]. In the 1980s, the single score approach was found to mask many important evaluative distinctions regarding children's competence or adequacy in various domains of their lives. Abstract reasoning was reported to begin at around 12 years of age, with abstraction of self traits also beginning in early adolescence (age 11–13 years) [7, 13, 14]. These findings, that pre-adolescents tend to express elaborate taxonomic attributes and focus on specific competencies, led to the development of a multi-dimensional or domain-specific approach to child development [15–17]. This resulted in the formulation of two determinants, with success in domains deemed important determined by self and the reflected appraisals of others [18, 19].

The Children's Perceived Competence Scale (CPCS) in this study is a revised Japanese version of the Perceived Competence Scale for Children (PCSC) developed by Harter which is a well-known worldwide multi-dimensional questionnaires [20]. Although several questionnaires in Japanese are used to assess self-perceived competence, quality of life, and self-esteem, few of these measures show good reliability and validity for children of both elementary and junior high school age [21, 22].

PCSC first developed in 1982 [17, 23], consists of seven items in each of four domains (cognitive, social, physical, and general self-worth) for children aged 8–15 years. Each of these 28 items utilized two-step dichotomous scales. Although the Japanese version of the PCSC was shown to have good validity and reliability [24], it was revised in 1992 because its two-step dichotomous scale is difficult to apply to elementary school children in a very large survey. This led to the development of a revised version of the Japanese PCSC version, CPCS [25]. This scale consists of 10 items in each of the four domains (cognitive, social, physical, and general self-worth). Although the contents of the PCSC and CPCS are similar, the CPCS is easier to understand due to its simplicity and clarity of sentences and contents and its four-point scale system. Harter developed various revised or new versions of the PCSC, including the Pictorial Scale of Perceived Competence and Acceptance for young children aged 4–7 years in 1983, the self perception profile for children (SPPC) for children aged 8–13 years in 1985 and 2012, the self-perception profile for adolescents for children and adolescents aged 14–18 years in 1988 and 2012 and others [26, 27].

The SPPC consists of the three subscales and general self-worth domain which are in CPCS, along with two additional subscales, physical appearance and behavioral conduct [20, 28–30].

Although the validity and reliability of the Japanese version of the SPPC has been evaluated [31–33], exploratory factor analysis by three different studies each reported different results and low factor loadings on many items, especially in behavioral conduct. Also only one of the three studies reported confirmatory factor analysis recommending different models for students in elementary and junior high school and the inclusion of only three of the six items in the behavioral conduct domain [31]. Therefore, we abandoned the idea of adopting SPPC in favor of the CPCS, the revised Japanese version of the PCSC. General self-worth scores on the CPCS are closely associated with overall self-esteem. Although the subscale reliability of the Japanese version of the CPCS was assessed using Cronbach's alpha, its validity was only partially evaluated [24, 25]. Also our previous study of CPCS scores in elementary school children found scores decreased significantly as children progressed from school grade four to school grade five (approximately age 10–11 years) [34]. This period, namely the beginning of adolescence, is very important for paying attention to the self-esteem of children, and it is desirable to follow up the situation during adolescence. In the present study, continuously applying the CPCS to students in elementary school through junior high school in Japan, we attempted to reevaluate the validity and reliability of the CPCS.

Methods

Participants

This study involved 698 students, 350 boys and 348 girls, enrolled in three elementary schools and 992 students, 524 boys and 468 girls, enrolled in four junior high schools in Aichi prefecture, Japan, between September and December 2014. Aichi has the fourth largest population of the 47 Prefectures in Japan, with a population of about 7.5 million. To sample a representative cross-section of the target-age population, three elementary schools were selected, one located in old downtown, one in a rural seacoast town and one in the largest city. Similarly, four junior high schools were selected, one located in old downtown, one in a rural seacoast town and two in the largest city.

Measures

CPCS

The CPCS is a Japanese questionnaire derived from the PCSC. This instrument was designed to measure children's self-perception of competence across the cognitive (scholastic) (10 items, e.g., "Are you among the best in your class at studying?"), social (peer relationship) (10 items, e.g., "Do you have many friends?") and physical (athletic) (10 items, e.g., "Are you good at sports?") domains, as well as general self-worth (self-esteem) (10 items, e.g., "Do you have self-confidence?"). General self-worth is regarded as self-esteem, a concept different from that in the other three competence domains. CPCS subscale scores indicate a child's perceived self-competence in each domain. Each item was scored on a four-point scale: true (4), relatively true (3), relatively false (2), and false (1). Therefore, the score on each domain ranged from 10 to 40, with higher scores indicating greater perceived self-competence. The CPCS was administered in a classroom setting and completed by the students themselves.

Kid-KINDL^R and Kiddo-KINDL^R

These tests are self-reported instruments for assessing generic health-related quality of life in children aged from 6 to 12 and 13 to 18 years old [35]. The questionnaire consists of 24 items addressing six subscales: physical well-being, emotional well-being, self-esteem, family, friends, and school life. Three versions of the KINDL are available, the kiddy-KINDL^R for children aged 4–6 years old, the Kid-KINDL^R for children aged 7–13 years and the Kiddo-KINDL^R for children aged 14–17 years. Japanese versions of the Kid-KINDL and Kiddo-KINDL were developed for elementary school [36] and junior high school [22] students. Self-esteem, friends and school life in the Kid-KINDL^R correspond to general self-worth, social, and cognitive domains, respectively, in the CPCS.

Rosenberg Self Esteem Scale

The Rosenberg Self Esteem Scale [37] (RSES), comprising 10 items, is the most commonly used instrument for measuring self-esteem in adolescents and adults. A Japanese version of the RSES [38] was administered to junior high school students in this study.

The grade of physical performance test

Japanese students undergo nationwide physical performance tests once a year. The grade of physical performance on these tests, graded as excellent (81–100 percentile), average (20–80 percentile), and poor (0–20 percentile), was provided by teachers at each school.

Chronic disease

Each school nurse answered yes or no about presence of chronic diseases based on the health information report of each student. Chronic diseases were defined as mental and physical illnesses requiring regular hospital stay or visits, or requiring special attention by teachers.

Procedure

Of the 698 elementary school students invited to participate, 697 (99.9%), 349 boys and 348 girls, retuned questionnaires. Similarly, of the 992 junior high school students invited to participate, 956 (96.4%), 498 boys and 458 girls, returned questionnaires. All completed the CPCS. To validate the CPCS, the Kid-KINDL^R was also administered to 450 elementary school students and the Kiddo-KINDLE^R and RSES were administered to 305 junior high school students. To assess the test–retest reliability of the CPCS, this test was administered twice to 336 students, at intervals of 7–14 days. Students selected for testing by the Kid-KINDL, Kiddo-KINDL and RSES and those selected for retesting with the CPCS were chosen by the principal of each school.

Statistical analysis

The sample was randomly divided into two groups, with the first group undergoing exploratory factor analysis (EFA) for the CPCS items. After determining the means, standard deviations, and skewness of the CPCS items, factors were extracted based on the maximum-likelihood method, with the number of factors determined by the scree plot method. Following Promax rotation, a diagonal rotation method, CPCS items belonging to three subscales, Cognitive, Social, and Physical, were entered into EFA. Because the General self-worth subscale was regarded as qualitatively different from the other specific domains of competence, the General self-worth subscale scores were regarded as a measure of construct validity.

The factor structure extracted through the EFA was cross-validated by a series of confirmatory factor analyses (CFAs) using the second group. Factor models were revised by adding correlations between error variables according to modification indices. These were added only to error variables belonging to the same factor. The fit of each model to the data was examined using Chi squared (CMIN), comparative fit index (CFI), and root mean square error of approximation (RMSEA). According to conventional criteria, a good fit would be indicated by CMIN/df < 2, CFI > .97, and RMSEA < .05, and an acceptable fit by CMIN/df < 3, CFI > .95, and RMSEA < .08 [39].

After determining factor structure, measurement invariance between elementary and junior high school students as well as between boys and girls was determined by weak factorial variance, in which loading of each factor was the same between groups. If weak factor invariance was not confirmed, the path and indicator with the greatest critical ratio for difference in factor loading were deleted, and the examination was repeated until weak factor invariance was obtained. After determining the factor structure of weak factorial invariance between elementary and junior high school students, it was subjected to examination of weak factorial invariance between boys and girls. Finally, a factor structure with weak factorial invariance between elementary and junior high school students and between boys and girls was obtained. The above treatment resulted in the creation of subscales of the CPCS, with each subscale calculated by adding scores of items belonging to each factor. The correlations between the scores of these CPCS subscales and demographic variables, Kid-KINDL (Kiddo-KINDL) scores and RSES scores were assessed.

The reliability of each CPCS subscale was examined by determining its internal consistency (Cronbach's alpha coefficient) and test–retest reliability (intraclass correlation coefficient: ICC). Finally, the distribution of CPCS subscale scores by age (grade) was determined separately in boys and girls.

Missing values were determined by adopting listwise deletion for EFAs and CFAs. Multiple imputations were used when analysing all data for validation of the CPCS subscales. Little's MCAR test showed that the null hypothesis (the data were missing completely at random) was rejected (Chi squared $= 4241.5$, $df = 3641$, $P < .001$). All statistical analyses were performed using SPSS version 20.

Results

CPCS: item scores and gender difference

The population of elementary and junior high school students was divided randomly into two groups. Evaluation of the first group ($n = 797$) showed that the distribution of all CPCS items was relatively non-skewed (Table 1). Boys and girls differed mainly in the physical and general self-worth subscales. Boys scored significantly higher than girls on physical items such as "good at sports" and "interested in trying new sports" and significantly lower on items such as "prefer watching rather than participating in sports" and "dislike PE". Boys also scored significantly higher on general self-worth items such as "have self-confidence", "have a lot of things to be proud of" and "have confidence in one's own opinions" and significantly lower on items such as "not a useful person" than girls.

Factor structure of the CPCS

The scree plot for EFA on data from the first group ($n = 797$) suggested a three-factor structure. The first factor included CPCS items belonging to the physical domain; the second factor included items belonging to the cognitive domain; and the third factor included items belonging to the social domain (Table 2).

Cross-validation of the factor structure of the CPCS was examined by a CFA on the second group of students ($n = 792$). The original three-factor model without correlations between error variables showed non-acceptable goodness-of-fit: Chi squared/$df = 4.7$, CFI $= .861$, and RMSEA $= .068$. The addition of inter-error correlations according to the modification indices resulted in a revised model (Fig. 1), which showed better

goodness-of-fit indices: Chi squared/$df = 3.7$, CFI $= .902$, and RMSEA $= .058$.

We also examined whether the 3-factor structure showed factorial invariance between elementary and junior high school students as well as between boys and girls. Multigroup analysis revealed a difference between elementary and junior high school students (increase of Chi squared $= 63.684$, $df = 27$, $P < .001$). Because weak measurement invariance was refuted, we searched critical ratios for differences between parameters in the two groups. We individually deleted parameters (factor loading) with the highest critical ratios until weak factor invariance appeared. This was obtained by deleting four CPCS items (items 2, 18, 25, and 27), yielding Chi squared/$df = 2.4$, CFI $= .901$, and RMSEA $= .044$ (Fig. 2).

Using this three-factor model with 26 items, we examined whether boys and girls differed in factor structure. Compared with the model without constraining parameters, the model that constrained factor loadings between boys and girls did not differ significantly in increased Chi squared (22.094, $df = 23$, $P = .515$). Weak factorial invariance between the two genders was confirmed by this model. Hence this final model showed weak factorial invariance both between elementary and junior high school students and between boys and girls. The first factor with nine items reflected physical domain, the second factor with nine items reflected cognitive domain, and the third factor with eight items reflected social domain.

The CPCS is usually used as a measure in children of grade 3 and higher. It is not usually administered to children in grades 1 and 2. Therefore, we repeated the test of factorial invariance between children in grades 1–2 and those in grades 3 and higher. The model of restricted parameters for all factor loadings did not exceed the model of free parameters for factor loadings in terms of Chi squared (32.065, $df = 23$, $P = .099$). Hence weak factorial invariance was confirmed between children in grades 1–2 and those in grades 3–9.

Concurrent and construct validity of the CPCS

To examine the concurrent and construct validity of the three subscales derived from the above EFA and CFA results, we assessed the 755 students administered the Kid-KINDL and Kiddo-KINDL instruments. We constructed three subscales by adding the scores of items belonging to each factor: cognitive, social and physical. All three subscale scores of the CPCS correlated significantly with general self-worth score (Table 3). In addition, the scores of all six Kid-KINDL and Kiddo-KINDL subscales correlated with the scores of their equivalent CPCS subscales. In the junior high school students, the scores on the RSES correlated with the scores of all three CPCS subscales. Therefore, the scores on the

Table 1 Exploratory factor analysis of the CPCS (N = 797)

Item no.	Contents	M (SD)				Skewness
		Total	Boys	Girls	Gender difference	
	Cognitive					
1	Among the best at studying	2.44 (1.00)	2.45 (1.01)	2.43 (1.00)	t (791) = .3	− .0
5	Poor at studying (R)	2.41 (1.11)	2.42 (1.13)	2.40 (1.09)	t (793) = .2	.1
9	You are one of the cleverest	2.20 (1.02)	2.19 (1.02)	2.21 (1.02)	t (794) = .2	.2
13	Your grades are bad (R)	2.51 (1.09)	2.45 (1.13)	2.57 (1.05)	t (791.9) = 1.5	− .1
17	Finish your homework quickly	2.71 (1.07)	2.73 (1.12)	2.68 (1.02)	t (791.2) = .6	− .3
21	Understand school lessons well	2.98 (.92)	2.97 (1.00)	2.99 (.85)	t (788.3) = .3	− .6
25	Unable to answer questions (R)	2.82 (.98)	2.77 (1.04)	2.88 (.91)	t (789.0) = 1.6	− .5
29	Attempt challenging problems	2.82 (1.07)	2.86 (1.09)	2.78 (1.05)	t (792) = 1.1	− .4
33	Get good scores in exams	2.32 (1.02)	2.33 (1.03)	2.31 (1.03)	t (794) = .4	.1
37	Express your opinions in class	2.41 (1.11)	2.54 (1.12)	2.27 (1.09)	t (795) = 3.5	.1
	Social					
2	Have many friends	3.36 (.83)	3.39 (.83)	3.31 (.82)	t (793) = 1.3	− 1.2
6	You are popular in your class	2.04 (.90)	2.11 (.94)	1.96 (.86)	t (794.6) = 2.4*	.4
10	Teased by your friends? (R)	3.32 (.94)	3.26 (1.00)	3.38 (.89)	t (790.8) = 1.8	− 1.2
14	Nobody worries when you are absent (R)	2.72 (1.00)	2.72 (1.00)	2.72 (1.00)	t (794) = .1	− .3
18	Easy to make friends	2.69 (1.11)	2.74 (1.09)	2.63 (1.13)	t (793) = 1.4	− .3
22	Friends invite you to play	3.08 (1.00)	3.09 (1.00)	3.07 (.95)	t (795) = .4	− .8
26	You are the hub of the class	2.12 (1.00)	2.16 (.98)	2.08 (.93)	t (791) = 1.3	.4
30	You are liked by your friends	2.65 (1.00)	2.65 (.97)	2.65 (.94)	t (792) = .0	− .4
34	People do not pay much attention to you (R)	3.25 (.86)	3.20 (.89)	3.31 (.83)	t (790) = 1.9	− 1.1
38	People will feel sad if change school	2.82 (1.00)	2.76 (1.02)	2.88 (.98)	t (791.8) = 1.7	− .5
	Physical					
3	Good at sports	2.81 (1.06)	2.95 (1.01)	2.65 (1.09)	t (780.0) = 4.0***	− .4
7	Confidence in new sports	2.43 (1.08)	2.53 (1.07)	2.32 (1.08)	t (793) = 2.8**	.1
11	Chosen for the sports meets	2.12 (1.15)	2.17 (1.18)	2.07 (1.11)	t (793.0) = 1.1	.5
15	Prefer watching rather than participating in sports (R)	2.94 (1.20)	3.05 (1.19)	2.82 (1.21)	t (785.4) = 2.7**	− .6
19	Interested in trying new sports	2.83 (1.16)	2.90 (1.15)	2.75 (1.17)	t (794) = 1.8	− .4
23	Dislike PE (R)	3.28 (1.00)	3.43 (.91)	3.13 (1.02)	t (771.9) = 4.3***	− 1.2
27	Poor at sports	2.94 (1.16)	3.12 (1.09)	2.76 (1.19)	t (776.3) = 4.5***	− .6
31	Not lose to friends at sports	2.33 (1.09)	2.43 (1.08)	2.23 (1.09)	t (793) = 2.7**	.2
35	Amongst the best at sports	2.53 (1.05)	2.60 (1.15)	2.33 (1.33)	t (792) = 3.3**	− 1.4
39	Prefer not to be seen by others when you do sports (R)	2.91 (1.14)	3.02 (1.13)	2.79 (1.14)	t (794) = 2.9**	− .6
	General self-worth					
4	Have self-confidence	2.48 (1.00)	2.54 (.89)	2.40 (1.00)	t (791) = 2.0*	.0
8	Do things better than others	2.34 (.92)	2.42 (.92)	2.25 (.92)	t (792) = 2.5*	.1
12	Have a lot of things to be proud of	2.20 (1.00)	2.29 (1.04)	2.10 (.94)	t (793.0) = 2.7**	.4
16	Does not go well whatever you do (R)	2.89 (1.01)	2.97 (1.03)	2.82 (1.00)	t (791) = 2.1*	− .6
20	Satisfied with the way you are now	2.39 (1.09)	2.45 (1.10)	2.34 (1.07)	t (795) = 1.4	.1
24	Will surely become a great person	1.84 (.94)	1.94 (1.00)	1.73 (.89)	t (791) = 3.1**	.9
28	Not a useful person (R)	2.63 (1.00)	2.68 (.88)	2.58 (.95)	t (795) = 1.4	− .3
32	Have confidence in your own opinion	2.51 (1.06)	2.60 (1.07)	2.42 (1.05)	t (788) = 2.4*	.0
36	Have few good points (R)	2.53 (1.06)	2.54 (1.09)	2.52 (.99)	t (792.8) = .2	− .1
40	Worried about whether or not you fail (R)	2.37 (1.15)	2.52 (1.17)	2.22 (1.10)	t (794.0) = 3.7***	.2

R reversed

* $P < .05$; ** $P < .01$; *** $P < .001$

Table 2 Exploratory factor analysis of the CPCS (N = 797)

Item no.	Contents	Factor		
		1	2	3
	Cognitive			
1	Among the best at studying	.03	.83	−.11
5	Poor at studying (R)	.03	.71	−.14
9	One of the cleverest	−.02	.86	−.04
13	Your grades are bad (R)	−.12	.74	−.00
17	Finish your homework quickly	.04	.46	.02
21	Understand school lessons well	−.04	.64	.02
25	Unable to answer teachers' questions (R)	−.05	.42	.14
29	Attempt challenging problems	.08	.58	.05
33	Get good scores in exams	−.04	.84	−.03
37	Express your opinions in class	.08	.44	.18
	Social			
2	Have many friends	.21	.02	.51
6	Popular in your class	.17	.13	.47
10	Teased by your friends (R)	−.11	−.16	.41
14	Nobody worries when you are absent (R)	−.10	.11	.59
18	Easy to make friends	.20	−.01	.32
22	Friends invite you to play	.09	−.11	.52
26	The hub of the class	.07	.17	.36
30	Liked by your friends	−.05	.02	.65
34	People do not pay much attention to you (R)	−.07	−.07	.62
38	People will feel sad if change school	−.01	.09	.69
	Physical			
3	Good at sports	.93	−.03	−.09
7	Confidence in new sports	.77	.08	−.04
11	Chosen for the sports meets	.61	.04	.02
15	Prefer watching rather than participating in sports (R)	.60	−.02	.01
19	Interested in trying new sports	.66	−.04	.07
23	Dislike PE (R)	.60	−.05	.04
27	Poor at sports	.87	−.11	−.08
31	Not lose to friends at sports	.72	.09	−.01
35	Amongst the best at sports	.85	.06	−.07
39	Prefer not to be seen by others when you do sports (R)	.38	−.12	−.19

Factor loadings of .30 or more are in italics

CPCS subscales assessed similar aspects of perception measured by the other scales.

The scores on the Social subscale did not correlate with the student's grades, whereas the scores on the Cognitive ($r = −.30$) and Physical ($r = −.23$) subscales were significantly negatively correlated with grade (Table 3). The Physical performance test scores were moderately correlated with Physical subscale. The comparison of the scores by gender and chronic diseases also indicated (Table 3). Boys showed significantly higher scores in Physical subscale than girls and three

CPCS subscale scores did not differ between students with and without chronic diseases.

Reliability of the CPCS

Cronbach's alpha coefficients were, .87, .79, and .88 for the cognitive, social, and physical subscales, respectively (Table 4). These were virtually the same when calculated for elementary and junior high school students separately and for boys and girls separately.

Test–retest reliabilities were, .89, .81, and .90 for cognitive, social, and physical subscales, respectively. These

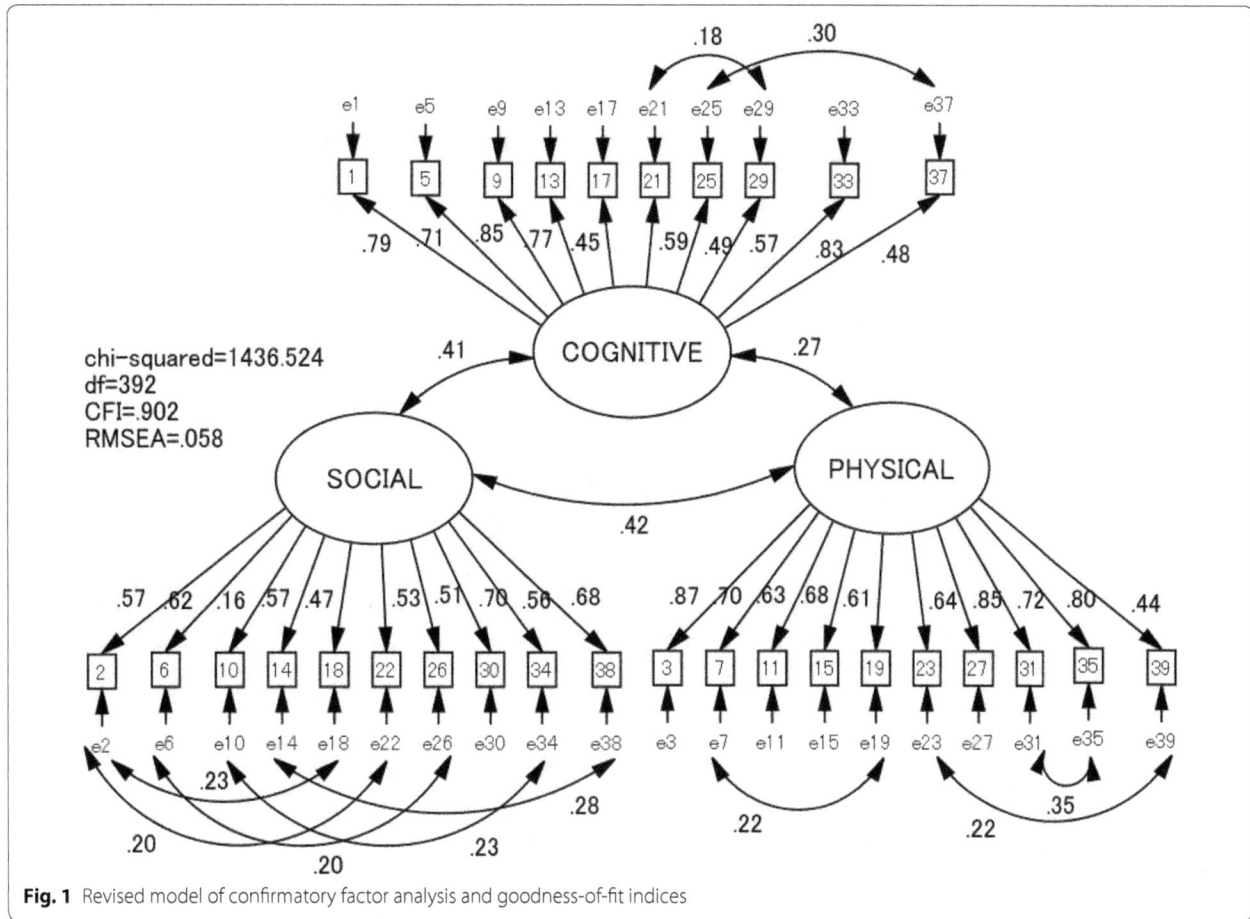

Fig. 1 Revised model of confirmatory factor analysis and goodness-of-fit indices

were virtually the same when calculated for elementary and junior high school students separately and for boys and girls separately.

Age distribution of the CPCS subscale scores

Because the scores of the physical subscale differed in boys and girls, we examined the distribution of scores of the CPCS subscales over age (grade) in boys and girls separately (Table 5).

All three CPCS subscale scores differed among the nine grades in boys, whereas both Cognitive and Physical subscale scores differed over these grades in girls. Post-hoc comparison (Tukey) showed that both boys and girls scored higher in lower than in higher grades, except for social subscale scores in boys.

Discussion

Validity and reliability

In the present study, we reevaluated the validity and reliability of the CPCS. All the CPCS items, except for General self-worth, were used for an EFA. The three factors extracted from the EFA were in agreement with theoretic

expectations. Our final model showed acceptable fit in a CFA. One strength of our study was its assessment of factor invariance. We identified the factor structure that was invariant between age groups and between genders. In most investigations examining different populations, the robustness of the measurement is of great concern. Researchers wish to ensure that the questionnaire items used in measurements did not greatly alter their relationship to the latent variables across populations with different attributes. Any observed difference would make the interpretation of the results derived from that measure difficult. We identified weak factorial invariance between age groups as well as between genders after deleting a few CPCS items. This means that a simple summation of items may distort the results of the data.

The validity of the three subscales derived from the EFA, CFA, and deletion of a few items that reduced factor invariance was examined for its relationship with General self-worth, as well as with Kid KINDLE, Kiddo KINDLE, and RSES scores. All results were as expected.

Reliability, as determined by internal consistency and test–retest formats, was also excellent. This is consistent

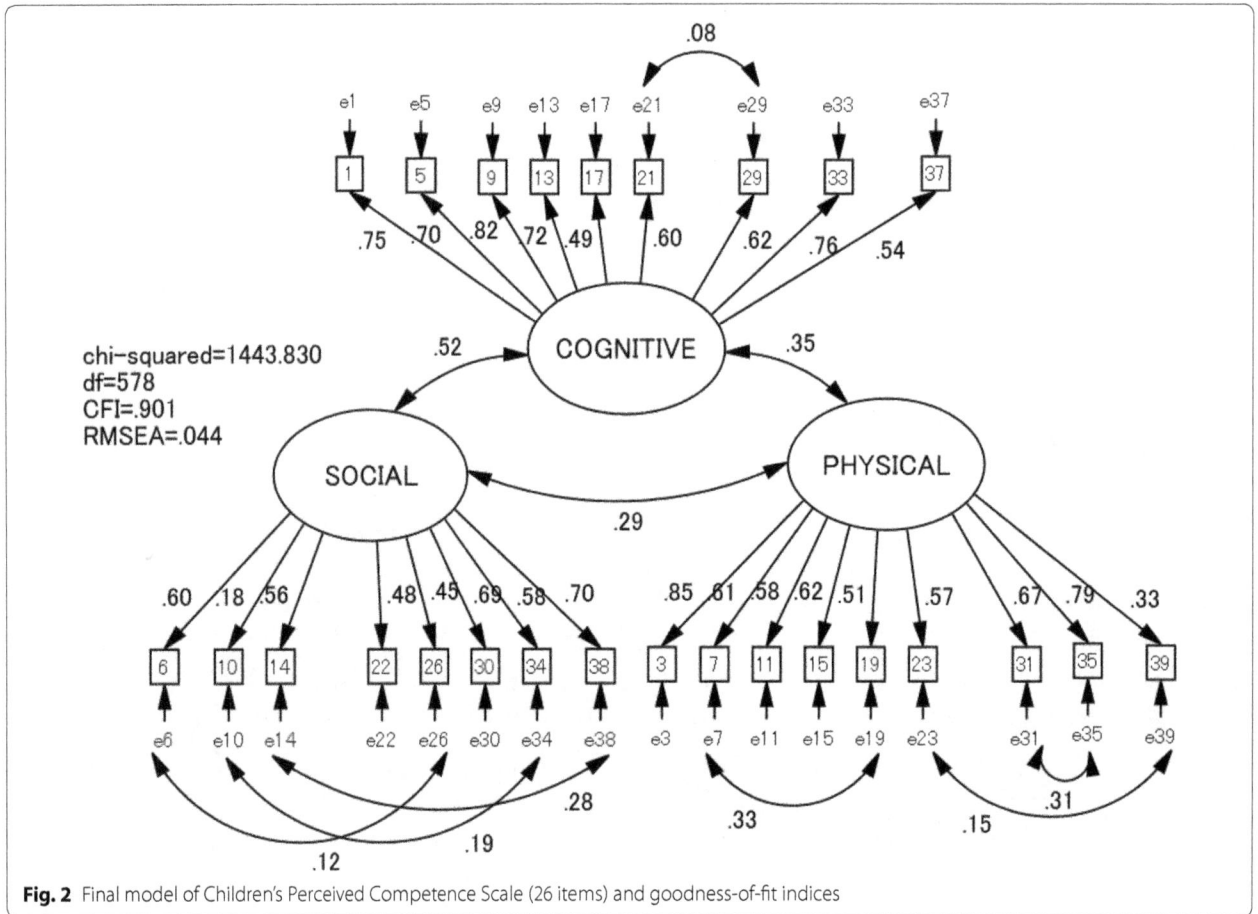

Fig. 2 Final model of Children's Perceived Competence Scale (26 items) and goodness-of-fit indices

with a report showing that Chronbach's alpha ranged between .75 and .87 [40].

Gender differences

Evaluation of students in grades 3–9 showed that boys consistently showed significantly higher scores than girls on the physical (athletic) subscale [17]. In addition, many studies have reported that boys score higher than girls on measures of self-esteem [22, 35, 41]. Our findings, that boys scored higher than girls on Physical and general self-worth subscales, were compatible with these previous reports. The higher Physical scores in boys than in girls, especially those in junior high school, may be due to gender differences in body composition among junior high school students varies, with boys having more muscle mass and girls having more fat mass [42]. Gender differences on the general self-worth subscale may be explained, at least in part, by girls expressing more self-conscious emotions, like shame and guilt, than boys [43, 44]. Moreover, the lower scores on Physical subscales in girls may also contribute to their lower scores on General self-worth.

Chronic diseases

In our study the three CPCS subscale scores did not differ between students with and without chronic diseases. Thus, all students were included in our analyses. Most of the students with chronic diseases in our study had mild allergic diseases, including allergic rhinitis and atopic dermatitis, allowing regular school attendance. The school nurse-provided information may have contributed to this result.

Grade differences

Several studies using self-administered questionnaires have assessed self-perception or self-esteem in students from elementary through junior high school. A study using Kid-KINDL and Kiddo-KINDL in Japanese elementary and junior high school students showed that school life (scholastic) and self-esteem domains decreased markedly with age, whereas friends (social) domain did not [21, 22]. In contrast, another study found no marked changes with age [17]. Scores on the Self Description Questionnaire I, which measures seven specific self-concept factors (physical ability, physical appearance, peer relationship, parent relationship, reading, mathematics

Table 3 Correlations of the CPCS subscales with other variables and the comparison of the scores by gender and chronic diseases (N = 755)

	CPCS subscales		
	Cognitive	Social	Physical
CPCS			
General self-worth (r)	.62***	.63***	.52***
Kid-KINDL^R/Kiddo-KINDL^R			
Physical health (r)	.26***	.29***	.23***
Emotional well-being (r)	.28***	.58***	.26***
Self-esteem (r)	.55***	.56***	.46***
Family (r)	.29***	.35***	.17***
Friends (r)	.30***	.61***	.32***
School life (r)	.60***	.34***	.27***
RSES (N = 305) (r)	.51***	.62***	.44***
Grade (r)	− .30***	.00	− .23***
Physical performance test (r)	− .10 ***	− .09***	.39***
Gender			
Boys (n = 385) (Mean (SE))	22.9 (.2)	21.9 (.2)	25.3 (.2)
Girls (n = 370) (Mean (SE))	22.6 (.2)	22.9 (.2)	23.2 (.3)
t test	− 1.0 NS	− .6 NS	6.2**
Chronic disease			
None (n = 619) (Mean (SE))	22.7 (.2)	22.0 (.1)	24.3 (1.9)
Present (n = 136) (Mean (SE))	23.3 (.4)	21.6 (.3)	23.9 (.4)
t test	− 1.4 NS	1.2 NS	.9 NS

* P < .05; ** P < .01; *** P < .001; () indicates standard error

Table 4 Internal consistency and test–retest reliability of each subscale in CPCS

	CPCS subscales		
	Cognitive	Social	Physical
Internal consistency			
Total (N = 755)	.87	.79	.88
Elementary school (n = 450)	.85	.77	.86
Junior high school (n = 305)	.89	.83	.91
Boys (n = 385)	.88	.80	.86
Girls (n = 370)	.86	.79	.90
Test–retest reliability (ICC)			
Total (n = 431)	.89***	.81***	.90***
Elementary school (n = 336)	.88***	.80***	.89***
Junior high school (n = 95)	.92***	.85***	.88***
Boys (n = 215)	.89***	.83***	.89***
Girls (n = 216)	.89***	.78***	.91***

* P < .05; ** P < .01; *** P < .001

and general school), declined linearly with age in all subscales in students in grades 2–9 [45]. We observed age-related reductions in cognitive, physical, and general self-worth subscale scores, with some fluctuation, but no consistent pattern, in social subscale scores.

Adolescents aged 11–16 years gradually evaluate their attributes via interactions with others and with regarded to different roles and relational contexts. They can recognize positive and negative attributes simultaneously, inter-coordinate their traits into single abstractions and form links between single abstractions. This process of preoccupation with others' thoughts of the self and cognition about contradictory characteristics of the self tends to lead to confusion and inaccuracies [14]. This view of adolescence provides an appropriate guide to understanding its description as "a period of crisis" [46].

Limitations

The present study has limitations. First, the population studied was selected from schools in Aichi prefecture, one of 47 prefectures in Japan. Although we tried to balance socio-economic variables by selecting elementary and junior high schools differing in academic level, local economy, industry, and population, a nationwide survey may yield different reference values. Generalization of our results to the entire Japanese population requires an expansion of the number of locations. Second, we used the CPCS, a Japanese revised version of the PCSC. Thus, it may be difficult to compare our data directly with data obtained using the PCSC in other countries. Studies have reported that self-esteem is much lower in Japanese children than in children in other countries. For example, almost all scores on QOL subscales, including self-esteem in Kid-KINDL, in elementary school children were lower in Japan than in Finland [47]. Scores on all subscales of the Self-Description Questionnaire, including general self-esteem, were found to be higher in elementary school children in the USA than in Japan [48]. Although the result of CPCS in our study cannot be used for research on international comparison, this study may provide insights on how to evaluate and create measures of self-esteem for children and adolescents.

Third, the validity of the information on presence of disease might be weak as some students may have had more slight symptoms than others and as the students with chronic disease were defined by a yes or no report regarding their health.

Fourth, the students selected by principals for test–retest reliability might have undergone selection bias. School events and education curriculum prevented the selection of a randomized sample.

Conclusion

This study reevaluated the validity and reliability of the CPCS. The results indicate that the CPCS can be applied to children and adolescents attending

Table 5 Means and standard errors in each subscale of CPCS

| | n | CPCS subscales | | | | | | | | |
| | | Cognitive | | Social | | Physical | | General | | |
	Boys:girls	Boys	Girls	Boys	Girls	Boys	Girls	Boys	Girls
1	27:34	28.2 (1.1)	28.4 (.8)	22.6 (1.0)	23.1 (.7)	28.1 (.9)	28.2 (1.1)	28.9 (1.5)	30.0 (.7)
2	28:41	24.4 (1.2)	26.0 (.9)	19.2 (1.2)	21.8 (1.0)	26.9 (1.2)	27.2 (1.0)	24.9 (1.3)	25.4 (1.1)
3	27:36	26.5 (1.2)	23.6 (1.0)	23.5 (1.0)	22.2 (.7)	30.0 (.9)	26.8 (1.1)	30.0 (1.4)	25.2 (.9)
4	47:26	23.5 (.9)	24.3 (1.1)	20.6 (.6)	21.3 (1.0)	25.6 (1.0)	23.5 (1.5)	24.0 (1.0)	23.4 (1.5)
5	44:31	22.7 (1.0)	22.2 (1.1)	20.1 (.8)	21.1 (.8)	25.0 (1.0)	21.8 (1.5)	22.6 (1.1)	22.1 (1.2)
6	52:57	24.7 (.9)	23.4 (.7)	23.4 (.6)	22.1 (.7)	26.5 (.8)	22.7 (.9)	26.0 (.8)	22.8 (.9)
7	49:51	22.1 (1.0)	21.4 (.9)	22.2 (.7)	21.4 (.7)	25.3 (1.0)	22.6 (1.2)	24.0 (1.1)	22.5 (.9)
8	73:58	20.8 (.8)	22.1 (.8)	22.0 (.6)	Grade	24.0 (.8)	22.8 (1.0)	23.6 (.8)	22.7 (.7)
9	38:36	20.6 (1.1)	20.6 (1.0)	21.3 (.6)	21.6 (.6)	23.4 (1.1)	22.9 (1.0)	22.9 (1.2)	21.8 (.8)
	F	5.66***	6.58***	3.40**	.58 ns	3.54**	4.45***	4.52***	6.43***
Post hoc comparison		1 > 5, 7–9 3 > 8, 9 6 > 8	1 > 3, 5, 6–9 2 > 7–9	2 < 6 5 < 6	–	3 > 5, 8, 9	1 > 5, 6–9 2 > 6, 7	1 > 5, 8, 9 3 > 4, 5, 7–9	1 > 2–9

() Standard error. * $P < .05$; ** $P < .01$; *** $P < .001$

elementary and junior high schools regardless of suffering from chronic diseases. The CPCS may be a useful measure to evaluate the mental state of students from age 6 through 15 years not only in a medical field but in an educational or social welfare field. Although the general self-worth subscale is not included in the CPCS model in our study, its three subscales (cognitive, social, physical) may effectively measure important aspects of self-esteem in children and adolescents.

Authors' contributions
YN, KN and MN conceptualized and designed the study and administered the questionnaire in each school. TK performed statistical analysis and gave us opinions from the statistical point of view. OU supervised the study and ensured we focused on the main purpose and feasibility of the study. All authors mentioned above agree to be accountable for all aspects of the work. All authors read and approved the final manuscript.

Author details
[1] Department of Pediatrics, Japanese Red Cross Nagoya Daini Hospital, 2-9 Myoken-cho Showa-ku, Nagoya, Aichi 466-8650, Japan. [2] Graduate School of Education and Human Development, Nagoya University, Furo-cho Chikusa-ku, Nagoya, Aichi 464-8601, Japan. [3] Department of Clinical Trial, Tokyo Metropolitan Children's Medical Center, 2-8-9 Musashidai, Fuchu, Tokyo 183-8561, Japan. [4] Department of Pediatric Nephrology, Aichi Children's Health and Medical Center, 1-2 Osakata Morioka-cho, Obu, Aichi 474-8710, Japan. [5] Present Address: Japanese Red Cross Toyota College of Nursing, Clinical Medicine, 12-33 Nanamagari, Hakusan-cho, Toyota, Aichi 471-8565, Japan.

Acknowledgements
The authors appreciate the teachers, parents and students of seven elementary and junior high schools in Aichi prefecture for their cooperation in our study. We also appreciate all people in the Japan Tapie Center who collected and processed the data from schools.

Competing interests
The authors declared that they have no competing interests.

Funding
No funding was secured for this study.

References
1. Erikson EH. Identity: youth and crisis. New York: WW Norton & Company; 1994.
2. Harter S. Issues in the assessment of the self-concept of children and adolescents. Boston: Allyn & Bacon; 1990.
3. Moksnes UK, Espnes GA. Self-esteem and emotional health in adolescents–gender and age as potential moderators. Scand J Psychol. 2012;53(6):483–9.
4. Perrin JM, Gnanasekaran S, Delahaye J. Psychological aspects of chronic health conditions. Pediatr Rev. 2012;33(3):99–109.
5. Cottenceau H, Roux S, Blanc R, Lenoir P, Bonnet-Brilhault F, Barthelemy C. Quality of life of adolescents with autism spectrum disorders: comparison to adolescents with diabetes. Eur Child Adolesc Psychiatry. 2012;21(5):289–96.
6. Macleod E, Woolford J, Hobbs L, Gross J, Hayne H, Patterson T. Interviews with children about their mental health problems: the congruence and validity of information that children report. Clin Child Psychol Psychiatry. 2017;22(2):229–44.
7. Deci EL. Intrinsic motivation: (by) Edward L. Deci. New York: Plenum Press; 1975.
8. Harter S. Effectance motivation reconsidered. Toward a developmental model. Hum Dev. 1978;21(1):34–64.
9. Charms Rd. Personal causation; the internal affective determinants of behavior. New York: Academic Press; 1968.
10. Piers EV, Harris DB. Age and other correlates of self-concept in children. J Educ Psychol. 1964;55(2):91.
11. Coopersmith S. The antecedents of self-esteem. Palo Alto: Consulting Psychologists Press; 1967.
12. Rosenberg M. Conceiving the self. New York: Basic Books; 1979.
13. Piaget J. The stages of the intellectual development of the child. Bull Menninger Clin. 1962;26:120–8.
14. Harter S. The Construction of the self: developmental and sociocultural foundations. New York: Guilford Press; 2012.

15. Bracken BA. Multidimensional self concept scale. Austin: Pro-ed; 1992.
16. Marsh HW. SDQ I manual & research monograph: self-description questionnaire. San Antonio: Psychological Corporation [and] Harcourt Brace Jovanovich; 1988.
17. Harter S. The perceived competence scale for children. Child Dev. 1982;53(1):87–97.
18. Cooley CH. Human nature and the social order. Piscataway: Transaction Publishers; 1992.
19. James W. Psychology, briefer course. Cambridge: Harvard University Press; 1984.
20. Butler RJ, Gasson SL. Self esteem/self concept scales for children and adolescents: a review. Child Adolesc Ment Health. 2005;10(4):190–201.
21. Furusho J, Kubagawa T, Satoh H, Shibata R, Nemoto Y, Matsuzaki K, et al. Study of the kid-kINDL questionnaire scores for children with developmental disorders in normal classes and their parents. No To Hattatsu. 2006;38(3):183–6.
22. Matsuzaki K, Nemoto Y, Shibata R, Morita K, Sato H, Furusho J, et al. A study of the Kiddo-KINDL^R (questionnaire for measuring quality of life in children, revised version for 13 to 16-years-old) in Japan. J Jpn Pediatr Soc. 2007;111(11):1404–10 **(in Japanese)**.
23. Harter S. Perceived competence scale for children. Denver: University of Denver; 1979.
24. Sakurai S. Development of the Japanese edition of the Harter's perceived competence scale for children. Jpn J Educ Psychol. 1983;31(3):245–9.
25. Sakurai S. The investigation of self-consciousness in 5th-and 6th-grade children. Jap J Exp Soc Psychol. 1992;32(1):85–94.
26. Harter S, Pike R. The pictorial scale of perceived competence and social acceptance for young children. Child Dev. 1984;55(6):1969–82.
27. Harter S. Susan Harter self-report instruments in DU Portfolio. https://portfolio.du.edu/SusanHarter/page/44342. Accessed 12 Oct 2017.
28. Shields N, Taylor NF, Dodd KJ. Self-concept in children with spina bifida compared with typically developing children. Dev Med Child Neurol. 2008;50(10):733–43.
29. Liu M, Wu L, Ming Q. How does physical activity intervention improve self-esteem and self-concept in children and adolescents? Evidence from a meta-analysis. PLoS ONE. 2015;10(8):e0134804.
30. Harter S. Self-perception profile for children: (revision of the perceived competence scale for children). Denver: University of Denver; 1985.
31. Tanaka M, Wada M, Kojima M. A Study of Japanese version of the scale for the self-cognition in childhood and early adolescence. Annu Bull Grad Sch Educ Tohoku Univ. 2005;54(1):315–37.
32. Maeda K. The modification and standardization of "self-perception profile for children" with Japanese school-age children. Ochanomizu Med J. 1998;46(2):113–23 **(in Japanese)**.
33. Maeshiro K. Structure of the self esteem in childhood. Bull Grad Sch Soc Sci Tokyo Int Univ. 2000;10:63–82 **(in Japanese)**.
34. Nagai Y, Nomura K, Nagata M, Ohgi S, Iwasa M. Children's Perceived Competence Scale: reference values in Japan. J Child Health Care. 2015;19(4):532–41.
35. Ravens-Sieberer U, Bullinger M. Assessing health-related quality of life in chronically ill children with the German KINDL: first psychometric and content analytical results. Qual Life Res. 1998;7(5):399–407.
36. Shibata RNY, Matsuzaki K, Tanaka D, Kawaguchi T, Kanda A, et al. A study of Kid-KIND questionnaire for measuring quality of life in elementary school children in Japan. J Jpn Pediatr Soc. 2003;107(11):1514–20.
37. Rosenberg M. Society and the adolescent self-image. Princeton: Princeton University Press; 1965.
38. Mimura C, Griffiths P. A Japanese version of the Perceived Stress Scale: cross-cultural translation and equivalence assessment. BMC Psychiatry. 2008;8:85.
39. Schermelleh-Engel K, Moosbrugger H, Müller H. Evaluating the fit of structural equation models: tests of significance and descriptive goodness-of-fit measures. Methods Psychol Res Online. 2003;8(2):23–74.
40. Nagai Y, Nomura K, Nagata M, Ohgi S, Iwasa M. Children's Perceived Competence Scale: reference values in Japan. J Child Health Care. 2014. https://doi.org/10.1177/1367493513519295.
41. Kling KC, Hyde JS, Showers CJ, Buswell BN. Gender differences in self-esteem: a meta-analysis. Psychol Bull. 1999;125(4):470–500.
42. Fukunaga Y, Takai Y, Yoshimoto T, Fujita E, Yamamoto M, Kanehisa H. Influence of maturation on anthropometry and body composition in Japanese junior high school students. J Physiol Anthropol. 2013;32(1):5.
43. Alessandri SM, Lewis M. Parental evaluation and its relation to shame and pride in young children. Sex Roles. 1993;29(5–6):335–43.
44. Walter JL, Burnaford SM. Developmental changes in adolescents' guilt and shame: the role of family climate and gender. N Am J Psychol. 2006;8(2):321–38.
45. Marsh HW. Age and sex effects in multiple dimensions of pre-adolescent self-concept: a replication and extension. Aust J Psychol. 1985;37(2):197–204.
46. Erikson EH. Identity and the life cycle: selected papers. Psychological issues. New York: International Universities Press; 1959.
47. Tuboi HMM, Keskinen S. Japanese children's quality of life (QOL): a comparison with Finish children. Jap J Child Adolesc Psychiatry. 2012;53:14–25.
48. Tomioka HI. Self-concepts in Japanese and American elementary school children: psychometric analysis of the self-description questionnaire I (SDQ-I). Jpn J Pers. 2011;19(3):191–205.

22

Determinants of early child development in rural Tanzania

Ingeborg G. Ribe[1], Erling Svensen[1,2], Britt A. Lyngmo[1], Estomih Mduma[2] and Sven G. Hinderaker[1*]

Abstract

Background: It has been estimated that more than 200 million children under the age of five do not reach their full potential in cognitive development. Much of what we know about brain development is based on research from high-income countries. There is limited evidence on the determinants of early child development in low-income countries, especially rural sub-Saharan Africa. The present study aimed to identify the determinants of cognitive development in children living in villages surrounding Haydom, a rural area in north-central Tanzania.

Methods: This cohort study is part of the MAL-ED (The Interactions of Malnutrition & Enteric Infections: Consequences for Child Health and Development) multi-country consortium studying risk factors for ill health and poor development in children. Descriptive analysis and linear regression analyses were performed. Associations between nutritional status, socio-economic status, and home environment at 6 months of age and cognitive outcomes at 15 months of age were studied. The third edition of the Bayley Scales for Infant and Toddler Development was used to assess cognitive, language and motor development.

Results: There were 262 children enrolled into the study, and this present analysis included the 137 children with data for 15-month Bayley scores. Univariate regression analysis, weight-for-age and weight-for-length z-scores at 6 months were significantly associated with 15-month Bayley gross motor score, but not with other 15-month Bayley scores. Length-for-age z-scores at 6 months were not significantly associated with 15-month Bayley scores. The socio-economic status, measured by a set of assets and monthly income was significantly associated with 15-month Bayley cognitive score, but not with language, motor, nor total 15-month Bayley scores. Other socio-economic variables were not significantly associated with 15-month Bayley scores. No significant associations were found between the home environment and 15-month Bayley scores. In multivariate regression analyses we found higher Bayley scores for girls and higher Bayley scores in families with more assets. Adjusted R-squared of this model was 8%.

Conclusion: We conclude that poverty is associated with a slower cognitive development in children and malnutrition is associated with slower gross motor development. This information should encourage authorities and other stakeholders to invest in improved welfare and nutrition programmes for children from early infancy.

Keywords: Child development, Mental development, Cognitive development, Bayley Scales of Infant, Toddler development

Background

It has been estimated that more than 200 million children under the age of five do not reach their full potential in cognitive development. This phenomenon is largely due to mechanisms that can be influenced; such as poverty, poor nutrition, and suboptimal care in the home [1]. We know that intervention programmes in the early years could prevent delay in development [2]. A life-course perspective shows that early child development affects future educational and occupational opportunities, and it may also determine a person's risk of physical health in terms of obesity, malnutrition and mental-health problems [3]. Failure to thrive cognitively not only adversely affects the individual, but collectively limits national development. The cycle continues as it may be passed

*Correspondence: Sven.Hinderaker@uib.no
[1] University of Bergen, Bergen, Norway
Full list of author information is available at the end of the article

on to future generations and the gap of health inequities grows.

The first years of life constitute a critical period in brain development and functions [4]. Certainly genetic disposition plays a role [5], but external environmental factors are also important, including [3] nutritional status, socioeconomic status, and home environment. Early interventions that influence these external factors may be effective in assuring children a good start [6], and may not only benefit the individual but also the society as a whole [7].

Much of what we know about early child development is based on research from high-income countries [8]. One study from rural Kenya analyzed the prevalence and risk factors of neurological disability and impairment in 6–9 year-olds. They found that moderate to severe cognitive impairment was present in 3% of children, and neonatal insult was the only risk factor identified [9]. However, to our knowledge, there is limited evidence on the determinants of early child development of the general population in low-income countries, and more specifically from rural sub-Saharan Africa.

A multicenter cohort study called MAL-ED (The Interactions of Malnutrition and Enteric Infections: Consequences for Child Health and Development) was started with one of the field sites in rural Tanzania. The study includes many items related to normal child development and aims to identify determinants of early child development in children. Specifically, the objectives of this paper were to find the associations between nutritional status, socio-economic status, and home environment—all at 6 months of age—and cognitive outcomes at 15 months of age in children living in villages surrounding Haydom, a rural area in north-central Tanzania.

Methods

This study is part of the MAL-ED (The Interactions of Malnutrition & Enteric Infections: Consequences for Child Health and Development) [10] multi-country consortium studying risk factors for ill health and poor development in children. In this paper, data from the Tanzanian site (TZH) was analyzed.

Study design

The study had a prospective cohort design. The outcome measurement was the score on the Bayley Scales of Infant and Toddler Development at 15 months of age. Independent variables were gender, WAMI index, HOME score, weight-for-age z-score, length-for-age z-score, and head circumference-for-age z-score.

Study setting

The setting is rural northern central Tanzania, in the Manyara region in villages surrounding Haydom (TZH). The population is mainly peasants living from mainly maize, beans farming and animal keeping. The village is of low economic status and without tarmac roads. Malnutrition is common among children under the age of five in the Manyara region, with a quarter of them underweight (weight-for-age below $-$ 2 SD) [11] The study site is described more in detail elsewhere [12].

The study population

The study's catchment area was defined geographically and all pregnant women in their third trimester over a period of 2 years were asked to participate. Exclusion criteria were if the family had plans to move outside the area, if the mother was younger than 16 years of age, twin pregnancy, born underweight (< 1.5 kg), or if they already had a child enrolled in the study. Infants participated in repeated household visits; 262 infants were enrolled within 17 days of birth. For the present analysis, 137 children with Bayley scores at age 15 months (455 ± 15 days) were included in the analysis.

Study instruments

The third edition of the Bayley Scales for Infant and Toddler Development was used to assess cognitive, language and motor development [13]. The test includes various questions, scenarios and tasks and takes approximately 45–60 min to complete. The test was administered by a trained person and conducted at 15 months of age. Details about translations and needed adaptations (e.g. replacing "foreign" items such as snow and vacuum cleaners) are described elsewhere [14].

Socioeconomic status was measured at the 6-month follow-up using a socioeconomic questionnaire. A WAMI index (scale from 0 to 1) [15], accounting for a household Water and sanitation type, various Assets, Maternal education and monthly Income is used in this analysis (Box 1).

The Home Observation for Measurement of the Environment (HOME) inventory, an instrument developed and validated by Caldwell and Bradley [16], was used to assess quality of the child´s home environment. The HOME inventory was also taken at 6 months of age (Box 2).

Box 1 Calculation of the Water/sanitation, Assets, Maternal education, and Income (WAMI) index (Psaki et al.)

	Description	Range
Water/ sanitation	Using WHO definitions of access to improved water and improved sanitation, households with access to improved water or improved sanitation are assigned a score of 4 for each. Households without access to improved water or improved sanitation are assigned a score of 0 for each. These scores were summed	0–8
Assets	Eight priority assets were selected. For each asset, households were assigned a 1 if they have the asset and 0 if they do not have the asset. These scores were summed	0–8
Maternal education	Each child's mother provided the number of years of schooling she had completed, ranging from 0 to 16 years. This number was divided by 2	0–8
Income	Monthly household income was converted to US dollars using the exchange rate from January 1, 2010. Income was divided into octiles using the following scores and cutoffs: 1 (0–26), 2 (26.01–47), 3 (47.01–72), 4 (72.01–106), 5 (106.01–135), 6 (135.01–200), 7 (200.01–293), 8 (293 +)	0–8
TOTAL	Scores in water and sanitation, assets, mother´s education, and income were summed then divided by 32	0–1

Box 2 Description of calculation of the adjusted HOME Inventory for the Tanzanian site

HOME category	Description	Range
Emotional and verbal responsivity	Caregiver tells the child the name of some object or says the name of a person or object in a teaching style during the visit. (0–1) Caregiver's speech is distinct, clear, and audible. (0–1) Caregiver initiates verbal exchanges with the observer—asks questions, makes spontaneous comments. (0–1) Caregiver expresses ideas freely and easily, and uses statements of appropriate length for conversation (i.e., gives more than brief answers). (0–1) Caregiver spontaneously praises child's qualities or behavior at least twice during visit. (0–1) Caregiver shows some positive emotional response or praise to the child offered by the observer. (0–1) Caregiver smiles at the child or laughs with the child. (0–1)	0–7

HOME category	Description	Range
Organization	When the primary caregiver is away, care is provided by one of three regular substitutes. (0–1) The child has a special place to keep his toys and "treasures." (0–1) The child's play area is relatively safe and free from hazards. (0–1) The stove is located in a relatively safe area. (0–1) The house is relatively light. (0–1) The house is relatively ventilated. (0–1) The house is relatively clean. (0–1) The house is relatively neat and orderly. (0–1)	0–8
Opportunities	The caregiver sings to the child everyday. (0–1) The family visits or receives visits from relatives at least once per month. (0–1) The family visits or receives visits from close friends at least once per month. (0–1)	0–3
Cleanliness of child	The child is relatively clean, with no offensive odor. (0–1) The child's hair is relatively clean. (0–1) The child's clothes are relatively clean. (0–1)	0–3

Nutritional status was assessed using anthropometric measurements. Weight at enrollment was examined and z-scores for length, weight and head circumference at enrollment and at 6 months of age were calculated using WHO child growth standards.

Data collection and analysis

Data was collected by trained local field staff. Statistical analyses were conducted using SPSS Version 23. The Bayley assessments were all video recorded and evaluated locally, and 10% of the videos were sent off-site for another quality check performed by a trained Bayley administrator. These evaluations revealed that one out of four of the local Bayley examiners did not have the necessary quality in the assessment. All included assessments were analyzed for psychometric properties in order to check for scale reliability. Bayley assessment was done at 15 months, because at 12 and 18 months there were too many other assessments in this "MALED" study. Some data was missing, and some was tested too late, and one field assistant for Bayley assessment was excluded.

Statistical analysis

Following the procedure described in length by Lyngmo et al. [17] the subscales of Bayley were revised as following. All items with zero variance were removed, thereafter all items with < 0.30 item-total correlation. This yielded a revised measurement consisting of four subscales: Cognitive (23 items, Cronbach alpha 0.85), Language (15 items, Cronbach alpha 0.89), Fine motor (12 items, Cronbach alpha 0.71), and Gross motor (22 items, Cronbach alpha 0.82). These four scales as well as the total score were used as the outcome measures. Using the same procedure with the HOME inventory psychometric properties were analyzed and adjusted in order to be more reliable in this setting. Items with no variance were excluded and correlations coefficients were calculated. All items with correlations coefficients less than 0.30 were excluded one by one until satisfactory correlations were obtained. As a result some subscales were omitted and we kept the following: seven items on emotional and verbal responsivity (Cronbach alpha 0.66), eight items on organization of physical and temporal environment (Cronbach alpha 0.72), three items on opportunities for variety in daily stimulation (Cronbach alpha 0.68), and three items on cleanliness of child (Cronbach alpha 0.83). Each item in both HOME and Bayley were scored as either 0 or 1, making the maximum score the same as the number of items for that scale.

Means and standard deviations were calculated for continuous data and proportions for categorical data. Variables were tested for normality. Potential associations between 15-month Bayley scores and selected determinants were analyzed by univariate linear regression analysis, with 5% significance level. The associations are presented as adjusted Beta regression coefficients.

A multivariate model was built for the cognitive scale of the Bayley, retaining potential explanatory variables where the p value in univariate regression was less than 0.1, and then running a forward stepwise linear regression. Gender and tribe were included in the multivariate model as a control factors. In our model male gender was 1 and "female" was 2, and for Iraq tribe was 1 and "others" was 2.

Ethical issues

The study was approved by the Tanzanian National Institute for Medical Research and Ministry of Health and Social Welfare. Parents or legal guardians signed an informed consent form after the study's objectives, procedures, risks, benefits, and confidentiality procedure were explained.

Results

We screened 274 pregnant women. None of these declined and all were over 16 years. Three mothers were not able to give informed consent, seven children were not healthy and two pregnancies were twins, hence not eligible. There were 262 presumably healthy singleton children enrolled into the study, and we included the 135 children who had data for 15-month Bayley scores; 77 (56.2%) were girls (Table 1). Mean weight at enrollment

Table 1 Baseline characteristics of 137 children in rural Tanzania

Variables	n	Mean	Standard deviation	%
Bodyweight at enrolment (0–17 days)	137	3.39 kg	0.49	
WAZ at enrolment (0–17 days)	137	− 0.13	0.91	
Gender	137			
Male	60			43.8
Female	77			56.2
Tribe				
Iraqw	103			85.8
Datog	10			8.3
Other	7			2.5
Missing	17			2.5
Nutritional status				0.8
LAZ at 6 months	137	− 1.24	1.05	
LAZ ≤ − 2 (stunted)	28			20.4
WAZ at 6 months	137	− 0.60	1.12	
WAZ ≤ − 2 (wasted)	14			10.2
WLZ at 6 months	137	0.32	1.20	
WLZ ≤ −2 (malnourished)	4			2.9
Socioeconomic status				
WAMI index	135[b]	0.21	0.12	
Sanitation[a]	135[b]	1.81	2.17	
Assets	135[b]	1.90	1.64	
Maternal education (years)	135[b]	5.20	2.78	
Income per month (TZH shilling)[a]	135[b]	42,861	58,699	
Mother's age (years)	121[c]	29.31	6.61	
Mother's number of pregnancies[a]	122[d]	4.70	2.81	
Home environment				
Emotional and verbal responsivity[a]	137	6.70	0.85	
Organization	137	3.04	2.18	
Opportunities[a]	137	2.77	0.58	
Cleanliness of child[a]	137	2.48	0.93	
Cognitive development at 15 months				
Bayley total score	137	43.15	8.55	
Bayley cognitive score	137	11.50	4.13	
Bayley language score	137	8.26	3.99	
Bayley fine motor score[a]	137	10.94	1.43	
Bayley gross motor score	137	12.45	2.45	

LAZ length-for-age z-score; WAZ weight-for-age z-score; WLZ weight-for-length z-score; WAMI index water, assets, maternal education, and income

[a] Not normally distributed

[b] Missing 2

[c] Missing 16

[d] Missing 15

(within 17 days after birth) was 3.36 kg (SD = 0.5) and 3.6% of the children had a bodyweight of 2500 grams or less at enrollment. Almost all of them (97%) started breastfeeding within 24 h. Apgar score was not available as most of the births were at home (54%).

Socioeconomic indicators showed that the mothers' mean years of schooling were 5.2 (SD = 2.8). The mean family income per month was 42,860 Tanzanian shillings (20 USD). The mean age of their mothers was 29.3 years (SD = 6.6) and they had a mean number of pregnancies of 4.7 (SD = 2.8). The children's mean 15-month Bayley scores are shown in Table 1.

In univariate regression analysis weight-for-age and weight-for-length z-scores at 6 months were significantly associated with 15-month Bayley gross motor score, but not with other 15-month Bayley scores (Table 2). Length-for-age z-scores at 6 months were not significantly associated with 15-month Bayley scores.

The cleanliness of child at 6 months from the HOME inventory scale was significantly associated with 15-month Bayley total score, but not with any of the other 15-month Bayley scores. The cleanliness variable was not normally distributed as it was strongly skewed to the right, meaning higher level of cleanliness. Other scores from the HOME inventory were not significantly associated with 15-month Bayley scores.

The WAMI index, assets component, and monthly income were significantly associated with 15-month Bayley cognitive score, but not with language, motor, nor total 15-month Bayley scores. Other socioeconomic variables in the WAMI index were not significantly associated with 15-month Bayley scores.

Multivariate regression analysis of cognitive Bayley, showed statistically significant associations with gender and socioeconomic status, with higher Bayley cognitive scores for girls, and higher Bayley cognitive scores in families with more assets and income from the WAMI index. Adjusted R-squared in this model was 8% (Table 3).

Discussion

Our analysis aiming at identifying factors thought to influence early child development shows that socioeconomic factors were associated with cognitive development, and nutritional status was associated with gross motor development.

Our analysis shows that the strongest factor correlated with child cognitive development at 15 months of age is the socioeconomic status of the household. The robust association between socioeconomic status and child

Table 2 Univariate linear regression analysis of determinants of Bayley scores at 15 months of age in 137 children in rural Tanzania

Determinants at 6 months	Bayley scores at 15 months									
	Cognitive score		Language score		Fine motor score		Gross motor score		Total score	
	Beta	p	Beta	p	Beta	p	Beta	p	Beta	p
Gender[a]	0.18	0.03	0.12	0.15	0.11	0.21	0.05	0.58	0.18	0.04
Tribe[b]	0.04	0.69	0.14	0.12	0.08	0.36	0.02	0.84	0.10	0.26
Nutritional status										
Length-for-age z-score	0.05	0.56	0.05	0.56	0.11	0.22	0.03	0.77	0.06	0.50
Weight-for-age z-score	0.01	0.95	0.05	0.60	0.01	0.91	0.18	0.03	− 0.03	0.73
Weight-for-length z-score	0.02	0.80	0.03	0.77	0.09	0.28	0.19	0.03	− 0.07	0.42
Socioeconomic status										
WAMI index	0.17	0.05	0.02	0.83	0.04	0.67	0.06	0.46	0.12	0.18
Sanitation	0.01	0.92	0.07	0.40	0.00	0.99	0.10	0.26	0.06	0.51
Assets	0.21	0.01	0.03	0.76	0.06	0.49	0.000	1.00	0.10	0.25
Maternal education	0.08	0.35	0.01	0.92	0.03	0.75	0.10	0.27	0.08	0.39
Monthly income	0.20	0.02	0.03	0.72	0.03	0.71	0.05	0.60	0.08	0.39
Home environment										
Emotional and verbal responsivity	0.05	0.60	0.09	0.28	0.06	0.50	0.05	0.53	0.06	0.49
Organization	0.12	0.17	0.05	0.58	0.09	0.28	0.07	0.42	0.07	0.42
Opportunities	0.04	0.67	0.08	0.38	0.05	0.55	0.07	0.39	− 0.08	0.34
Cleanliness of child	0.15	0.08	0.15	0.09	0.05	0.60	0.16	0.07	− 0.19	0.02

Beta is the regression co-efficient

[a] In the regression model male = 1 and female = 2

[b] In the regression model Iraqw = 1 and others = 2

Table 3 Multivariate linear regression analysis of determinants of Bayley cognitive score at 15 months of age in 137 children in rural Tanzania

Determinants	Bayley cognitive score at 15 months	
	Beta	p
Gender[a]	− 0.20	0.03
Tribe[b]	0.06	0.51
Assets	0.24	0.01

Adjusted r-squared 7.6%

[a] In the regression model male = 1 and female = 2

[b] In the regression model Iraqw = 1, others = 2

development is well known [1, 18–20]. The Lancet series on children's development in low-income countries concluded that low socioeconomic status was a determinant of poor development [1]. This effect can be seen before birth and continue into adulthood [21]. Socioeconomic factors may affect childhood brain development through a variety of mechanisms, such as prenatal factors, parental care, cognitive stimulation, toxin exposure, nutrition, and stress [22, 23]. A study from Greece showed that maternal education, which is a component of the WAMI index, and which is often itself associated with socioeconomic status, was positively correlated with child development [24]. A study on the effects of socioeconomic status on neurocognitive systems showed that the association is most pronounced with language and memory [25]. One study using magnetic resonance imaging of the brain found that lower family socioeconomic status was associated with smaller volumes of gray matter in the brain [26], and consequently environmental factors may have detrimental effects on brain structure and function.

Stunting and wasting are indicators that reflect nutritional status. Stunting (length-for-age z-score (LAZ) < -2) is an indicator of chronic malnutrition and wasting (weight-for-length z-score (WLZ) < -2) is an indicator of acute malnutrition [27]. Our analysis suggests that both stunting and wasting at 6 months of age are associated with poorer motor development at 15 months of age. A study from Pemba, Tanzania showed that higher LAZ scores were significantly associated with better motor and language development [28]. Many other studies from Africa to Asia show that better nutrition is positively correlated with child development [27, 29–32].

Lower socioeconomic status is associated with lower nutritional status, poor sanitary and hygiene conditions, which in turn is associated with higher rates of infections and stunting in children. All of these factors intertwine and contribute to a child's development [33, 34]. This demonstrates the interaction between socioeconomic

status and nutritional status, and it also highlights the complex interaction between environmental factors on child development.

Cleanliness of one's child was associated with total Bayley score. We do not have any clear explanation for this; there could be some information bias as the pregnant women learn about cleanliness in schools and at mother-and-child clinics and may respond correspondingly, but we also speculate that in poor households like these the cleanliness of the child is the last thing to give up.

In this study there was a significant association between girls' and cognitive Bayley score, also reflected in the total score. We do not have any good explanation for this. Some information bias is possible, as items used for measuring these Bayley scores may have been more familiar to female infants and hence influencing the score. The difference between tribes is also difficult to explain; some have different culture and habits like hygiene and hence the items used for Bayley scores may turn out somehow biased. The Iraqw tribe may have more of their extended family close to home and hence potentially more support from extended family.

We observed a better nutritional status was associated with better gross motor Bayley score, but not fine motor Bayley score. We do not have any explanation of this but speculate that gross motor score is more influenced by undernutrition because of less physical strength, whereas fine motor score is less dependent on this.

Strengths and limitations

This study has several strengths. It is part of a large multi-centre research project studying determinants of child development, and with a strong research group coordinating the study sites [10]. The study tools used were acknowledged and tested, and data collection was done under close continuous supervision [14].

Some limitations of this study should be noted. First, in this observational study we cannot prove any causal relationships, only statistical associations. Second, some determinants of child development were not examined; for example, genetic factors, neighborhood processes, conflict and violence [23]. Third, the Bayley and the HOME inventory were modified in order to be more applicable in the local rural Tanzanian setting, and hence their validity was not yet evidence-based in all aspects. Fourth, unfortunately, as explained in Methods, a substantial proportion (52%) of the enrolled participants did not have their Bayley test taken at 15 months of age and were excluded from analysis, limiting the sample size and statistical power. As this also posed a risk of selection bias we compared the excluded and included participants by sex (p = 0.27), initial bodyweight (p = 0.57), initial z-score (p = 0.52) and 12 m WAMI (p = 0.27), and concluded that the excluded participants were very probably comparable to those included. The minimal sex difference among the participants included and those excluded causes slight concern as this sex is a weak risk factor, and could slightly affect the associations studied. Finally, in this area all households were poor to some degree and the variation in SES was not large; consequently this results in low statistical power in analysis of these associations.

Conclusions and implications

We conclude that lower socioeconomic status is associated with poor cognitive development in children and malnutrition is associated with reduced gross motor development. This information should encourage authorities and other stakeholders to invest in improved welfare and nutrition programmes for children from early infancy.

Abbreviations

MAL-ED: The Interactions of Malnutrition & Enteric Infections: Consequences for Child Health and Development; Bayley: Bayley Scales of Infant Development; TZH: Tanzanian site; WAMI: Water and sanitation type, various Assets, Maternal education and monthly Income; HOME: Home Observation for Measurement of the Environment inventory; LAZ: length-for-age z-scores; WAZ: weight-for-age z-scores; WLZ: weight-for-length z-score.

Authors' contributions

IR drafted the protocol, analysed the data, drafted the paper, wrote the last version. ES supervised all steps, supervised data collection, drafted the paper, wrote the last version. BAL collected data, adjusted the Bayley for the Tanzanian site, edited the last version. EM supervised the site, collected data, edited the last version. SGH supervised all steps, drafted the paper, wrote the last version. All authors read and approved the final manuscript.

Author details

[1] University of Bergen, Bergen, Norway. [2] Haydom Lutheran Hospital, Haydom, Mbulu District, Tanzania.

Acknowledgements

The Etiology, Risk Factors and Interactions of Enteric Infections and Malnutrition and the Consequences for Child Health and Development Project (MAL-ED) is carried out as a collaborative project supported by the Bill & Melinda Gates Foundation, the Foundation for the NIH, and the National Institutes of Health, Fogarty International Center. The authors thank the staff and participants of the MAL-ED Network for their important contributions. The University of Bergen supported the study, including the publication fee.

Competing interests

The authors declare that they have no competing interests.

References

1. Grantham-McGregor S, Cheung YB, Cueto S, Glewwe P, Richter L, Strupp B. Developmental potential in the first 5 years for children in developing countries. Lancet. 2007;369(9555):60–70.
2. Engle PL, Black MM, Behrman JR, Cabral de Mello M, Gertler PJ, Kapiriri L, et al. Strategies to avoid the loss of developmental potential in more than 200 million children in the developing world. Lancet. 2007;369(9557):229–42.
3. Marmot M, Friel S, Bell R, Houweling TAJ, Taylor S. Closing the gap in a generation: health equity through action on the social determinants of health. Lancet. 2008;372:1661–9.
4. Rosenzweig MR. Effects of differential experience on the brain and behavior. Dev Neuropsychol. 2011;24:523–40.
5. Bouchard TJ Jr, McGue M. Genetic and environmental influences on human psychological differences. J Neurobiol. 2003;54(1):4–45.
6. Shonkoff JP, Phillips DA. From neurons to neighborhoods: the science of early childhood development. Washington D.C.: National Academy Press; 2000.
7. Marmot M, Bell R. Health equity and development: the commission on social determinants of health. Eur Rev. 2009;18(01):1.
8. Britto PR, Ulkuer N. Child development in developing countries: child rights and policy implications. Child Dev. 2012;83(1):92–103.
9. Mung'ala-Odera V, Meehan R, Njuguna P, Mturi N, Alcock KJ, Newton CR. Prevalence and risk factors of neurological disability and impairment in children living in rural Kenya. Int J Epidemiol. 2006;35(3):683–8.
10. MAL-ED. The MAL-ED study: a multinational and multidisciplinary approach to understand the relationship between enteric pathogens, malnutrition, gut physiology, physical growth, cognitive development, and immune responses in infants and children up to 2 years of age in resource-poor environments. Clin Infect Dis. 2014;59(Suppl 4):S193–206.
11. National Bureau of Statistics, ICE Macro. Tanzania Demographic and Health Survey 2010. Dar es Salaam, Tanzania; 2011.
12. Mduma ER, Gratz J, Patil C, Matson K, Dakay M, Liu S, et al. The etiology, risk factors, and interactions of enteric infections and malnutrition and the consequences for child health and development study (MAL-ED): description of the Tanzanian site. Clin Infect Dis. 2014;59(Suppl 4):S325–30.
13. Bayley N. The Bayley scales of infant and toddler development. 3rd ed. Agra: Psychological Corporation; 1993.
14. Murray-Kolb LE, Rasmussen ZA, Scharf RJ, Rasheed MA, Svensen E, Seidman JC, et al. The MAL-ED cohort study: methods and lessons learned when assessing early child development and caregiving mediators in infants and young children in 8 low- and middle-income countries. Clin Infect Dis. 2014;59(Suppl 4):S261–72.
15. Psaki SR, Seidman JC, Miller M, Gottlieb M, Bhutta ZA, Ahmed T, et al. Measuring socioeconomic status in multicountry studies: results from the eight-country MAL-ED study. Popul Health Metr. 2014;12(1):8.
16. Caldwell B, Bradley RH. Home observation for measurement of the environment (HOME). Little Rock: University of Arkansas Press; 1984.
17. Lyngmo BA, Kvestad I, Svensen E. Is Bayley-III a feasible tool for investigating early child development in rural Tanzania? University of Bergen; 2014.
18. Ronfani L, Vecchi Brumatti L, Mariuz M, Tognin V, Bin M, Ferluga V, et al. The complex interaction between home environment, socioeconomic status, maternal iq and early child neurocognitive development: a multivariate analysis of data collected in a newborn cohort study. PLoS ONE. 2015;10(5):e0127052.
19. Rindermann H. African cognitive ability: research, results, divergences and recommendations. Personal Individ Differ. 2013;55(3):229–33.
20. Contreras D, González S. Determinants of early child development in Chile: health, cognitive and demographic factors. Int J Educ Dev. 2015;40:217–30.
21. Bradley RH, Corwyn RF. Socioeconomic status and child development. Annu Rev Psychol. 2002;53:371–99.
22. Hackman DA, Farah MJ, Meaney MJ. Socioeconomic status and the brain: mechanistic insights from human and animal research. Nat Rev Neurosci. 2010;11(9):651–9.
23. Neisser U, Boodoo G, Bouchard TJ Jr, Boykin AW, Brody N, Ceci SJ, Halpern

DF, Loehlin JC, Perloff R, Sternberg RJ, Urbina S. Intelligence: knowns and unknowns. Am Pyschol. 1996;51(2):77–101.

24. Koutra K, Chatzi L, Roumeliotaki T, Vassilaki M, Giannakopoulou E, Batsos C, et al. Socio-demographic determinants of infant neurodevelopment at 18 months of age: mother-child cohort (Rhea Study) in Crete, Greece. Infant behav Dev. 2012;35(1):48–59.

25. Farah MJ, Shera DM, Savage JH, Betancourt L, Giannetta JM, Brodsky NL, et al. Childhood poverty: specific associations with neurocognitive development. Brain Res. 2006;1110(1):166–74.

26. Jednorog K, Altarelli I, Monzalvo K, Fluss J, Dubois J, Billard C, et al. The influence of socioeconomic status on children's brain structure. PLoS ONE. 2012;7(8):e42486.

27. Sudfeld CR, McCoy DC, Fink G, Muhihi A, Bellinger DC, Masanja H, et al. Malnutrition and its determinants are associated with suboptimal cognitive, communication, and motor development in Tanzanian children. J Nutr. 2015;145(12):2705–14.

28. Olney DK, Kariger PK, Stoltzfus RJ, Khalfan SS, Ali NS, Tielsch JM, et al. Development of nutritionally at-risk young children is predicted by malaria, anemia, and stunting in Pemba, Zanzibar. J Nutr. 2009;139(4):763–72.

29. Yousafzai AK, Rasheed MA, Rizvi A, Armstrong R, Bhutta ZA. Effect of integrated responsive stimulation and nutrition interventions in the Lady Health Worker programme in Pakistan on child development, growth, and health outcomes: a cluster-randomised factorial effectiveness trial. Lancet. 2014;384(9950):1282–93.

30. Siegel EH, Stoltzfus RJ, Kariger PK, Katz J, Khatry SK, LeClerq SC, et al. Growth indices, anemia, and diet independently predict motor milestone acquisition of infants in South Central Nepal. J Nutr. 2005;135:2840–4.

31. Kitsao-Wekulo P, Holding P, Taylor HG, Abubakar A, Kvalsvig J, Connolly K. Nutrition as an important mediator of the impact of background variables on outcome in middle childhood. Front Human Neurosci. 2013;7:713.

32. Olney DK, Pollitt E, Kariger PK, Khalfan SS, Ali NS, Tielsch JM, et al. Young Zanzibari children with iron deficiency, iron deficiency anemia, stunting, or malaria have lower motor activity scores and spend less time in locomotion. J Nutr. 2007;137:2756–62.

33. Duncan GJ, Brooks-Gunn J. Family poverty, welfare reform, and child development. Child Dev. 2000;71(1):188–96.

34. Linver MR, Brooks-Gunn J, Kohen DE. Family processes as pathways from income to young children's development. Dev Psychol. 2002;38(5):719–34.

Permissions

The contributors of this book come from diverse backgrounds, making this book a truly international effort. This book will bring forth new frontiers with its revolutionizing research information and detailed analysis of the nascent developments around the world.

We would like to thank all the contributing authors for lending their expertise to make the book truly unique. They have played a crucial role in the development of this book. Without their invaluable contributions this book wouldn't have been possible. They have made vital efforts to compile up to date information on the varied aspects of this subject to make this book a valuable addition to the collection of many professionals and students.

This book was conceptualized with the vision of imparting up-to-date information and advanced data in this field. To ensure the same, a matchless editorial board was set up. Every individual on the board went through rigorous rounds of assessment to prove their worth. After which they invested a large part of their time researching and compiling the most relevant data for our readers.

The editorial board has been involved in producing this book since its inception. They have spent rigorous hours researching and exploring the diverse topics which have resulted in the successful publishing of this book. They have passed on their knowledge of decades through this book. To expedite this challenging task, the publisher supported the team at every step. A small team of assistant editors was also appointed to further simplify the editing procedure and attain best results for the readers.

Apart from the editorial board, the designing team has also invested a significant amount of their time in understanding the subject and creating the most relevant covers. They scrutinized every image to scout for the most suitable representation of the subject and create an appropriate cover for the book.

The publishing team has been an ardent support to the editorial, designing and production team. Their endless efforts to recruit the best for this project, has resulted in the accomplishment of this book. They are a veteran in the field of academics and their pool of knowledge is as vast as their experience in printing. Their expertise and guidance has proved useful at every step. Their uncompromising quality standards have made this book an exceptional effort. Their encouragement from time to time has been an inspiration for everyone.

The publisher and the editorial board hope that this book will prove to be a valuable piece of knowledge for researchers, students, practitioners and scholars across the globe.

List of Contributors

Arnold Lohaus, Sabrina Chodura, Christine Möller and Tabea Symanzik
Faculty of Psychology and Sports Sciences, University of Bielefeld, 33501 Bielefeld, Germany

Daniela Ehrenberg, Ann-Katrin Job and Nina Heinrichs
University of Braunschweig, Institute of Psychology, Humboldtstr. 33, 38106 Brunswick, Germany

Vanessa Reindl and Kerstin Konrad
Department for Child and Adolescent Psychiatry, University Hospital Aachen, Neuenhoferweg 21, 52074 Aachen, Germany

Andreas Jud
Child and Adolescent Psychiatry/Psychotherapy, University of Ulm, Ulm, Germany
School of Social Work, Lucerne University of Applied Sciences and Arts, Lucerne, Switzerland

Tanja Mitrovic and Rahel Portmann
School of Social Work, Lucerne University of Applied Sciences and Arts, Lucerne, Switzerland

Céline Kosirnik, Hakim Ben Salah and René Knüsel
Observatory on Child Maltreatment, University of Lausanne, Lausanne, Switzerland

Etienne Fux and Jana Koehler
School of Information Technology, Lucerne University of Applied Sciences and Arts, Rotkreuz, Switzerland

Luuk J. Kalverdijk
Department of Psychiatry, University of Groningen, University Medical Center Groningen, Groningen, The Netherlands

Christian J. Bachmann
Freelance Researcher, Marburg, Germany

Lise Aagaard
Life Science Team, IP and Technology, Bech-Bruun Law Firm, Copenhagen, Denmark

Mehmet Burcu and Julie M. Zito
Department of Pharmaceutical Health Services Research, University of Maryland, Baltimore, MD, USA

Gerd Glaeske
Division of Health Long-term Care and Pensions, University of Bremen, SOCIUM Research Center on Inequality and Social Policy, Bremen, Germany

Falk Hoffmann
Department of Health Services Research, Carl von Ossietzky University, Oldenburg, Germany

Irene Petersen
Department of Primary Care and Population Health, University College London, London, UK

Catharina C. M. Schuiling-Veninga
University of Groningen, Pharmacotherapy, Epidemiology and Economics, Groningen, The Netherlands

Linda P. Wijlaars
Department of Primary Care and Population Health, University College London, London, UK
Population, Policy and Practice, University College London Great Ormond Street Institute of Child Health, London, UK

L. E. W. Leenarts, T. Pérez, K. Schmeck and M. Schmid
Forschungsabteilung, Kinder-und Jugendpsychiatrische Klinik, Universitäre Psychiatrische Kliniken (UPK), Schanzenstrasse 13, 4056 Basel, Switzerland

C. Dölitzsch and J. M. Fegert
Klinik für Kinder- und Jugendpsychiatrie/Psychotherapie, Universitätsklinikum Ulm, Steinhövelstrasse 5, 89075 Ulm, Germany

George Nikolaidis and Kiki Petroulaki
Department of Mental Health and Social Welfare, Centre for the Study and Prevention of Child Abuse and Neglect, Institute of Child Health, 7 Fokidos Str., 11526 Athens, Greece

Altin Hazizaj
Children's Human Rights Centre of Albania, Tirana, Albania

Jelena Brkic-Smigoc and Emir Vajzovic
Faculty of Political Sciences, University of Sarajevo, Sarajevo, Bosnia and Herzegovina

Vaska Stancheva and Stefka Chincheva
Department of Medical Social Sciences, South-West University "N. Rilski", Blagoevgrad, Bulgaria

Marina Ajdukovic and Miro Rajter
Department of Social Work, Faculty of Law, University of Zagreb, Zagreb, Croatia

Marija Raleva and Liljana Trpcevska
University Clinic of Psychiatry, University of Skopje, Skopje, Former Yugoslav Republic of Macedonia

Maria Roth and Imola Antal
Social Work Department, Faculty of Sociology and Social Work, Babes-Bolyai University, Cluj-Napoca, Romania

Veronika Ispanovic
Faculty for Special Education and Rehabilitation, University of Belgrade, Belgrade, Serbia

Zeynep Olmezoglu-Sofuoglu and Ismail Umit-Bal
Association of Emergency Ambulance Physicians, İzmir, Turkey

Donata Bianchi
Instituto degli Innocenti, Florence, Italy

Franziska Meinck
Centre for Evidence-Based Interventions, University of Oxford, Oxford, UK
School of Behavioural Sciences, North-West University, Vanderbeijlpark, South Africa

Kevin Browne
Centre for Forensic and Family Psychology (Division of Psychiatry and Applied Psychology), School of Medicine, University of Nottingham, Nottingham, UK

Foteini Zarokosta
Department of Mental Health and Social Welfare, Centre for the Study and Prevention of Child Abuse and Neglect, Institute of Child Health, 7 Fokidos Str., 11526 Athens, Greece
Department of Applied Mathematics and Computer Science, Technical University of Denmark, Copenhagen, Denmark

Antonia Tsirigoti
Department of Mental Health and Social Welfare, Centre for the Study and Prevention of Child Abuse and Neglect, Institute of Child Health, 7 Fokidos Str., 11526 Athens, Greece
"The Smile of the Child", Athens, Greece

Enila Cenko
Children's Human Rights Centre of Albania, Tirana, Albania
Humanities and Social Sciences Department, University of New York Tirana, Tirana, Albania

Natasha Hanak
Faculty for Special Education and Rehabilitation, University of Belgrade, Belgrade, Serbia
AWO Clearinghaus for Unaccompanied Minor Refugees, Dortmund, North Rhine-Westphalia, Germany

Katri Maasalo, Jaana Wessman and Eeva T. Aronen
University of Helsinki and Helsinki University Hospital, Children's Hospital, Child Psychiatry, Tukholmankatu 8 C 613, 00290 Helsinki, Finland
Helsinki Pediatric Research Center, Laboratory of Developmental Psychopathology, Helsinki, Finland

Ricardo Orozco, Corina Benjet, Guilherme Borges, Diana Fregoso Ito, Clara Fleiz and Jorge Ameth Villatoro
Department of Epidemiology and Psychosocial Research, National Institute of Psychiatry (Mexico), Calzada Mexico-Xochimilco No. 101, Col. San Lorenzo Huipulco, 14370 Mexico City, Mexico

María Fátima Moneta Arce
General Office of Psychiatric Services, Ministry of Health (Mexico), Av. Paseo de la Reforma No. 450 Piso 1, Col. Juárez, 06600 Mexico City, Mexico

Rikuya Hosokawa
School of Nursing, Nagoya City University, Mizuho-cho, Mizuho-ku, Nagoya 467-8601, Japan
Graduate School of Medicine, Kyoto University, Kyoto, Japan

Toshiki Katsura
Graduate School of Medicine, Kyoto University, Kyoto, Japan

Kathrin Schuck and Silvia Schneider
Mental Health Research and Treatment Center, Ruhr-University Bochum, Massenbergstrasse 9-13, 44787 Bochum, Germany

Simone Munsch
Department of Psychology, Clinical Psychology and Psychotherapy, University of Fribourg, Rue P.A. de Faucigny 2, 1700 Fribourg, Switzerland

Seo Ah Hong
ASEAN Institute for Health Development, Mahidol University, Salaya, Phutthamonthon, Nakhon Pathom 73170, Thailand
Institute for Health and Society, Hanyang University, Seoul, Republic of Korea

Karl Peltzer
Department for Management of Science and Technology Development, Ton Duc Thang University, Ho Chi Minh City, Vietnam
Faculty of Pharmacy, Ton Duc Thang University, Ho Chi Minh City, Vietnam

Bum-Sung Choi
Department of Psychiatry, Medical Research Institute, Pusan National University Yangsan Hospital, 20 Geumo-ro, Yangsan, Mulgeum-eup 50612, Republic of Korea

Johanna Inhyang Kim and Bung-Nyun Kim
Division of Child and Adolescent Psychiatry, Department of Psychiatry, Seoul National University College of Medicine, 101 Daehak-no, Chongno-gu, Seoul 03080, Republic of Korea

Bongseog Kim
Department of Psychiatry, Sanggye Paik Hospital, Inje University College of Medicine, 1342 Dong-il Street, Seoul 01757, Republic of Korea

Jingjing Lu, Feng Wang, Lu Li and Xudong Zhou
The Institute of Social and Family Medicine, School of Public Health, Zhejiang University, 866 Yuhangtang Rd., Hangzhou 310058, Zhejiang, People's Republic of China

Pengfei Chai
Yinzhou District CDC, 1221 Xueshi Rd., Ningbo 315199, Zhejiang, People's Republic of China

Dongshuo Wang
Oxford Road, SG16 Samuel Alexander Building, Manchester M13 9PL, UK

Kirsten Hauber
De Jutters B.V, Centre for Youth Mental Healthcare Haaglanden, The Hague, The Netherlands
Department of Child and Adolescent Psychiatry, Curium-Leiden University Medical Centre, Leiden, The Netherlands

Albert Eduard Boon
De Jutters B.V, Centre for Youth Mental Healthcare Haaglanden, The Hague, The Netherlands
Lucertis, Child and Adolescent Psychiatry Rotterdam, Rotterdam, The Netherlands
Department of Child and Adolescent Psychiatry, Curium-Leiden University Medical Centre, Leiden, The Netherlands

Robert Vermeiren
Department of Child and Adolescent Psychiatry, Curium-Leiden University Medical Centre, Leiden, The Netherlands
Department of Child and Adolescent Psychiatry, VU University Medical Centre, Amsterdam, The Netherlands

Tanya van de Water and Soraya Seedat
Department of Psychiatry, Stellenbosch University, Cape Town, South Africa

Elna Yadin
Department of Psychiatry, University of Pennsylvania, Philadelphia, PA, USA

Jaco Rossouw
Department of Psychiatry, Stellenbosch University, Cape Town, South Africa
Faculty of Medicine and Health Sciences, Stellenbosch University, Cape Town 8000, South Africa

C. S. Barendregt and A. M. Van der Laan
Research and Documentation Centre (WODC) of the Dutch Ministry of Justice and Security, 2500 EH The Hague, The Netherlands

I. L. Bongers and Ch. Van Nieuwenhuizen
GGzE Center for Child and Adolescent Psychiatry, 5600 AX Eindhoven, The Netherlands
Scientific Center for Care and Welfare (Tranzo), Tilburg University, 5000 LE Tilburg, The Netherlands

Kenneth J. Zucker and Susan J. Bradley
Department of Psychiatry, University of Toronto, Toronto, ON M5T 1R8, Canada

A. Natisha Nabbijohn, Alanna Santarossa and Joanna Matthews
Department of Psychology, University of Toronto Mississauga, Mississauga, ON, Canada

Hayley Wood
Psychological Services, Toronto District School Board, Toronto, ON, Canada

Doug P. VanderLaan
Department of Psychology, University of Toronto
Mississauga, Mississauga, ON, Canada
Underserved Populations Research Program, Child,
Youth and Family Division, Centre for Addiction
and Mental Health, Toronto, ON, Canada

Ed L. B. Hilterman
GGzE Center for Child and Adolescent Psychiatry,
Eindhoven, The Netherlands
Tilburg University, Scientific Center for Care and
Welfare (Tranzo), Tilburg, The Netherlands
Justa Mesura, Consultancy and Applied Research,
Barcelona, Spain

Ilja L. Bongers and Chijs van Nieuwenhuizen
GGzE Center for Child and Adolescent Psychiatry,
Eindhoven, The Netherlands
Tilburg University, Scientific Center for Care and
Welfare (Tranzo), Tilburg, The Netherlands

Tonia L. Nicholls
Department of Psychiatry, University of British
Columbia, Vancouver, Canada
BC Mental Health and Substance Use Services,
Forensic Psychiatric Services Commission,
Coquitlam, Canada

**Sabine Loos, Naina Walia, Thomas Becker and
Bernd Puschner**
Section Process-Outcome Research,
Department of Psychiatry II, Ulm University,
Ludwig-Heilmeyer-Str. 2, 89312 Günzburg, Germany

Ramesh P. Adhikari
Padma Kanya Multiple Campus, Tribhuvan
University Kathmandu, Bagbazar, Kathmandu,
Nepal
Research Department, Transcultural Psychosocial
Organization (TPO), Baluwatar, Kathmandu, Nepal

Nawaraj Upadhaya and Emily N. Satinsky
Research Department, Transcultural Psychosocial
Organization (TPO), Baluwatar, Kathmandu, Nepal

Matthew D. Burkey
Global Mental Health and Addiction Program, University of Maryland College Park, College Park, USA
Johns Hopkins University, Baltimore, MD, USA

Brandon A. Kohrt
Department of Psychiatry and Behavioral Sciences,
George Washington University, Washington, DC,
USA

Mark J. D. Jordans
Centre for Global Mental Health, Institute of
Psychiatry, Psychology and Neuroscience, King's
College London, London, UK

**Egil Haga, Berit Grøholt, Anita J. Tørmoen and
Lars Mehlum**
National Centre for Suicide Research and Prevention,
University of Oslo, Sognsvannsveien 21, Bygg 12,
0372 Oslo, Norway

Eline Aas
Department of Health and Health Economics,
University of Oslo, Oslo, Norway

Yukiyo Nagai and Kayo Nomura
Department of Pediatrics, Japanese Red Cross
Nagoya Daini Hospital, 2-9 Myoken-cho Showa-ku,
Nagoya, Aichi 466-8650, Japan

Masako Nagata
Graduate School of Education and Human
Development, Nagoya University, Furo-cho
Chikusa-ku, Nagoya, Aichi 464-8601, Japan

Tetsuji Kaneko
Department of Clinical Trial, Tokyo Metropolitan
Children's Medical Center, 2-8-9 Musashidai,
Fuchu, Tokyo 183-8561, Japan

Osamu Uemura
Department of Pediatric Nephrology, Aichi
Children's Health and Medical Center, 1-2 Osakata
Morioka-cho, Obu, Aichi 474-8710, Japan
Japanese Red Cross Toyota College of Nursing,
Clinical Medicine, 12-33 Nanamagari, Hakusan-cho,
Toyota, Aichi 471-8565, Japan

**Ingeborg G. Ribe, Britt A. Lyngmo and Sven G.
Hinderaker**
University of Bergen, Bergen, Norway

Estomih Mduma
Haydom Lutheran Hospital, Haydom, Mbulu
District, Tanzania

Erling Svensen
University of Bergen, Bergen, Norway
Haydom Lutheran Hospital, Haydom, Mbulu
District, Tanzania

Index

www.ingramcontent.com/pod-product-compliance
Lightning Source LLC
Chambersburg PA
CBHW061300190326

41458CB00011B/3726